Primary Maternal and Neonatal Health
A Global Concern

Primary Maternal and Neonatal Health

A Global Concern

Edited by

Fe del Mundo, M.D.

The Children's Medical Center
Quezon City, Philippines

Elena Ines-Cuyegkeng, M.D.

Association of Philippine Medical Colleges
Manila, Philippines

and

Domingo M. Aviado, M.D.

Atmospheric Health Sciences, Inc.
Short Hills, New Jersey

PLENUM PRESS · NEW YORK AND LONDON

Library of Congress Cataloging in Publication Data

International Congress on Maternal and Neonatal Health (1st: 1981: Manila, Philippines)
Primary maternal and neonatal health.

"Proceedings of the First International Congress on Maternal and Neonatal Health, held November 2-7, 1981, in Manila, Philippines" — verso t.p.
Bibliography: p.
Includes index.
1. Maternal health services — Congresses. 2. Child health services — Congresses. 3. Birth control — Congresses. 4. Medical personnel — Training of — Congresses. I. Mundo, Fe del. II. Ines-Cuyegkeng, Elena. III. Aviado, Domingo M. IV. Title. [DNLM: 1. Maternal welfare — Congresses. 2. Neonatology — Congresses. W3 IN 629 1st 1981p / WA 310 I61 1981p]
EG940.I57 1981   362.1'982   82-18947

ISBN-13:978-1-4613-3610-5   e-ISBN-13:978-1-4613-3608-2
DOI: 10.1007/978-1-4613-3608-2

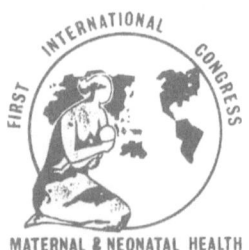

MATERNAL & NEONATAL HEALTH

Proceedings of the First International Congress on Maternal
and Neonatal Health, held November 2-7, 1981, in Manila, Philippines

©1983 Plenum Press, New York
Softcover reprint of the hardcover 1st edition 1983

A Division of Plenum Publishing Corporation
233 Spring Street, New York, N.Y. 10013

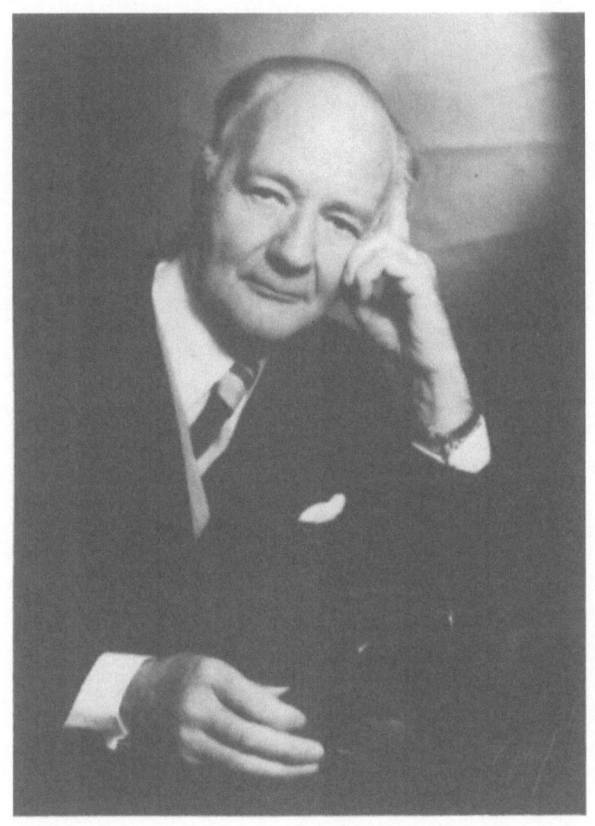

PROFESSOR HUBERT DE WATTEVILLE, M.D.
Beloved Accoucheur
Respected Clinician, Teacher, and Scientist
Benefactor of Mothers and Children
Especially in Developing Countries

DEDICATORY FOREWORD

   The First International Congress on Maternal and
Neonatal Health (IAMANEH) chose as its theme <u>Primary
Maternal and Neonatal Health Care: A Global Concern</u>. If
the primary goal of all World Health Organization member
states of "Health For All By The Year 2000" is to be met,
the most difficult challenge lies in the area of maternal
and neonatal health care. Indeed, the preventable mortality of mothers and their newborns related to the quality
of maternity care extracts a greater toll in life expectancy than any specific disease category. Such mortality
is but the tip of an iceberg of morbidity that saps the
quality of life of a majority of this world's citizens.
They are the less privileged by accident of birth only.
An intolerable situation exists.

   These <u>Proceedings</u> reflect a world concern by minis-
ters of health, academicians, scientists and providers of
maternal and neonatal care. No blueprint is offered for
solution of this world's greatest health problem. But the
<u>Proceedings</u> do contain an accurate description of the
problem and revealing epidemiological diagnoses that both
lay bare deficiencies in care and suggest the way to improve "health for all". The implications of these papers
will not bring comfort to those responsible for the
allocation of scarce resources for health. They rather
suggest radical changes are needed and that failure to
make these changes could mean a catastrophic and meaning-
less loss of life during the balance of this century.

   No doubt additional research in fertility and sterility and improved skills of obstetricians, gynecologists
and pediatricians can make significant contributions to
improved maternal care. The International Federation of
Fertility Societies (IFFS) and the International
Federation of Gynecology and Obstetrics (FIGO) are leading
international non-governmental organizations contributing
greatly to these areas of expertise. The contents of

these _Proceedings_ suggest the need for an additional service oriented organization that can lead a crusade for
improved maternal and neonatal health, an organization
that will involve all persons interested in the provision
of maternal and neonatal care, including professionals,
community leaders and the mothers themselves. Only a
social movement will do, if we are to create both the
political will and community involvement to break the
present acceptance of poor maternal and neonatal care, a
component of the more general accommodation to poverty.
Progress from now on will increasingly require needed
changes. The _International Association for Maternal and
Neonatal Health_ (IAMANEH) is dedicated to the task of
creating this social movement.

     Research, professional development and social action
will be needed to accomplish our objectives. It is fortunate that IFFS, FIGO and IAMANEH hold their Congresses
every third successive year. For each international
group, six more Congresses can yet be held from now to the
year 2000. Their contents must increasingly be focused in
a time-bound manner to reach our objective of "health for
all" for that year.

     It is no accident that one person wrote the consti-
tutions and nurtured the early development of all three of
these international organizations and had the vision for
their complementary roles. These _Proceedings_ are
dedicated in gratitude to that man, Professor Hubert de
Watteville.

                    Elton Kessel, M. D.
                    On behalf of the Editors, Officers,
                    Contributors and Participants

ORGANIZATIONS

International Association for Maternal and Neonatal Health

IAMANEH OFFICERS

President:	Prof. Silvio Aladjem, M.D., Chicago, U. S. A.
1st Vice-President:	Prof. Yutaka Moriyama, M.D., Tokyo, Japan
2nd Vice-President:	Ambassador Andre Dominice, Geneva, Switzerland
Secretary-General:	Prof. Hubert de Watteville, M. D., Geneva, Switzerland
Treasurer:	Dir. Eduard Berchten, Geneva, Switzerland
Executive Director:	Me. Evelyn Reymond, Geneva, Switzerland
Secretariat:	11, rue de'Italie, CH-1204, Geneva, Switzerland

Maternal and Child Health Association of the Philippines

Host: IAMANEH Philippine National Section

MCHAP OFFICERS

President:	Remedios G. Arellano, M.D.
Vice-President:	Trinidad A. Gomez, M.D.
Secretary:	Eustacia M. Rigor, M.D.
Treasurer:	Carmelita B. Cayugan, M.D.
Public Relations:	Jose R. Relacion, Jr., M.D.
Auditor:	Aquilino B. Esguerra, M.D.
Past President:	Fe del Mundo, M.D.
Directors:	Alice O. Caspellan, M.D., Estrella P. de Leon, M.D., Minerva B. Inciong, M.D., Augusto M. Manalo, M.D., Perla D. Santos-Ocampo, M.D.

First International Congress Organizing Committee

President:	Fe del Mundo, M.D.
Vice-President:	Remedios G. Arellano, M.D.
Secretary:	Lucrecia R. Castillo, M.D.
Asst. Secretary:	Eustacia M. Rigor, M.D.
Treasurer:	Carmelita B. Cuyugan, M.D.
Asst. Treasurer:	Martina T. Certeza, M.D.
Secretariat:	11 Banaue, Quezon City, Philippines
Arrangements:	Julita U. Denoga, M.D., Victorina G. Leus, M.D.
Awards:	Felix Estrada, M.D., Estrella P. de Leon, M.D.
Documentation:	Trinidad A. Gomez, M.D., Stella Gonzales, M.D.
Exhibits:	Ramon Arcadio, M.D., Orpha K. Abrigo, M.D.
Hospitality:	Salud A. Angala, M.D., Victoria A. Sanvictores, M.D.
Invitation and Reception:	Esperanza F. Rivera, M.D., Lucrecia R. Castillo, M.D., Eustacia M. Rigor, M.D.
Publicity:	Isidora Y. Zalamea, M.D., Jose R. Relacion, M.D.
Registration:	Alice O. Caspellan, M.D., Juanita S. Yadao, M.D.
Socials:	Carmelita B. Cuyugan, M.D., Jesus Tomacruz, M.D.
Souvenir Program:	Arturo Ludan, M.D., Miguel Noche, M.D.
Program:	Aquilino B. Esguerra, M.D., Perla D. Santos-Ocampo, M.D.
Ways and Means:	Remedios G. Arellano, M.D., Nena Eng Tan, M.D., Nenita Lee Tan, M.D.
Government Participation	Evangeline G. Suva, M.D., Esperanza de Castro, M.D.

PREFACE

In recent years there has been an increasing interest in and concern for women and children during the vulnerable period around birth. Thus the International Association of Maternal and Neonatal Health (IAMANEH) has expressed its deep and global concern in its First International Congress. This is understandable as a worldwide view shows that millions of women every year suffer serious complications during pregnancy.

It is a fact that numerous problems remain unsolved in saving the precious lives of mothers and newborns; yet most of the causes of morbidity and mortality are preventable and controllable with the present day remarkable achievements and amazing advances in technology, medicine and public health.

It is further reported that because of maternal ill-health and malnutrition, 21 million low birth weight babies accounted for four percent of all births, but caused 4 to 74 percent of all prenatal deaths (deaths between the 28th week of gestation and the end of the first week of life).

In a sincere desire to reduce mortality and morbidity and to reach the goal of improved health of neonates, the IAMANEH convened experts from 25 countries and 40 speakers accepted to cover the convention theme in five main topics, namely: (a) Interrelations between maternal and neonatal health and family planning); (b) Future aspects of the family planning program; (c) Prevention and cure of prevalent infections in the mother and newborn; (d) Monitoring of maternal and neonatal health within and outside clinical settings; and (e) Strategies for implementation of recent knowledge and technology relative to maternal and neonatal health within primary health care.

After the conclusion of the Congress, all contributors were requested to revise their presentations for
publication in these Proceedings. They were encouraged
to submit only essential text material, illustrations,
tables and references. The overwhelming consideration was
that these Proceedings would be available to professors,
students and practitioners of Obstetrics and Gynecology,
Pediatrics, Perinatology, Reproductive Toxicology, Epidemiology, Public Health, and Primary Health Care. For the
benefit of readers with such a varied background and   '
interest, the Proceedings have been regrouped into nine
sections, namely:

Section I: Keynote Reviews, including a brief
history of IAMANEH and its primary concern for improving
maternal and neonatal health.

Section II: Maternal Health, Neonatal Care and
Family Planning, including discussions of their interrelationships and cross benefits.

Section III: Future Prospects of Family Planning
Programs, reviewing contraceptive practices, both in
current use and under research investigation.

Section IV: Prevention and Cure of Prevalent
Infections, such as bacterial, parasitic and viral in
origin. These are the only maternal and neonatal diseases
that the etiology can be unequivocally demonstrated.

Section V: Search for Risk Factors Influencing
Reproduction. The studies on incomplete abortion and
postpartum ovulation illustrate the limitations of
epidemiologic studies in proving causes of diseases involving reproduction. The discussions on environmental
factors and cigarette smoking illustrate the difficulties
in proving causal relationship. Abnormalities in the
neonates are associated with several risk factors
influencing the mother. Therefore it is not possible to
attribute any form of abnormality or disease to a single
risk factor such as cigarette smoking or exposure to an
environmental factor.

Section VI: Maternal and Neonatal Health Care
Monitoring in Indonesia and the Philippines, by computer-
ized techniques. The contributors to this section have
been requested to submit additional material collected
even after the Congress concluded, because the Editors
felt that the subject had not been hitherto covered in
monographs devoted to perinatology and epidemiology.

Section VII: <u>Stragegies for Implementation of Recent Knowledge and Technology</u>, with descriptions of primary health care in Pakistan, Hong Kong, Ghana, Sri Lanka, Japan, Nigeria and the People's Republic of China. It should be noted that most of the information on maternal and neonatal health from these countries are being reported for the first time and serve to supplement earlier publications from the World Health Organization.

Section VIII: <u>Strategies for Training Primary Health Care Persons</u>, with special reference to meeting the manpower needs of developing countries.

Section IX: <u>Concluding Remarks</u> by Professor Hubert de Watteville and by the Editors.

The Editors acknowledge the help of Asuncion Guevara for supervising all phases of finalizing the mauscripts of these <u>Proceedings</u>, and Domingo Guevara Aviado for the preparation of the Index. The Editorial Staff of Plenum Press, particularly Messrs. James R. Busis and John Matzka, deserve a debt of gratitude for printing and distributing a truly professional book commemorating the first official publication of the International Association for Maternal and Neonatal Health. Let us hope that the Editors of the next <u>Proceedings</u> will find an equally sympathetic publishing firm.

Fe del Mundo, M.D.
Elena Ines-Cuyegkeng, M.D.
Domingo M. Aviado, M.D.
July 25, 1982

CONTENTS

REPORT OF THE EXECUTIVE BOARD TO THE GENERAL ASSEMBLY

ON THE DEVELOPMENT AND ACTIVITIES OF IAMANEH

H. de Watteville

Secretary General
IAMANEH
Geneva, Switzerland

GROWTH OF THE ASSOCIATION

At present, a national section is affiliated to
IAMANEH in 25 countries, which are: Argentina, Austria,
Bangladesh, Belgium, Brasil, Columbia, Egypt, Germany,
Greece, Hong Kong, India, Indonesia, Japan, Korea, The
Netherlands, Pakistan, Peru, Philippines, Spain, Sudan
Switzerland, Tunisia, Turkey, United States and Venezuela.

The Executive Board has remained unaltered since the
Extraordinary General Assembly held in Tokyo in October
1979. The new president of FIGO, Professor Keith Russel
(Los Angeles, USA) has replaced the outgoing President,
Professor R. Caldeyro Barcia, in the Scientific Council.

In over 30 countries, contacts have been established
with colleagues who are interested in IAMANEH and who will
try to form a national section of this organization. It
is hoped that in several of these countries such a section
will become affiliated to our organization in the near
future.

The cooperation of members of national sections for
the recruitment of new national affiliates or individual
members of IAMANEH (persons and/or body corporates) in
countries where no national section exists is urgently
requested.

National Sections

Those fostering the creation of a national section of IAMANEH should bear in mind the following objectives:

(a)   The great progress of modern medicine in the field of obstetrics and pediatrics is documented by an impressive drop of maternal and perinatal mortality and morbidity, mainly in the industrialized countries. However, in certain parts of Latin America, Africa and Asia, these figures are still up to 100 times higher. This is due to the fact that in highly populated areas of the world, women deliver without assistance by medically trained personnel during pregnancy, confinement and after delivery. Most governments have also included in their program for developing primary health care in the rural and suburban areas of their countries, some projects to improve mother and child health. However, the task is of such magnitude and the financial burden so heavy that the cooperation of non-government organizations may considerably accelerate the improvement of maternal and child health in many parts of the world.

(b)   The national sections of IAMANEH should pursue the goal of elaborating and supporting projects for improved obstetrical and neonatal care mainly on the primary health care level. Wherever necessary and feasible, family planning counseling and services should be included in these programs. It appears that no one is better placed for family planning activities than those who take care of the women during pregnancy and child birth and of their new born babies, be it even a traditional birth attendant. On the other hand, the mother will more easily accept methods for spacing deliveries if less of her children die after delivery and during the first year of their lives.

(c)   The national sections should encourage cooperation between obstetricians, pediatricians and family planners working in the field of obstetrical and neonatal care since such a cooperation is often missing.

(d)   The national sections should consider social aspects in reproduction which are often neglected by scientific and/or professional associations. Affiliates of IAMANEH should give priority to the implementation of projects dealing with obstetrical and neonatal care at the primary health care level. Sections in industrialized countries may contribute to the realization of such a project in developing countries.

(e) The national sections should try to raise private funds from donors and members of their section for the implementation of their programs. The fund-raising campaigns should be organized with the help of influential businessmen and philanthropic societies like the Lion's or Rotary Clubs. Furthermore, interested persons may help the implementation of the national program by becoming an ordinary or life member of the national section. Banks, insurance companies and commercial firms may become body corporates. To reach this goal, public opinion must be sensitized for the great need of better obstetrical and neonatal care by adequate publicity.

(f) In countries where an organization pursuing goals similar to the ones of IAMANEH already exists, this organization may become its affiliate rather than having a new national section created.

(g) No project should be realized in a developing country when not approved or even better, requested by the health authorities of the country; and no help should be offered to a community without its consent and active participation. By acting along these lines, IAMANEH and its national sections will play a specific role and not duplicate the efforts of other already existing groups. A national section which is conducting projects by cooperation between health officials, physicians, midwives and social workers would be useful even in countries where only little or no private funds can be raised by the section for the implementation of its project. Should the project be realized with the help of another section of IAMANEH or its headquarters, then it could nevertheless be presented as a IAMANEH action of the national section receiving the aid.

Recognition of IAMANEH by UNFPA

On the request of its Executive Board, IAMANEH has been recognized on October 2, 1980 by the United Nations Fund for Population Activities in New York as a non-governmental organization maintaining official relations with UNFPA.

Executive Board Meeting

At the occasion of the World Congress on Fertility and Sterility, the Executive Board of IAMANEH met in Madrid on July 8, 1980. The Board discussed several modifications of the constitution and by-laws concerning the full autonomy of national affiliates, the scheduling of General Assemblies and the composition of the Scientific

Council. It was decided to submit these modifications for approval to the General Assembly. The affiliated sections have been informed of the modifications within the time limits laid down in the constitution.

The Board has nominated Dr. Elton Kessel as honorary Deputy Secretary General and has changed the title of Mr. Reymond from Executive Director to Legal Advisor for reasons which have been explained to IAMANEH's constituency in a circular letter. The Board furthermore decided that part of the money deposited in IAMANEH's central account in Geneva will be used for offering surgical instruments and equipment to the Health Service of Mali. This material will be used in a small peripheral hospital (Hôpital du Cercle in Kolondjeba), where a general practitioner is dealing with many obstetrical emergency cases, since this hospital is a referral station for a large rural area.

At the conclusion of the Board meeting, a general discussion on the organization of maternal and neonatal care at the primary health care level took place. Colleagues from many countries where no section of IAMANEH exists attended the meeting in the capacity of observers and participated in this discussion which apparently aroused great interest for IAMANEH and the goals it pursues. Therefore time has been allotted for a similar discussion at the General Assembly of the First Congress held in Manila. The discussion offered the delegates of national affiliates an opportunity for reporting on the activities of their sections. This interchange of experience and ideas contributed to the development and implementation of new projects for improving maternal and neonatal care.

IAMANEH'S HEADQUARTERS IN GENEVA

With the growth of IAMANEH and the expansion of its activities, the burden of its Secretariat in Geneva has increased. Many hundreds of letters have been dispatched and numerous telephone calls and cables handled by the private office of the Secretary General, Professor H. de Watteville, and by the Legal Adviser, Mr. E. Reymond, without any cost for IAMANEH. The activity of the Secretariat was hampered by lack of sufficient staff and its effectiveness could be considerably increased by the appointment of an Executive Director, at least half-time. This would become mandatory if the General Assembly decides to organize at the occasion of each of the forthcoming General Assemblies an International Congress, and in

connection with the annual meetings of the Excutive Board
a workshop or symposium, since the Secretariat would have
to cooperate with the host society in the preparation of
such a scientific meeting.

Therefore, steps have been undertaken to find in
Switzerland financial support which will make it possible
to establish an annual budget for the Secretariat and to
run it with a sound financial basis. Nevertheless, voluntary contributions of the national affiliates to the
central account of IAMANEH will be most welcome and will
certainly foster the activities and growth of our
Association.

Once a worldwide network of national sections of
IAMANEH exists, its headquarters in Geneva will have to
accomplish important tasks which include the following:

(a)   To communicate with the officers, members of
the Board and Scientific Council and furthermore with the
national sections and body corporates.

(b)   To foster the creation of new national sections
and the recruitment of individual members in countries
where no national section exists and also of new body
corporates.

(c)   To prepare agenda for meetings of the Executive
Board and the General Assemblies.

(d)   To participate in the preparation of special
activities of IAMANEH as for instance, the 1979 Workshop
on Social Obstetrics in Tokyo and the 1981 Congress on
Maternal and Neonatal Health in Manila.

Relations Between the National Sections and the
Headquarters in Geneva.

The objectives of IAMANEH have been described in
paragraph 4 of its constitution. However, the structure
of the Association has undergone a decisive change since
its foundation in 1977. The national sections have become
fully autonomous and from a highly centralized organization, IAMANEH has thus become a loose federation of
national sections which have one thing in common, and that
is, their interest for the promotion of maternal and neonatal care as well as family planning wherever necessary
and feasible.

Whereas each national section should try to establish close contacts with the health authorities of their country, IAMANEH's headquarters should do the same with international governmental organizations in order to link private initiative and humanitarian work to the government action on an international level, for instance, by close cooperation with the United Nations Fund for Population Activities (UNFPA), the World Health Organization (WHO) and UNICEF.

Furthermore, IAMANEH can discuss, develop or implement certain of its projects together with other non-governmental organizations like the International Planned Parenthood Federation (IPPF), the International Federation of Gynecology and Obstetrics (FIGO), the International Federation of Pediatrics (IFP), the International Federation for Family Health (IFFH) or the World Federation of Health Agencies for the Advancement of Voluntary Surgical Contraception (WFAVS).

Furthermore, the headquarters should establish contacts between the national sections and the Scientific Council of IAMANEH, as well as between the national sections themselves, acting thus as a center for the evaluation and comparison of national projects. As far as the funds available in the central account in Geneva permit, the Executive Board may decide to support, with part of this money, a national project.

CONCLUSION

It must be stated that the usefulness of IAMANEH depends first of all on the number and strength of its national sections and on their effectiveness in the implementation of their national projects.

MATERNAL ASPECTS OF MATERNAL AND NEONATAL HEALTH

A GLOBAL CONCERN

S. Surjaningrat

Minister of Health and Chairman of the
National Family Planning Coordinating Board
Jakarta, Indonesia

INTRODUCTION

We are all aware that "Health For All By the Year 2000" has now become the official target for all WHO (World Health Organization) member states. "Health for all" means health is to be brought within reach of everyone in a given country. The word "health" implies a personal state of well being that enables a person to lead a socially and economically productive life. This means that health should be regarded as an objective of broad socio-economic development and not merely as one of the means of attaining it. This concept is better understood if one relates it with the definition of health embodied in the WHO constitution, which formulates health as a state of complete physical, mental and social well-being, and not merely the absence of disease or infirmity. Health is in fact an outcome of interrelated and interdependent factors, namely, environment, behavior, health services and heredity. The influence of these four factors on maternal and neonatal health is now widely accepted (1-6).

Maternal and neonatal health is a body of science and practice dedicated to alleviating problems that are uniquely affecting these vulnerable groups. These groups are considered vulnerable because of the special characteristics of pregnancy and infancy in relation to growth and development.

CHALLENGES TO MATERNAL AND NEONATAL CARE

We should be aware of the magnitude of maternal and neonatal health problems including factors that influence them, so that appropriate ways and means to reduce these problems can be developed. Although some information on developed countries is mentioned in this presentation, it will mainly focus on problems faced by developing countries.

The proportion of women in reproductive age is approximately the same in all parts of the world, i.e., 24 percent of the total population. However, data on mortality and morbidity are seriously inadequate in countries where health problems are most widespread and severe. Data inadequacies are most striking for pregnant women and children, especially the newborn. This observation should be taken into consideration when reviewing data on maternal mortality and morbidity.

In developed countries with well-developed health care delivery system, maternal mortality rate is at 5 to 30 per 100000 live births, and is continuously decreasing. In most developing countries, special studies conducted seeking information on maternal mortality rates suggest that it is in excess of 500 per 100,000 live births; rates of over 1000 per 100,000 live births has been reported in parts of Africa. A preliminary report from a maternal care monitoring project conducted in West Java registers a maternal mortality rate of 100 per 100,000 live births.

Common causes of maternal deaths include postpartum hemorrhage with anemia as an underlying or associated cause, and sepsis. These are directly related to the absence or inadequacy of prenatal and delivery care. Hypertensive disorders of pregnancy are important both in developed countries (where they account for 25 to 35 percent of maternal deaths) and in developing countries. The etiology of toxemia is not well known. However, this condition is more frequently associated with the first pregnancy, very young mothers, and women over 35 years old, especially in very high parity women.

Illegally induced abortion as a cause of maternal death is well recognized, but the importance of its role is difficult to estimate because of the secrecy surrounding abortion as a cause of death. In Latin America where abortion is usually illegal, it has been estimated that induced abortion is the cause of 20 to 50 percent of all maternal deaths.

As regards to maternal morbidity, reliable data are even more scarce than for maternal mortality. However, it is observed that malnutrition and anemia, which is closely interrelated with acute and chronic infections such as malaria, urinary tract infections and pulmonary tuberculosis, are common among women associated with prenatal, delivery and postnatal care. Anemia is widespread among women of child-bearing age, both in developed and developing countries. In developing countries, non-pregnant women with hemoglobin levels showing anemia account for 10 to 100 percent. Chronic diseases such as hypertension, heart and renal diseases and diabetes are aggravated by pregnancy. Addictive drugs, alcohol and smoking during pregnancy can lead to intrauterine growth retardation or even malformation.

Involuntary infertility is a condition of deep personal distress and has social implications. In most parts of the world, about 2 to 10 percent of couples are affected, but data from certain areas of Africa suggest that infertile couples amount to as high as 40 percent. Sexually transmitted diseases resulting in tubal obstruction and sequelae from obstetric conditions are reponsible for this observation.

Information on the frequency of teenage pregnancies in developing countries is limited. However, where the minimum legal age at marriage is low, the first pregnancy can be expected to occur during the midteens and repeated pregnancies are likely to occur before the age of 20. In some countries, 50 percent of the first births occur to mothers aged less than 20 years, as do 25 percent of second births, and 10 percent of third births. Early teenage pregnancies pose special health risks not only for the mother but also for the child. Evidence clearly shows that maternal mortality rates are considerably higher for younger women and that teenage mothers also run a higher risk of losing their babies in infancy.

As mentioned before, there are a number of factors which affect maternal health status. Environment is one of the most important factor, under which the socio-economic conditions of the country, physical and biological environment and cultural background is implied.

Inclusive in this concept is the level of economic development which influences the health status of mothers. Agricultural policy and land ownership have a direct

bearing on maternal nutritional status. Unsanitary
environment, including unsafe and insufficient water,
overcrowding, transport and communication difficulties,
have substantial influence on maternal health status.
Urbanization, with its accompanying breakdown of
traditional structures causes health problems, such as
pollution, mental problems, etc., that affect maternal
health.

Another factor is socio-cultural values and education. A society's cultures, philosophies and religions
all shape and are shaped by its people's understanding and
conception of health, sickness and death. Various harmful
effects have been observed as a result of food taboos in
the treatment of sickness in children, and eating practices of pregnant women, child marriages, etc. On the other
hand, there are also positive aspects, such as the traditional bonding or close contact of mother and infant, and
the value attached to cleanliness and personal hygiene in
many religions. Changes in traditional family life-styles
are inevitable; however, valuable practices such as
breast feeding should be maintained and promoted. The
relationship between education and health is often reflected in the association of a high infant mortality rate
and low level of education.

Other factors affecting the health status of mothers
and children also include community and social support
measures, such as neighborhood day-care centers or organized health care delivery systems. The extent to which
these are provided and utilized and the quality of their
services have some bearing on maternal and child health
status. To illustrate this observation, the following
findings are presented.

In a household survey conducted in 1980 involving
24,000 households in over 6 provinces in Indonesia, it was
revealed that 66 percent of the pregnant women were aware
of prenatal care facilities provided by the government.
However, only half of them sought and received prenatal
care, the reason being that they felt it unnecessary and
that the distance between homes and the facilities was
considered too far. Further, it was revealed that 60 percent of mothers who delivered babies were aware of the
government facilities, but only 25 percent of them used
it. The rest of the deliveries were helped by "dukun" the
traditional birth attendant (55 percent) and by privately
practicing midwives (15.5 percent).

Former patterns of maternal and child health care

were designed and provided in the form of vertical programs based on models from a few developed countries.
These models were designed on the provision of continuous
supervision and preventive care for mothers and children
in affluent societies where basic needs were satisfied and
where coverage by other health programs was almost universal. Because of their costs, such vertical programs were
unable to provide even minimal coverage when applied in a
different socio-economic conditions such as in less
developed countries.

Current trend requires that maternal and child health
care be integrated in the primary health care approach applied in an increasing number of countries. The strategy
is based on self-care and organized community participation with the primary health care or community health
worker providing maternal and child care in an integrated
manner and as a major and essential element of primary
health care. Activities at this level stress on prevention and are based heavily on health education and income-
generating activities. The goal is to teach mothers and
family members to provide much of this care themselves.

Community resources must be mobilized and utilized.
Communities will be more likely to commit their own
resources (time, labor, money) to activities that they
personally and collectively consider important. The
system should also build upon existing community structures and channels. In this regard, school teachers are
the most numerous workers at the community level. Other
categories include agricultural extension officers, members of voluntary agencies, women's groups or other local
organizations. This set-up requires intersectoral
approach to community involvement and emphasizes the need
for intersectoral training of personnel working at the
community level.

Development and adaptation of appropriate technologies at this level include among others, upgrading the
knowledge and skill of traditional birth attendants,
monitoring the growth and nutritional status of children
using growth charts, use of oral rehydration in diarrhea,
etc. The level of care described above should be supported by advice, guidance and in-service training required by
the peripheral level workers, the logistic support needed
by these workers and the necessary facilities for referral
and support in the case of problems that cannot be dealt
with at the primary level of contact. The health facilities for referral care of mothers and children consist
of health centers and obstetric and pediatic out-patient

facilities or hospital beds at intermediate level of care.

At a more central level, maternal and child health services should be managed in relation to the overall socio-economic development plan and be fully integrated into the health and family planning service system as a whole. This level is responsible for defining policies for the health and welfare of mothers and children with clear priorities and targets, establishing strong commitment to these policies and priorities through realistic budgeting support, carrying out systematic planning and conducting training and research in MCH services.

The "risk approach" being promoted by WHO provides more effective maternal and child health care. In this way, the more skilled health worker will attend to the high-risk groups and maximum utilization of community resources is obtained through mobilization of unconventional personnel resources, such as traditional birth attendants, women's groups, school teachers, etc., to perform health tasks for those who are not at high risk. First pregnancy, high parity, too frequent pregnancies, pregnancy at the extremes of reproductive age, previous loss of a child, and malnutrition are examples of universal high risk factors for the mother that increase the chances of poor outcome of pregnancy. Some factors are easily detected even by untrained health workers as age, parity, maternal height and previous loss of fetus or child.

Maternal and child health care programs may vary from one country to another as they are adapted to local problems and means for solutions. However, they should include the following essential elements: prenatal and childbirth care, promotion of breast feeding and appropriate infant and child nutrition, monitoring of growth and development, immunization, prevention and management of infant and childhood diarrhea including oral rehydration, family health education in support of family self-reliance and family planning. In the past decade, family planning has increasingly been considered an integral part of maternal and child health. It is recognized as one of the effective methods of reducing risk factor related to maternal health.

CONCLUSION

The knowledge and technology required to reduce the death rates of mothers and children and alleviate their

suffering are now available. For example, maternal deaths
could be brought to an acceptable level and complications
during pregnancy and childbirth could be reduced through
prenatal care for every woman and identification of those
needing extra care, nutritional supplementation when
required, and attendance during delivery by a person
trained in appropriate techniques. Moreover, maternal and
neonatal health care could be improved with the use of
effective methods to regulate the spacing and timing of
pregnancies.

        What a country needs is a firm political. decision to
set aside approrpriate amounts of resources to break the
vicious circle of poverty, ignorance and ill-health.
Community participation, cross-sectoral cooperation and
appropriate technology are pre-requisites of the primary
health care approach which has been accepted as the key
for achieving the goal of "health for all by the year
2000". I sincerely hope that this Congress will give its
full support to the achievement of the goal.

REFERENCES

1. Blum HL (1978): Expanding health care horizons. In:
    A General Systems Concept of Health to a National
    Health Policies, Third Party Associates Inc.,
    Oakland, California.
2. WHO (1980): Towards a better future - maternal and
    child health. WHO, Geneva.
3. Puffer RR, Griffiths GTW (1967): Patterns of urban
    mortality. PAHO, Washington.
4. WHO (1980): Sixth report on the world health
    situation, Part I. WHO, Geneva.
5. Ministry of Health (1981): 1980 Household Survey.
    Unpublished Report, Ministry of Health, Republic of
    Indonesia.
6. WHO (1976): New trends and approaches in the delivery
    of maternal and child care in health services. WHO
    Technical Report Series, No. 600, Geneva.

PRIMARY MATERNAL AND NEONATAL HEALTH: A GLOBAL CONCERN –

PEDIATRIC ASPECTS

M. Gabr

Professor of Pediatrics,
University of Cairo and Minister of Health
Cairo, Egypt

INTRODUCTION

The theme of this congress, "Primary Maternal and
Neonatal Health: A Global Concern", is of interest to the
clinician, the researcher and the policy maker. It requires the close collaboration of obstetricians,
pediatricians and public health professionals. The two
principal beneficiaries or victims are the mother and the
child. Mothers and children are at especially high risk
of morbidity and mortality. The child is particularly
vulnerable during certain states of development while the
mother is exposed to certain physical, physiological and
psychological stresses.

DATA SOURCES

There is no question that the level of child mortality and morbidity is unacceptably high in the Third World
compared to that of more developed countries. Unfortunately, details of child mortality are not uniformly
available for all countries due to incomplete reporting on
the part of the community and/or inadequate registration
systems on the part of the government. We are therefore
obliged to use estimates of child mortality or to extra-
polate from the statistics of a few developing countries
with relatively reasonable registration systems.

LEVELS AND TRENDS IN CHILD MORTALITY

Despite the limitation of statistics from developing countries, it can be inferred that the risk of infant mortality in such countries is 10 to 12 times as high as in more developed countries. It has been estimated, for example, that the infant mortality rate in many developing countries exceed 100 and may reach 200 per 1000 live births (1). The rate in more developed countries ranges from 8 to 15. The neonatal component of infant mortality is even harder to obtain from several countries. It can be estimated however that it may reach 120 per 1000 live births in some less developed countries compared to 10 per 1000 live births in more developed countries.

It should be noted, that regardless of the level of infant and child mortality, the probability of dying is at its highest about the time of birth and during the early neonatal period with a relative decline thereafter (1).

Of importance is the impact of mortality on certain major factors. These factors are:

(a) Biological factors - including maternal age and health, genetic factors, and birth weight.
(b) Family planning factors - namely the spacing, timing and number of pregnancies.
(c) Social and environmental factors - including education of the mother, the standard of living, the level of environmental sanitation, sources and modes of infection.
(d) Medical care factors - including genetic counseling, prenatal care, natal and neonatal care of the mother and care of the child, including nutrition and immunization.

CHILD MORTALITY TRANSITION

In order to understand the dynamics of interaction between these four categories of factors and child mortality, the following five points can be made, based on the theory developed by the Egyptian scientist A. R. Omran in his "Theory of Epidemiologic Transition" (14):

Point One. Considerable decline has occurred in infant and child mortality in both the more developed and the less developed countries; however, the rate of decline in the more developed countries has been spectacular, reaching a level of 10 or less per 1000 in some countries in Northern Europe which is very close to the irreducible minimum of 7 per 1000 for infant mortality rate.

Point Two. The fact that this reduction has been achieved at all should be an encouragement for the less developed countries. However, the dynamics of decline is different in more developed countries than that of the less developed. In Western countries, infant mortality declined starting the 19th century, due mainly to social and environmental factors as well as child spacing and fertility limitations. These factors were augmented in the 20th century by medical care factors including innovations in medical intervention. In less developed countries however, infant mortality decline was delayed until the 20th century, taking place mostly after World War II. The major factors involved were more medical than social due to the introduction of child care programs by national and international agencies. These included better child nutrition programs, immunization and the use of antibiotics.

Point 3. It seems that the influence of these factors in reaching a plateau and infant mortality decline in the Third World is slackening. For the decline to continue, there must be reinforcement of social factors (particularly the mother's education), environmental factors (particularly sanitation), medical care factors (particularly nutrition and immunization), and family planning.

Point 4. There was a differential decline in child mortality such that mortality at 1 to 4 years declined first and foremost. Post-neonatal infant mortality declined faster than neonatal mortality. Thus we find that in more developed countries, the ratio of neonatal to post-neonatal mortality has been increasing. Most of the decline has been in the group of preventable diseases including infectious diseases, nutritional disorders, diseases related to birth weight and diseases related to poor medical care. Breakthroughs in neonatology are expected to influence the hard core of diseases prevalent at birth or during the first month of life. It is expected that gradually the less developed countries will achieve great declines in child mortality.

Point 5. Child mortality levels have a crucial factor in determining how long a particular population is expected to live. In areas with high child mortality, life expectancy at birth is modest, only about 40 to 50 years, whereas in more developed countries, due to increased child survival, this may reach 70 years or more.

CERTAIN ASPECTS OF CHILD MORTALITY

Low Birth Weight

Defined as a birth weight below 2500 g, is a main contributing factor to perinatal mortality and morbidity. In a Pan-American Health Study (11) it was shown that neonatal mortality rises with the lowering of birth weight. In a recent World Health Organization Review (6), it was estimated that nearly 21 million infants of low birth weight are born each year. Globally this means that about 1 in every 6 infants has a low birth weight; however the incidence is not evenly distributed. In some parts of Asia, the ratio is almost 1 in 2, while in some parts of Europe it is 1 in 17. Between these extremes, the incidence ranges from 31 percent in Asia as a whole, 15 percent in Africa, 11 percent in Latin America and the Caribbean, to 8 percent in Europe and 7 percent in North America. Of the 20.6 million low birth weight infants born in 1979, over 19 million, or 90 percent were born in developing countries (mostly among the least privileged populations). These babies contribute to a large proportion of deaths and childhood morbidity - the risk of mortality being up to 20 times higher than for normal weight infants, both in neonatal period and later (3).

The distribution of birth weights of infants in two contrasting communities - the privileged and the poor, was illustrated in data presented to a workshop on birth weight organized by the Swedish Agency for research and cooperation with developing countries and the WHO in 1977 (7, Table 1).

Apart from gestational age, the birth weight depends on factors related to the mother: weight, height, age, parity, socio-economic status, education, smoking habits and nutritional status. Pathological factors related to complications during pregnancy may also influence the birth weight; these are toxemias of pregnancy and anemias (8).

In developing countries, the majority of low birth weight babies are born at term i.e., they are small-for-date mainly because of poor maternal health and nutrition before and during pregnancy (8).

In view of the significance and magnitude of immediate and long term effects of low birth weight, attention has been given in recent years to ways and means of its prevention through care and intervention during pregnancy rather than to treatment of preterm and low birth weight

Table 1.   Distribution of Birth Weights Expressed in
           Percentage in Two Contrasting Communities.

Birth Weight in grams	Privileged Communities	Poor Communities
0 - 1999	2	8
2000 - 2499	5	35
2500 - 2999	18	47
3000 - 3499	38	10
3500 - 3999	27	-
4000+	10	-

babies later on. One views with considerable skepticism
the rapid growth in many countries of the specialty of
clinical neonatology and the proliferation of neonatal
intensive care units. Not only is the necessary sophisticated equipment very difficult to maintain in working
order in developing countries, but also could only serve a
tiny fraction of those in need. Prevention of low birth
weight is of greater importance in promoting the full
development of children as well as avoiding the high costs
associated with immediate and long-term care of low birth
weight infants. Prenatal care and family planning in
general help to reduce the number of low birth weight
babies born in developing countries (3). Effective family
planning programs would help by influencing the mothers to
space their children and educating them against high
parity (9). In a WHO study in rural India (1), it was
found that mortality rates were more than twice as high
among neonates and infants born less than two years after
the preceding pregnancy terminated (whether by abortion,
fetal death, or live birth) than among those born more
than 4 years later.

Other Preventable Causes of Child Mortality

     Apart from low birth weight, many other causes of
neonatal mortality in developing countries are preventable. Proper maternal, antenatal, natal and postnatal
care effectively reduce death and morbidity from a variety
of well known traumatic, metabolic and infectious causes,
such as cerebral and other vital organ injuries, maternal
diabetes, blood group incompatibilities and neonatal
sepsis. The establishment of easily accessible primary
health care facilities are more cost-effective in improving neonatal health than the purchase of more
sophisticated neonatal equipment. A limited number of
well-equipped centers in developing countries are however

needed for special postgraduate training in order to
develop a cadre of specialists ready to carry on such
responsibilities as socio-economic standards improve.

Late neonatal mortality (after the first week of
life) is uncommon in developed countries but accounts for
almost two-thirds of all infant mortality in developing
countries. In many areas, tetanus may account for up to
10% of all neonatal mortality (1). Diarrheal diseases,
closely followed by respiratory infections, are the leading causes of morbidity and mortality in the first year of
life. Malnutrition as an underlying cause is also important. Neonatal tetanus could be controlled in all
societies by immunization of women twice before parturition (1). Deaths due to diarrheal diseases could also be
reduced significantly. The immediate application of oral
rehydration therapy could save millions of lives and give
young children a chance to survive the crucial weaning
period. Rehydration can be performed within the family,
thus greatly facilitating its widespread use.

Breast-feeding

The most effective measure for the prevention of
malnutriton and for the protection against infection
during infancy is breast-feeding. Evidence from developing countries indicates that infants breast-fed for less
than 6 months or not at all have a mortality 5 to 10 times
higher in the second 6 months of life than those breast-
fed for 6 months or more. In developing countries, data
gathered by the WHO collaborative study on breast-feeding
indicate that in some urban areas, relatively larger proportions of mothers are not establishing breast-feeding.
The prevalence and duration of breast-feeding among the
rural populations of developing countries continue to be
high. In some cases, problems of nutrition and health
status in infancy appear to be associated with the late
introduction of appropriate and regular supplementary
feeding (12).

CONCLUSION

Remedial programs to prevent neonatal mortality and
morbidity are unfortunately receiving little priority in
many developing nations. For such a program to succeed it
should be multisectoral and should be phased to fit within
the socio-economic constraints of each country. The child
health aspect should include:

(a) The spread of easily accessible primary health care
     services with a strong preventive maternal and child
     health component.
(b) The inclusion of family planning services as an es-
     sential component of the child's and mother's care.
(c) The establishment of a simple but effective informa-
     tion system for better registration and the analysis
     of births and deaths related to the most important
     causes with maternal and neonatal mortality being
     specifically categorized.
(d) Training should be a major component of the remedial
     remedial programs. Three main groups should be in-
     volved in this. The first group should be made of
     families, communities and the public at large. The
     second group should include workers in various de-
     velopmental sectors including policy-makers and
     planners. The third group should include the diff-
     erent categories of health workers: traditional
     birth attendants, health professionals and special-
     lists working at supervisory or referral levels.
(e) Research which is needed to fill in gaps in certain
     areas of our knowledge on neonatal mortality and
     morbidity. Evaluation of new or modified approaches
     as well as monitoring of maternal and neonatal
     health is also very essential.

REFERENCES

1. World Health Organization (1980): Towards a better
        future. Maternal and Child Health Book, WHO,
        Geneva.
2. World Health Organization (1969, 1975): World
        Health Statistics, Report 22:6; World Health
        Statistics Annual, Volume 1. Vital statistics
        and causes of death. WHO, Geneva.
3. World Health Organization (1976): New trends and
        approaches in the delivery of maternal and child
        care in health services. Technical Report
        Series 600, WHO, Geneva.
4. Maternal Child Health (1979): MCH Services in
        Egypt. MCH General Department, Ministry of
        Health, Egypt.
5. World Health Organization (1980): Report of
        scientific working group meeting on maternal
        health in the Eastern Mediterranean Region.
        WHO, EMRO, Geneva, 3-7.
6. World Health Statistics Quarterly (1980):33:197-224.
7. Swedish Agency for Research Cooperation (1978):
        Report No. R:2.

8. Ibrahim GI (1979): In: Care of the Newborn in
    Developing Countries. Macmillan Press, Ltd.,
    London.
9. World Health Organization (1970): Health aspects
    of family planning. Technical Report Series No.
    442, WHO, Geneva.
10. Omran AR and Standley CC (1976): In: Family
    formation patterns and health, WHO, Geneva.
11. Puffer RR and Serrano CV (1973): Patterns of
    mortality in childhood. Pan American Health
    Organization, Scientific Publication No. 262,
    Washington D.C.
12. World Health Organization (1981): Contemporary
    patterns of breast feeding. WHO, Geneva.
13. Gabr M (1981): Malnutrition during pregnancy and
    lactation. World Review of Nutrition and
    dietetics, 36:90-99.
14. Omran AR (1971): The theory of epidemiologic
    transition. Milbank Memorial Fund Quarterly.

INTERRELATIONS BETWEEN MATERNAL AND NEONATAL HEALTH

AND FAMILY PLANNING: CONCEPTUALIZATION OF THE THEME

A. R. Omran

Professor of Epidemiology
University of North Carolina
Chapel Hill, North Carolina

INTRODUCTION

When the "Health Theme in Family Planning" was formulated by this author ten years ago (1), most of the data came from the more developed countries. Evidence for the theme, based on data from developing countries, became available or newly discovered during the decade of the seventies. Furthermore, several major studies in the less developed countries were carried out and provided additional support for the theme. One prominent example is the World Health Organization (WHO) sponsored collaborative study of family planning and health in ten countries. The report on studies in India, Iran, Lebanon, Philippines and Turkey was published by WHO in 1976 (2). The report on studies in Colombia, Egypt, Pakistan and Syria was published in 1981 (3), while the Taiwan report is soon to be published by the Provincial Institute of Maternal and Child Health (4). Another prominent example is the study in several Latin American countries by the Pan American Health Organization (PAHO) in 1975 (5). Furthermore, analysis of data collected by the International Fertility Research Program (IFRP) has provided additional support (6).

One reason for emphasizing the significance of the evidence from less developed countries is that most of the leaders and policymakers, particularly those in Muslim and/or African communities, conveniently dismiss health rationale as being based on the experience of Western society. They require instead, and legitimately so,

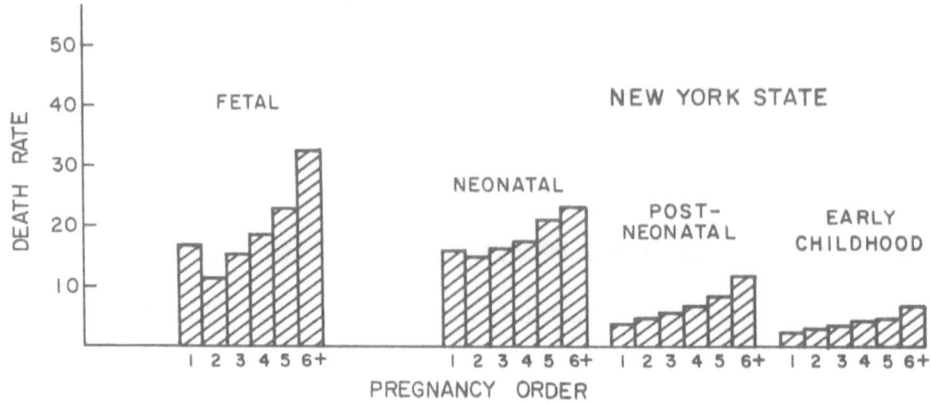

Figure 1.   Fetal, infant and child mortality
            by order of   pregnancy.

evidence from their own health experience. Such evidence
has been the focus of concern in our Center and perhaps in
other Centers as well.

     The purpose of this paper is to present in brief
terms selected concepts of the health theme in family
planning as recently revised. Each concept will be
illustrated by studies in both the more and less developed
countries, as far as space allows, with no attempt at
comprehensive coverage of the literature.

CONCEPTS OF THE HEALTH THEME IN FAMILY PLANNING RELATED TO
MATERNAL AND NEONATAL HEALTH

Parity and Child Mortality

     The risk of child mortality (including late fetal
death, perinatal, neonatal, infant and early childhood
mortality) tend to increase with succeeding parity of
the mother or birth order of the child. For some of the
categories, the risk may also be high for the first child
which gives the relationship with parity a J- or U-shape.

     Although a strong inverse relationship exists between
mortality and social class, the variations in mortality
with birth order are maintained within each social class.
These patterns also occur among all cultures and racial
groups, and persist over time despite considerable decline
in mortality levels.

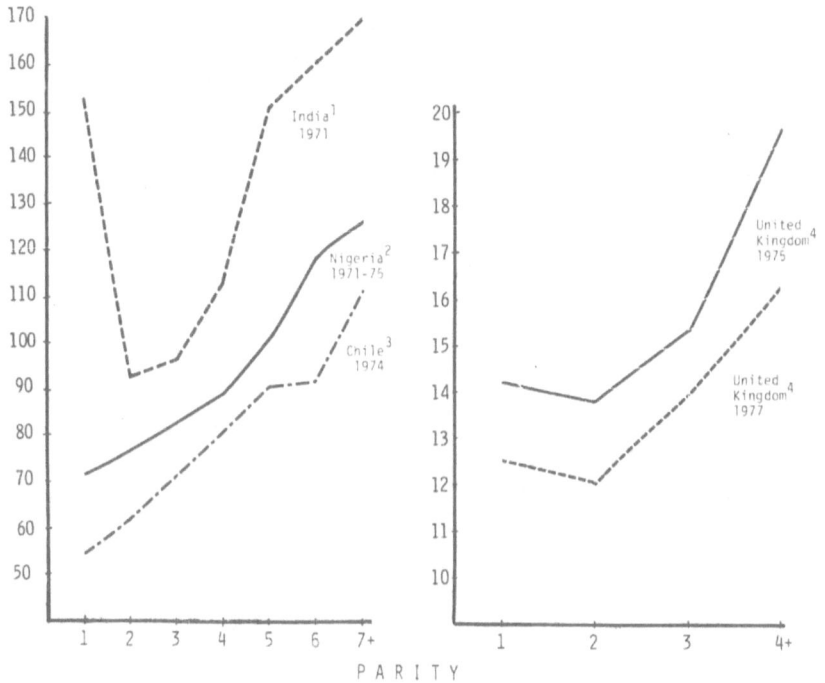

Figure 2. Infant mortality by parity for selected
          countries. [Sources: Pathak (10), Ayeni
          and Odutan (12), Cabrera (13) and
          Adelstein et al (14)

  Selected illustrations. An illustration of the
various child mortality risks in a more developed country
is provided by a study based on the outcome of nearly half
a million births reported in the New York State, exclusive
of New York City, for the period 1950 to 52 (8). While
the post-neonatal and early childhood mortality rates rose
steadily with birth order (parity), fetal and neonatal
death rates had a J-shaped relationship with birth order
(Fig. 1).

  Several studies demonstrate the persistence of this
pattern in various national settings, at different levels
of child mortality, and in different social classes in the
same area. Thus, the J-shaped relationship of late fetal
death with parity was found for several countries (9).

  The increased risk of infant mortality is shown in
Figure 2 for several countries at various levels of mortality ranging from 131 infant deaths per 1000 live births

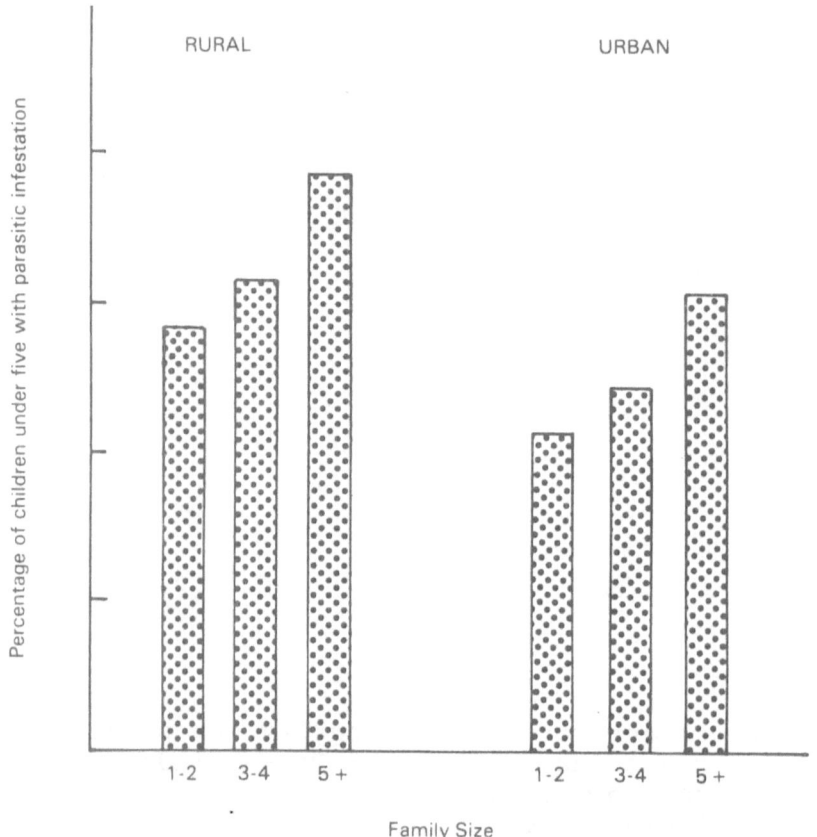

Figure 3. Parasitic infestation in children under
5, by family size. (Egypt)

in an Indian study (10), 89 per 1000 in Nigeria for 1971
to 75 (12), 69 per 1000 in Chile for 1974 (13), and in
England and Wales (14) 15.4 and 13.5 per 1000 for 1975 and
1977 respectively. It is to be noted that when the mortality risk is unusually high for first order births (as in
the Indian study), the relationship is more like a U-
shape. These data demonstrate the persistence of the risk
pattern in various geographic, cultural, and social
settings.

Parity and Child Health and Development

A large family (or sibship) size and high birth order
may exert a detrimental effect on physical and intellectual development. However, in view of the many competing

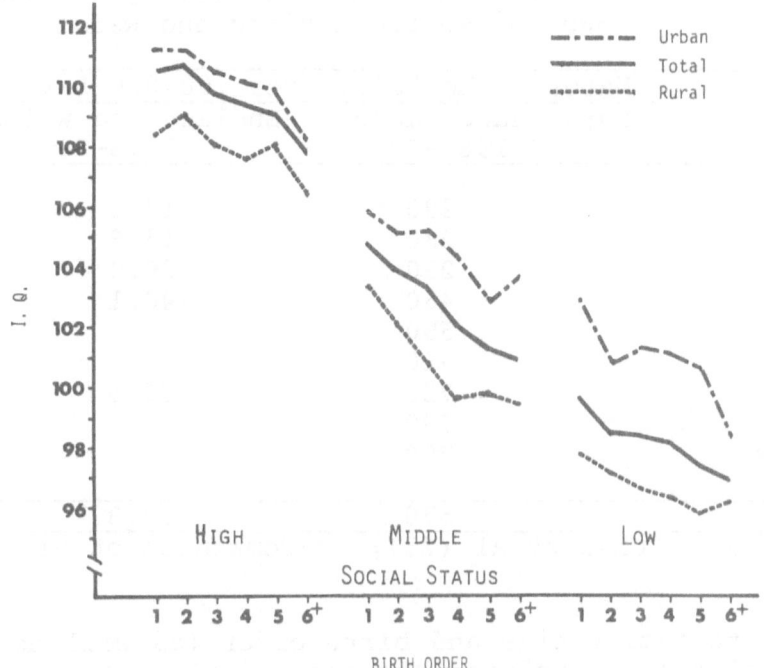

Figure 4. I.Q. by birth order, residence, and
social status (Taiwan). [Source: Omran
and Fan, (4)]

variables (genetic and environmental) and the difficulties
of assessing intellectual attainment in developing
societies, these data must be interpreted cautiously.

Birth weight and prematurity provide measures of
infant physical development. Controversy exists about the
relationship of birth weight and prematurity to birth order. Mean birth weight seems to increase with birth order
(although not consistently), while the rates for prematurity (defined as a birth weight of 2500 g or less)
have either a linear or a J-shaped relationship to birth
order.

As measured by weight, height, and sexual maturity,
the physical growth of children from large families
compares unfavorably with that of children from small
families. The difference, however, is small and is
evident mainly in large studies.

A number of child health conditions have also been

Table 1. Maternal Mortality by Parity: Rural
          Bangladesh and England and Wales

Parity	Maternal Mortality per 100,000 Live Birth	
	Rural Bangladesh* 1968-70	England and Wales** 1973-75
1	990	17.3
2	280	13.8
3	230	26.0
4	480	40.1
5	590	
6	520	
7	720	66.6
8	730	
9+	780	
All	570	20.3

Sources: *Chen et al (23); **Tomkinson et al (24).

linked to family size and birth order (as well as to
maternal age). Included are congenital malformation, physical handicaps, malnutrition, dental problems, infectious
diseases, emotional problems, and mental illness. Some
conditions, such as malnutrition, are probably directly
related to increased strain on family and maternal resources with each additional child. In the case of common
infections, larger family size may simply lead to more
frequent exposure to infectious agents through other
family members.

    Selected illustrations. An illustration of
prematurity in relation to parity is provided by an international maternity study in Dacca, Indonesia, Cairo,
Khartoum, Ibadan, Italy and Unea in Sweden (6). For example, in Dacca prematurity rates are relatively high for
primiparas (25 percent), decrease somewhat for parity 2-4
(20 percent), and increase again for grandmultiparities
(24 percent).

    Another illustration can be given for parasitic
infection from an Egyptian study (3) whereby the incidence
of parasitic infection increases with family size as shown
in Figure 3.

Sibling Size and Intelligence

    With regards to intellectual development, increasing
evidence shows that children from large families obtain

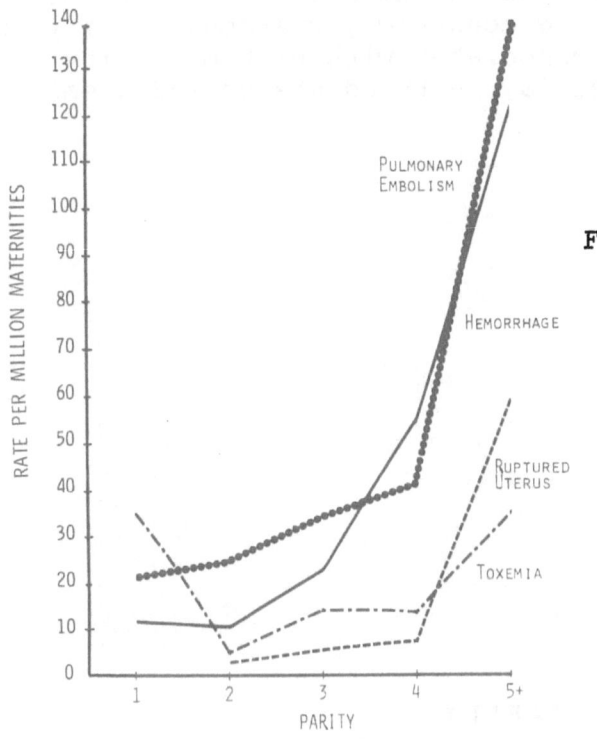

Figure 5. Maternal death by parity and cause, England and Wales, 1970 to 1972. [Source: Tomkinson et al (24).]

relatively lower intelligence scores than those from small families. Mental retardation also is positively associated with family size. This area, however, will require further research, especially in the developing world. This effect is independent of social class.

    Selected illustrations. The decline of intelligence scores with increasing birth order of family size is shown in Figure 4 of a Taiwanese study (15). This study shows the expected negative association of intelligence scores and social class, but within each social class, the decline of scores with parity is maintained.

Parity and Maternal Health

    Multiparity, especially grandmultiparity, carries increased risks of maternal mortality. The classical triad of maternal mortality in industrialized countries used to be toxemia, hemorrhage and sepsis. These conditions have been on the decline in recent years and are being displaced by complications of anaesthesia and

ammiotic fluid embolism, with toxemia continuing to be a
problem. In the developing countries, grandmultiparity is
still prevalent and is associated with high mortality from
hemorrhage, sepsis, toxemia, ruptured uterus and anemia.

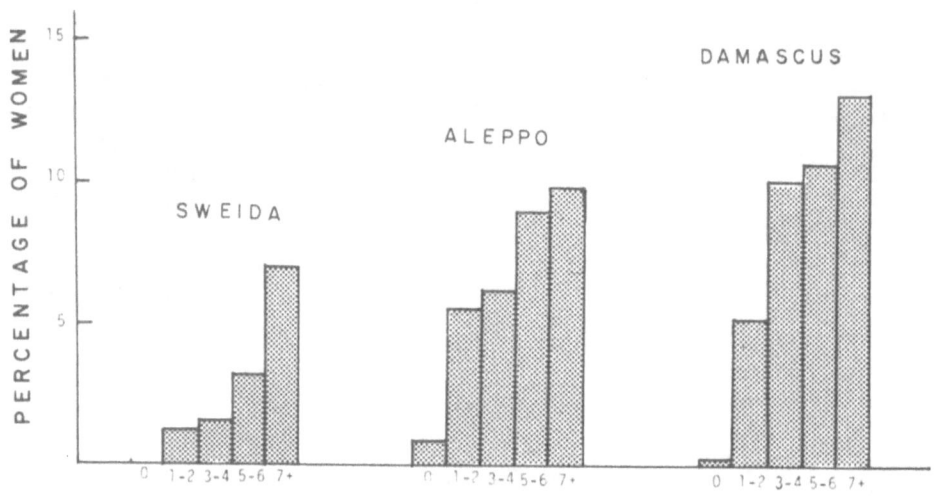

PARITY

Figure 6. Utero-vaginal prolapse by parity (Syria)
[Source: Omran and Standley (3)]

Selected illustrations. A J-shaped relationship of
maternal mortality to parity is evidenced in rural Bangladesh, and England and Wales, as shown in Table 1. The
British study provides also details for individual major
causes as shown in Figure 5. Maternal mortality rates
from pulmonary embolism, hemorrhage, and ruptured uterus
shows increase with parity, while toxemia show a U-shaped
relationship.

Parity and Maternal Morbidity

High parity, particularly grandmultiparity, is linked
with gynecological problems, such as prolapse, cervicitis,
cervical erosion, cancer of cervix, as well as non-obstet-
ric problems, particularly diabetes and rheumatic disease.
The evidence for hypertension in relation to parity is
still equivocal, while breast and ovarian cancer may be
inversely related to parity.

Selected illustrations. An International Maternity
Center Study (6) demonstrated an increase with parity of

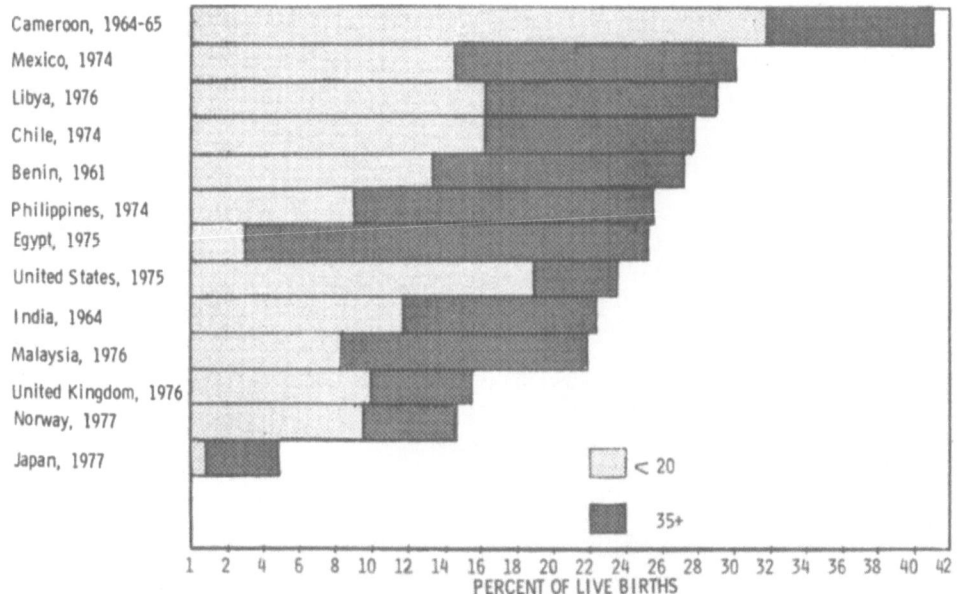

Figure 7.   Percent of live births born to women under age
            20 and age 35 and over, for selected countries
            and years. [Source: U. N. Demographic Yearbook
            (25)]

both the pregnancy complications or antenatal conditions
(including anemia, prepartum hemorrhage, toxemia and
hypertension). This study also demonstrated an increase
in the need for blood transfusion which was used as a
proxy indicator of labor complications.

     Ruptured uterus stands out as an important complica-
tion associated with parity as indicated by several
African and Asian studies. The increased incidence of
ruptured uterus with parity was reported by Armon (16) fo
Malawi and Tanzania, and Gurovsky (17) in Addis Ababa.

     Uterine prolapse is another gynecological condition
which increases with parity, as demonstrated by a Syrian
study (3) in Fig. 6. Diabetes is one of the non-
gynecological diseases associated with parity and this is
demonstrated for England (18) and the United States, 1960
to 62.

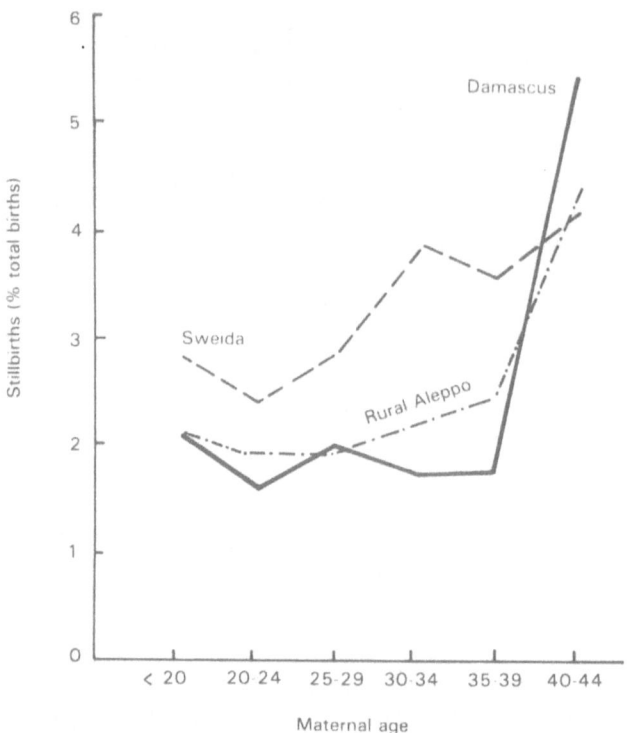

Figure 8.   Stillbirths as a percentage of total births, by
            residence and maternal age (Syria). [Source:
            WHO Collaborative Study, Omran and Standley (3)]

Maternal Age and Child Mortality

     There seems to be an age-band in the fertility span
of a woman during which the reproductive risks are at a
minimum;   on either side of this relatively safe age-band,
the risks progressively increases, described either by a
J-shaped, a U-shaped or occasionally a reversed J-shaped
curve. These patterns are particularly typical for late
fetal deaths, perinatal mortality, infant mortality,
prematurity, and maternal mortality.

     Selected illustrations. A substantial proportion
of children in the less developed countries, and in some
of the more developed countries, are born to mothers at
the risky age groups. Both teenage pregnancies and pregnancies at ages older than 38 are prevalent in Africa,

Table 2. Infant Mortality per 1000 Live Births by
          Maternal Age in Ghana, Chile, and Eng-
          land and Wales.

Maternal Age	GHANA* 1971	CHILE** 1975	ENGLAND AND WALES*** 1975	1977
Under 20	84.3	87.5		
Under 20	84.3	87.5	22.7	21.2
20 - 24	74.1	68.7	16.3	14.8
25 - 29	83.7	59.0	12.5	11.4
30 - 34	83.3	61.5	12.9	11.0
35+	108.2	76.3	17.1	13.2
All ages	87.0	69.4	15.1	13.4

[Source: *Tawiah, 1979; **Cabrera, (13); ***Adelstein, (14)]

Table 3. Incidence of Down's Syndrome per 100,000
          by Maternal Age in 16 Countries.

Maternal Age	Incidence per 100,000
Under 15	30
15 - 19	50
20 - 24	32
25 - 29	38
30 - 34	163
35 - 39	211
40 - 44	634
45+	1,665

[Source: Stevenson et al (21)]

Asia and Latin American as illustrated in Figure 7.
Teenage pregnancies may still be disproportionately high
in countries like the United States. Japan appears to be
one of the countries where women manage to restrict their
pregnancies to the safe band of reproductive age.

The relative increase of infant mortality at young
maternal ages (under 20) and at advanced maternal ages
(35+) is demonstrated in Table 2 for several countries at
different levels of infant mortality, ranging from 87 per
1000 in Ghana (26)), 69 per 1000 in Chile (13), and 15.4
for 1975 and 13.4 for 1977 in England and Wales (14). A
J-shaped relationship is found also (Fig. 8) for stillbirth ratios as demonstrated in the Syrian study (3).

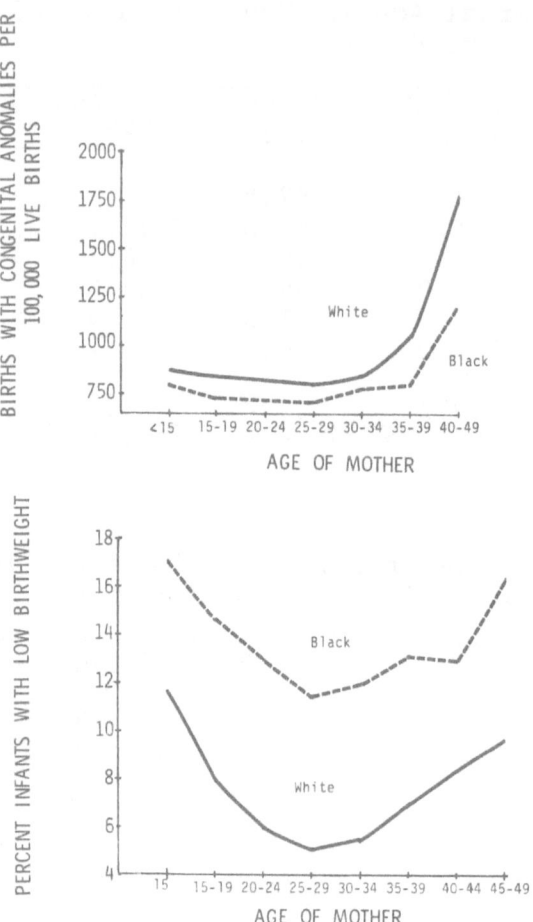

Figure 9.   Congenital anomaly rates by age of mother
(top)   and race, 1973 to 74, United States Average.
           [Source: Taffel (19)]

Figure 9.   Percent of infants of low birth weight by age of
(bottom)   mother and race, United States, 1976. [Source:
           Taffel (20)]

Maternal Age and Child Health and Development

     Maternal age has been found to be the family forma-
tion variable most strongly correlated with congenital
malformation and handicapping conditions in children. The
incidence of these conditions, especially Down's Syndrome,

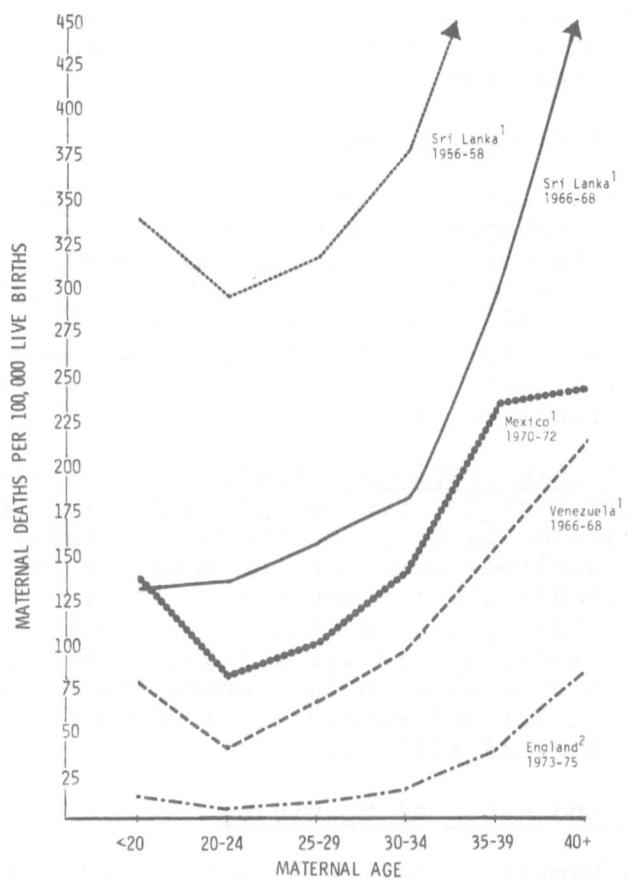

Figure 10.   Maternal deaths by age. [Source:
             Tietze (22) and Tomkinson (24)]

increases with advancing maternal age, especially after
age 30.

     In regard to birth weight and prematurity, teenage
girls and older mothers have been found to be more likely
to bear a low weight baby.

     Selected illustrations. The increase of congenital
malformation with maternal age is illustrated for the
United States (19) in Figure 9, top. A U-shaped relationship is depicted in Figure 9, bottom for low birth weight
and age for the United States (20).

     In a large WHO-sponsored study of congenital mal-

formation in 24 medical centers in 16 countries (both
developed and less developed), the most prominent finding
was the spectacular increase of Down's Syndrome with
advancing maternal age (21) as shown in Table 3.

Maternal Age and Maternal Mortality

The risk of maternal mortality usually describes a
parabolic, or J-shaped curve with maternal age. Minimal
high risk occurs for maternal ages in the early twenties,
with high risk for teenage pregnancies, and higher risk
for mothers over 35. This relationship with maternal age
is found for all major causes of mortality, including
sepsis, toxemia, and hemorrhage, and in countries at all
levels of maternal mortality.

Selected illustrations. Maternal mortality rates
are relatively high for teenage pregnancies in most countries as indicated in a recent WHO Report (22). The risk
of mortality declines somewhat for ages 20 to 29 or 20 to
34, then increases significantly with age in all countries
at various mortality levels (Fig. 10). This is true for
extrmely high maternal mortality rates in Sri Lanka, from
1956 to 58 and from 1966 to 68, intermediate rates in
Mexico (1970 to 72) and Venezuela (1966 to 68), and very
low rates in England (1973 to 75).

Maternal Age and Maternal Morbidity

A large number of maternal health conditions are
associated with maternal age. Antenatal complications,
obstetrical problems, diabetes, and hypertension have all
been shown to increase at older maternal ages. Teenage
pregnancies have increasingly become a major source of
concern and have been shown to carry a high risk of
toxemia, prolonged labor, caesarian section, cervical
laceration, and other obstetrical complications and
maternal health problems.

Figure 11. Pregnancy wastage by duration of preceding
(top)   pregnancy interval for all residential areas
           combined in Egypt. [Source: Omran and
           Standley (3)]

Figure 11. Infant deaths (<1 year of age) according to
(bottom)   birth interval and parity in Ghana. [Source:
           Addo and Goody (26)]

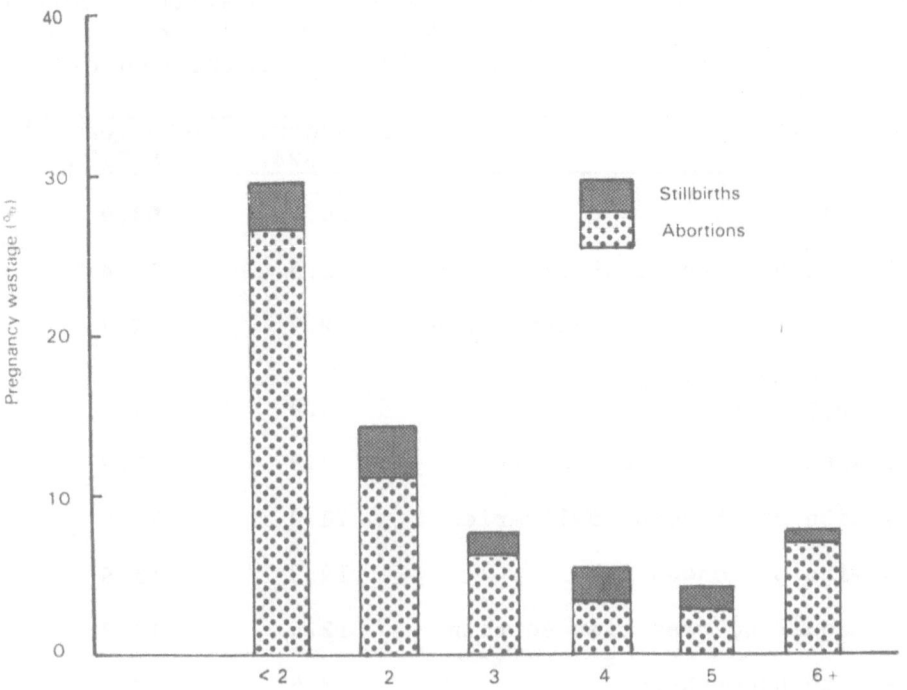

Preceding pregnancy interval (years)

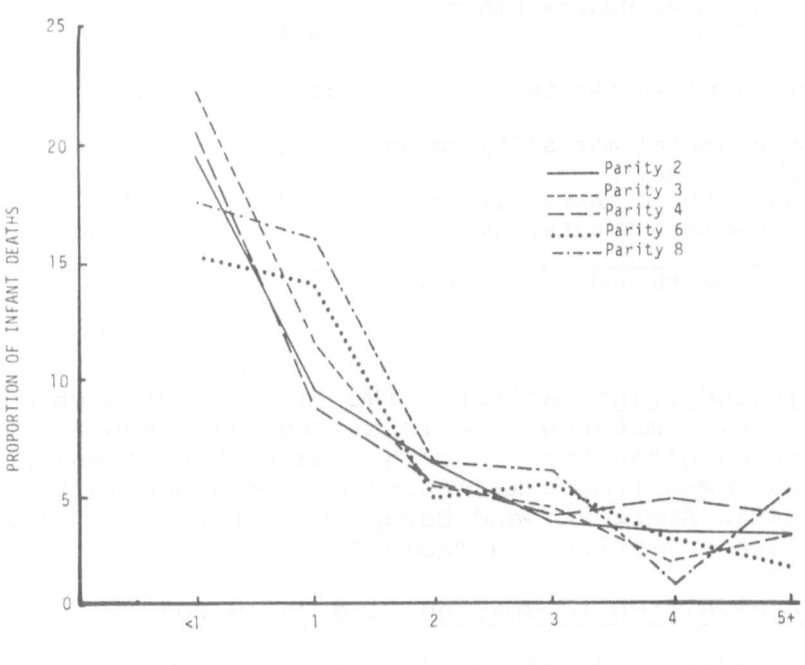

BIRTH INTERVALS IN YEARS

Table 4.   Reproductive Performance and Delivery Outcome
           for Teenagers and Women Ages   20 to 24 years in
           Seven African and Asian Maternity Centers.

Condition	Teenagers N=624	20-24 Year Olds N=2273
% multiparas	25.3	53.9
% with history of abortion	5.9	12.4
% with anemia during pregnancy	2.9	2.7
% with pre-eclampsia and hypertension	6.8	7.9
% with pre-term deliveries	17.9	13.2
% with spontaneous deliveries	78.4	71.9
% with prolonged labor	19.3	18.8
% requiring caesarian section	12.6	10.3
% with hemorrhage	3.5	2.5
% with puerperal complication	6.5	4.2
% with neonatal deaths among their babies	4.5	3.5
% with premature babies	19.6	12.2
% with perinatal mortality among their babies: those with no antenatal care those with antenatal care	6.1 7.4	5.7 3.3

[Source: Omran and Omran (7)]

Selected illustrations. The increase of morbidity
with advancing maternal age is all too well known. The
illustration given here concerns the risk of teenage pregnancy and comes from a maternity center study in Afro-
Asian, Latin American, and European centers (7). The
results are summarized in Table 4.

Birth Interval (Child Spacing) and Child Health

Prevailing medical opinions favor spacing of
pregnancies in order to allow restoration of health of

mothers, to safeguard the health of the offspring and to enable mothers to breast feed their children without the added burden of a new pregnancy.

Short birth intervals are associated with higher risks of poor outcome of subsequent pregnancy, child mortality and malnutrition, poor physical and intellectual development as well as high maternal risks. The effects do not relate only to the preceding, but also the succeeding intervals. It follows that both the displaced child and the displacing child are affected. Birth interval effects are by no means entirely independent of those of age and parity.

Selected illustrations. Illustrations for birth interval effect can be found in several studies. For this paper, we choose the following (Fig. 11 top, and 11 bottom):

(a)   A recent study in Egypt (27) of fetal wastage was extremely high for intervals of less than one year. Again the small rise at intervals of 6 or more years is also evident.

(b)   A study in Ghana (26) demonstrated the high risk of infant mortality associated with short intervals. This is demonstrated for all parities.

CONCLUSION

The overall conceptualization of the health theme in family planning can be stated as follows:

1.   A child's chances of being born alive, surviving the first five years of life, enjoying good health and adequate physical and intellectual development are reduced by:

(a)   Poor pregnancy timing, i.e., being conceived at an early maternal age of less than 20 years, or conversely at an advanced maternal age of 35+ years.
(b)   A large sibship size of three or more, i.e., high parity in regard to the mother and high birth order in regard to the child.
(c)   Inadequate spacing between the child and his preceding or succeeding sibs.
(d)   Multiparity.

(e)   Poor prenatal and natal care for the mother and poor
      child care.
(f)   Any combination of the above, particularly high pari-
      ty at a young age, or grandmultiparity at any age.

      2. A mother's chance of surviving pregnancy and
labor, of being free from obstetrical and gynecological
problems, of enjoying good health and having normal and
healthy children, are reduced by the same factors
affecting a child's health.

      The prescription of family planning will reduce
substantially health risks to children and mothers and
hence, should become a part of routine medical care for
responsible health professionals everywhere in the world.

      The provision of family planning services, including
effective information, education and communication programs is a basic responsibility of all governments and
policy makers, regardless of the level of demographic
pressures in the concerned countries.

REFERENCES

1. Omran AR (1971): The health theme family planning.
      Population Center Monograph No. 16, Chapel Hill,
      North Carolina.
2. Omran AR and Standley CC (1976): Family formation
      patterns and health. World Health Organization,
      Geneva.
3. Omran AR and Standley CC (1981): Family formation
      patterns and health, Volume II.   World Health
      Organization, Geneva.
4. Omran AR and Fan KY (1982): Family formation
      patterns and health in Taiwan. (In Press)
5. Puffer RR and Serrano CV (1975): Birth weight,
      maternal age, and birth order, Three important
      determinants in infant mortality. Pan American
      Health Organization Scientific Publication No. 294,
      WHO, Washington.
6. Omran AR (1978): Health consequences of high risk
      pregnancies in Muslim women. A cross-national
      maternity center study. Presented at the Pan
      Islamic Conference on Motherhood, Cairo, December
      11-13.
7. Omran AR and Omran KF (1977): International
      experience with teenage pregnancies, A preliminary
      report. Presented at the First International
      Conference of the Society of Gynecology and

Obstetrics of Nigeria, Ibadan, October 16-22.
8. Chase HC (1961): The relatioship of certain biologic
    and socioeconomic factors to fetal, infant and
    early childhood mortality. I. Father's
    occupation, parental age, and infant's birth rank.
    New York State Department of Health, Albany.
9. World Health Statistics Report (1971): 24:43-55.
10. Pathak SKB (1971): Infant motality, birth order, and
    contraception in India. J Family Welfare,
    25:12-21.
11. Omran AR (1975): Health rationale for family
    planning. In: Population change, a strategy for
    physicians, LS Block, Editor. World Fedration for
    Medical Education, Bethesda.
12. Ayenti O and Odutan SO (1978): The effects of sex,
    birth weight, birth order and maternal age on
    infant mortality in a Nigerian community. Ann
    Human Biol, 5:353-358.
13. Cabrera R (1980): The influence of maternal age,
    birth order and socioeconomic status on infant
    mortality in Chile. Am J Pub Health 70:174-177.
14. Adelstein AM, Davies IMM and Weatherall JAC (1980):
    Perinatal and infant mortality. Social and
    biological factors 1975-77. Studies on Medical
    and Population Subjects No. 41, Office of
    Population Censuses and Surveys, Her Majecty's
    Stationery Office, London.
15. Omran AR, Fan KY and Riad M (1982): Birth order,
    family size and intelligence. (In Press)
16. Armon PJ (1977): Rupture of the uterus in Malawi and
    Tanzania. East African Med J, 54:462-471.
17. Gurovsky S (1971): Rupture of the gravid uterus.
    Ethiopian Med J, 9:193-196.
18. Pyke DA (1956): Parity and the incidence of diabetes.
    Lancet, 1:818-821.
19. Taffel S (1978): Congenital anomalies and birth
    injuries among live births: United States,
    1973-74. Vital and Health Statistics, Series 21,
    No. 31.
20. Taffel S (1980): Factors associated with low birth
    weight, United States, 1976. Vital and Health
    Statistics, Series 21, No. 37.
21. Stevenson AC et al (1966): Congenital malformations.
    Bull WHO, 34 (suppl.): 5-127.
22. Tietze C (1977): Maternal mortality excluding
    abortion mortality. World Health Statistics
    Report, 30:312-338.
23. Chen LC et al (19747): Maternal mortality in rural
    Bangladesh. Studies in Family Planning,
    5:334-341.

24. Tomkinson J (1979): <u>Report on confidential enquiries
    into maternal deaths in England and Wales 1973-75</u>.
    Report on Health and Social Subject 14, Her
    Majesty's Stationery Office, London.
25. United Nations (1979): <u>Demographic Yearbook</u> 1978,
    New York.
26. Addo NW and Goody JR (1974): <u>Siblings in Ghana</u>.
    University of Ghana Population Studies No. 7,
    Legon.
27. Watson W et al (1979): Health, population and
    nutrition. Interrelations, problems and possible
    solutions. In: <u>World population and development,
    challenges and prospects</u>, P. Hauser, Editor,
    United Nations Fund for Population Activities, New
    York.
28. Wray JD (1971): Population pressure on families:
    Family size and child spacing. In: <u>Rapid
    Population Growth, Vol. II</u>, National Academy of
    Sciences, Baltimore, 403-461.

HEALTH BENEFITS OF APPROPRIATE TIMING, SPACING AND
AVOIDING HIGH PARITY AND RISKS OF UNPLANNED
FERTILITY FOR THE MOTHER

S. S. Ratnam and R. L. TambyRaja

Department of Obstetrics and Gynaecology
National University of Singapore
Singapore

INTRODUCTION

Childbirth in developing countries remains the main
cause of death in females between the ages of 15 and 45
and considerably affects female life expectancy. Differences in maternal mortality in the developed and
developing world are shocking (Table 1). Between 4 to 40
deaths per 100,000 births occur in developed countries
compared to 40 to 120 in developing countries, and 150 to
300 in underdeveloped or least developed countries. A
recent summary of maternal mortality from India shows a
mortality rate of 750 per 100,000 while in Denmark it is
only 4 per 100,000. Morbidity in the form of anemia from
repeated pregnancies and intercurrent infections have
contributed to obstetrical complications adding to the
heavy penalty of motherhood in the developing world (1-9).

Singapore has seen a dramatic decline in population
with a fall in total births from 50,000 in 1967 to
39,000 in 1978. The crude birth rate decreased from 42.7
to 16.9 and was accompanied by an unequivocal fall in
maternal mortality. More interesting is the decrease in
multiparous women in the last 15 years with the median
birth order falling to 1.75. The distribution of live
births by birth order, the numerical order of the child in
relation to all live-born issues of the mother, is shown
in Table 2. A distinct increase in the number and proportion of first and second order births since 1967 was
noted. The percentage of first order births increased from
23 percent in 1967 to 28 percent in 1970 and to almost

43

Table 1.   Comparison of Some Indicators Related to
           Health in Countries of Varying Levels of
           Development.

Health-Related Indicator	Countries		
	Developed	Developing	Underdeveloped
Maternal mortality rate per 100,000	4 - 40	40 - 120	150 - 300
Health manpower			
Health workers	1:130	1:500	1:220
Physicians	1:520	1:2700	1:1500
Nurses	1:220	1:1500	1:6500
Infant mortality rate per 1000 live births	<10-20	100 - 200	>200
Death rate (1 to 5 years) per 1000	1	20	30
Per capita daily energy supply (kilo cal)	3,400	2,400	<2000
Gross National Product (in U.S.$)	5000-10000	100-1000	<200
Health expendture in percent GNP	5 -9	2 - 3	
Literacy rate in percent/population	<100		28

42 percent in 1978. The second order births increased from
19 percent in 1967 to 23 percent in 1970 and 33 percent in
1978. Third order births increased, but at a slower pace
from 14 percent in 1967 to approximately 16 percent for the
1975 to 78 period.

Higher order births, on the other hand, showed a persistent decline. This decline is attributed to literate
and health conscious young mothers in Singapore in
contrast to neighboring countries.

DEMAND FOR IMPROVED MATERNAL AND NEONATAL HEALTH

The total population of the world increased in the
1970s at an annual rate of approximately 1.9 percent. If
this rate of increase continues, the total world population will exceed 6000 million by the year 2000. In 1980
the developing countries accounted for almost 75 percent
of the world population; by the year 2000, ths figure is
likely to increase to about 80 percent.

Table 2. Distribution of Live Births by Birth Order in
Singapore.

Birth Order	1967	1970	1978
1st	11,692	12,911	16,424
2nd	9,620	10,538	12,962
3rd	6,902	7,256	6,463
4th	5,394	4,588	2,181
5th and over	16,631	10,490	1,33
Not stated	321	151	78
Total	50,560	45,934	39,441
		Percent	
1st	23.1	28.1	41.6
2nd	19.0	23.0	32.9
3rd	13.7	15.8	16.4
4th	10..7	10.0	5.5
5th and over	32.9	22.8	3.4
Not stated	0.6	0.3	0.2
Total	100.0	100.0	100.0
Median Birth Order	3.7	2.45	1.75

Changes in age structure are also foreseen. In the
developed countries, 23 percent of the population are
below the age of 15, whereas 11 percent are aged 65 and
over; projections for the year 2000 in these countries
show a reduction of less than 22 percent in the population
below 15 and an increase to 13 percent in the population
aged 65 and over. As for developing countries, an average
of 40 percent of the population is below the age of 15 and
4 percent are aged 65 and over; projections for the year
2000 show a reduction to about 34 percent in those under
15 and an increase to about 5 percent in those aged 65 and
over. This is illustrated in the age pyramid for
Singapore.

Nearly 1000 million people of the developing
countries are trapped in the vicious cycle of poverty,
malnutritions, disease and despair that reduces their work
capacity and limit their ability to plan for the future
(Fig. 1). For the most part they live in rural areas and
urban slums of the developing countries. The depth of
their deprivation can be expressed by a few statistics
comprraring the developed, developing and underdeveloped
countries (Table 1).

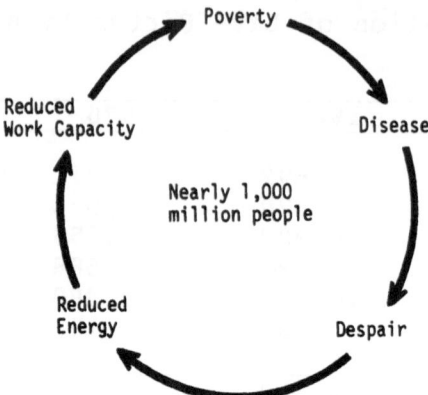

Figure 1.   Health and socio-economic status of nearly
            1000 million people in the developing world.

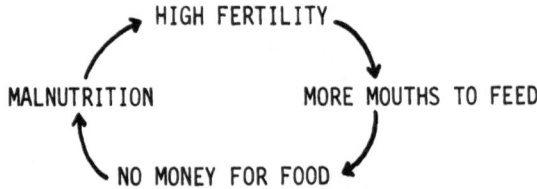

Figure 2.   Viscious cycle of poverty, malnutrition and
            high fertility.

     The health manpower availability in terms of total
health workers, physicians and nurses per population, show
gross disparity between developed and developing countries.
In some rural areas in the least developed countries, there
is only one doctor per 200,000 population compared to 1 per
300 in the metropolitan areas of some developed countries.
Infant mortality rate is only between 10 and 20 out of
every 1000 infants born in developed countries while it
ranges from nearly 100 to over 200 per 1000 in developing
and underdeveloped countries. Death rate for children
between 1 and 5 years old is about 1 per 1000 in most
developed countries; it averages about 20 in many developing countries and more than 30 in Africa. Of every 1000
children born into poverty in the least developed countries, 200 die within a year, another 100 die before the
age of 5 years, and only 500 survive to age 40. Hardly
half of the children reach the age of five. This wastage
of human life could be prevented by limiting family size
and spacing births. In the foreground are are three major

causes of this high mortality which are interacting in the
vicious circle: malnutrition, infectious diseases and
high fertility (Fig. 2).

In developing countries, malnutrition afflicts hundreds of millions of people. In these countries as many
as one-fourth of the people have food intake below the
critical minimum level. The average per capita daily
energy supply in developed countries is about 3400 kilo-
calories, a figure far in excess of standard requirements;
it is about 2400 for most developing counries and 2000 in
the least developed.

The economic situation of a country has a direct
bearing on health. Gross national product (GNP) is still
the economic indicator in most common use. In general,
countries with high GNP have low infant mortality rate and
a high life expectancy; the opposite high infant mortality rate and low life expectancy is the situation in
countries with a low GNP. The GNP ranges from US $5000 to
US $10,000 in most developed countries while it is from US
$200 to US $1000 in most developing countries. The health
expenditure expressed in percent GNP in developed countries is 5 to 9 percent and in developing countries is 2
to 3 percent.

Literacy is of major importance for health. It
enables people to understand their health problems and
ways of solving them, and facilitates their active involvement in community health activities. Whereas the
adult literacy rate is almost 100 percent in industrialized countries, it is 28 percent in the least developed
countries, and only 13 percent among women in those
countries. Some 900 million adults in developing countries cannot read or write, and only 4 out of every 10 of
their children complete more than three years of primary
schooling.

Singapore, compared to that of neighboring countries,
is now dealing with a more sophisticated, affluent and educated population. A few indicators illustrate this change.
The per capita GNP increased from US $995 in 1968 to US
$2990 in 1978. The total literacy rate increased from 72.2
percent in 1970 to 77.4 percent in 1978. The rate of
participation in the labor force has also increased considerably among Singapore females; only 28.4 percent of the
female population aged 15 years and over were working in
1966; this increased to 34.6 percent in 1978.

Singapore is one of the world's most densely populated

country. The population density is 3.784 persons per sq.
km. The population of Singapore is multi-ethnic in
structure with the Chinese contributing 76 percent of the
population, Malays 15 percent, Indians 7 percent and other
races 2 percent. In the late 1960's, the Singapore Family
Planning and Population Board was established to clearly
define population policy and set targets. This has had a
dramatic effect on the birth rate. Despite the increase
in the proportion of female population in the reproductive
age group, there is a drop in the live births and crude
birth rate from 1957 to 1980 (Fig. 3).

The population policies, incentives and disincentives, abortion and sterilization laws contributed to the
fall in the crude birth rate. The higher crude birth rate
from 1970 to 1973 is the result of a significant increase
among child bearing age group of 20 to 29 years. The
general decrease in crude birth rate is clearly reflected
in a drop of annual growth rate from 3.3 percent in 1966,
to 1.6 percent in 1978 and 1.4 percent in 1980. From 1966

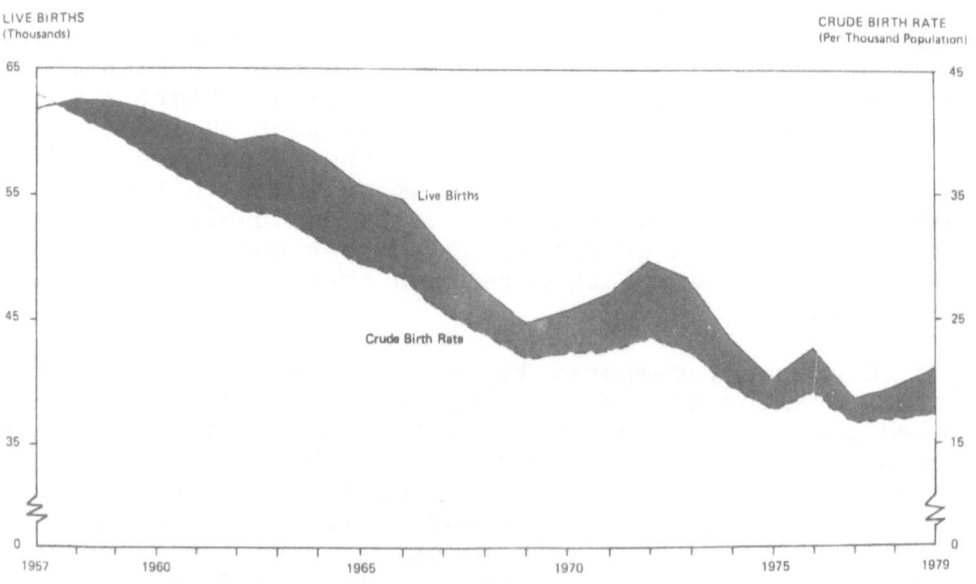

Figure 3.   Live Births and Crude Birth rates in
            Singapore, 1957-1979.

to 1977, the fertility rate also fell by 31 percent, and
this fall continued till 1976. The fertility rate dropped
sharply in 1974 to 75 because of the introduction of
legalized abortion, sterilization and social disincentives.
The social disincentives are in the form of higher delivery
fees, reduction of paid maternity leaves, lower priority
for choice of school for children and removal of income tax
relief for children of higher parity.

THE SINGAPORE EXPERIENCE

In Singapore, an effective sterilization program
accounting to nearly 7000 to 8000 sterilizations a year
and control of fertility (1400 to 5000 per year), has led
to one of the most effective means of avoiding high parity
and limiting family size. The liberalized abortion laws
has led to one of the most effective means of fertility
control; this, coupled with advice on contraception and
provision of heavily subsidized contraceptives by trained
personnel, have complemented other methods of fertility
control.

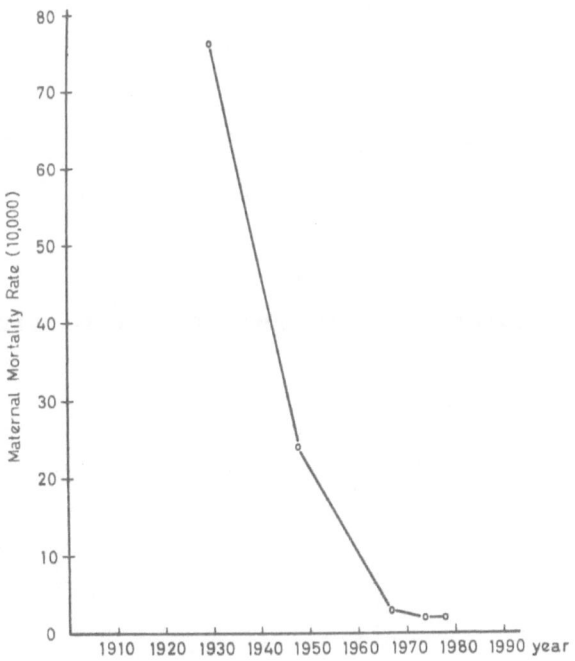

Figure 4. Maternal mortality in Singapore (1930-1978).

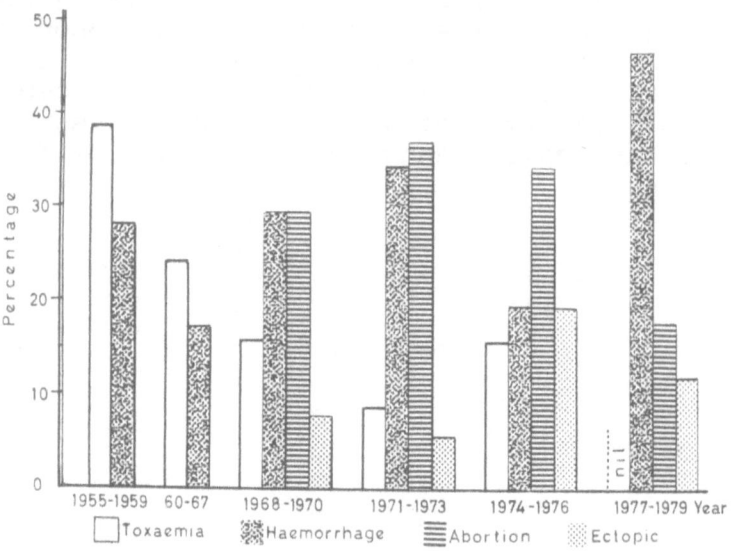

Figure 5.   Causes of maternal deaths in Singapore.

RESULTS OF FAMILY LIMITATION IN SIGNAPORE

The most important result of family limitation perhaps is the decline in maternal mortality reaching figures as low as 2 per 10000 births, comparing well or better than most industrialized nations (Fig. 4). Prior to liberalization of abortion laws in Singapore, maternal mortality from abortion was 40 per 10000 births; the reduction of abortion deaths from 1972 has contributed significantly to the reduction in maternal mortality (Fig. 5). It is paradoxical however that despite decreasing parity, hemorrhage has become the leading killer in Singapore.

With the well-known association of lower perinatal mortality in paragravida 2 and 3, we are now dealing with the ideal obstetric population against this background in the University Department of Obstetrics with ancillary aids of staff, drugs and biochemical and biophysical techniques like ultrasound and cardiotachography. Thus perinatal mortality has been reduced to nearly 10 per 1000 with a decrease in maternal mortality and morbidity. There could have been a reduction in perinatal morbidity by way of mental handicaps and subnormal infants.

CONCLUSION

Close surveillance is necessary even in Singapore because the rising number of young men and women in the population is an inevitable demographic fact. The only way in which the number of births can remain low over the next few years is for women to postpone having their babies. This can be achieved by:

(a) delaying the age of marriage;
(b) dalaying the birth of the first child; and
(c) spacing children.

This has to be applied to the rest of Southeast Asia.

Legislative changes like the liberalization of abortion and sterilization and making contraceptives easily available to an educated motivated population will reduce the number of high risk pregnancies and bring about a healthy family unit.

REFERENCES

1. SFPPB (1979): Fourteenth Report of Singapore Family
    Planning and Population Board.
2. TambyRaja RL, Ratnam SS (1981): The small fetus,
    preterrm and growth retarded. In: Clinics in
    Obstetrics and Gynaecology, RM Philpott, Editor,
    (In Press) 9:3.
3. Wong HB (1965): Perinatal mortality in Kandang Kerbau
    Hospital. Bulletin of Kandang Kerbau Hospital
    4:42-46.
4. Wong HB (1979): Perinatal morbidity and mortality in
    Southeast Asia. In: Problems in Perinatology,
    SMM Karim, Editor, MTP, Lancaster 129-146.
5. WHO (1970): The prevention of perinatal mortality and
    morbidity. Wold Health Organization Technical
    Series, 457, 60.
6. WHO (1973-79): World Health Organization Statistical
    Annual.
7. WHO (1976): New trends and approaches in the delivery
    of maternal and child care. Sixth Report, World
    Health Organization Technical Report Series, No.
    600, 98.
8. WHO (1978): Risk approach for maternal and child
    health care. World Health Organization Offset
    Publication, 39, Geneva.
9. World Health Statistics (1979): World Health
    Organization, Geneva, 17.

THE EFFECT OF PARITY, BIRTH INTERVALS AND

MATERNAL AGE ON THE HEALTH OF THE CHILD

O. Ransome-Kuti

Professor of Pediatric and Primary Care
College of Medicine, University of Lagos
Lagos, Nigeria

INTRODUCTION

When a group of mothers in Lagos were asked why they practiced sexual abstinence during lactation, the replies of the majority of both parents referred to the need for "the child to develop well" and also "to prevent the child from becoming ill". Asked if they would like the custom changed, the most frequent answer (29.6 percent) was that they would not because "it would adversely affect the child's health" (1).

Although the reasons given above relate to their perceived effect of breast milk "poisoned" by sexual intercourse on the child's health, they however indicate that this community realizes that early resumption of sexual activity which may result in a pregnancy could adversely affect the health of the child.

In spite of this, many communities in Africa and other developing countries, the birth of many children continues with dire consequences. Much of the argument and exhortation in favor of limiting family size has fallen on deaf ears because the propaganda runs counter to their fundamental belief.

FACTORS AFFECTING HEALTH OF THE CHILD

Parity

Many examples of high neonatal and infant death rates as a result of high parity can be cited from different parts of the world. Among women over the age of 25 of the Ibos of Ebendo village, Bendel State of Nigeria, 13 percent of babies born of mothers of parity three or under die during the first year of life compared with 10 percent of the births to women of parity four to seven and about 22 percent of the births to women of parity eight or over. In this village, due to environmental deprivation, the average mother has seen 1.5 of her children die and 80 percent of all the women have experienced at least one infant or child death before they reach the end of the reproduction period (2).

In Rwanda, 20 percent of infants who are fifth-born in their families die within a year of birth. Among the ninth born and succeeding children, the risk of death is doubled so that 40 percent die by age one (3). In El Salvador and Chile (4), infant deaths during the first year of life increase sharply after the third pregnancy.

Although the proportion of children who die is several times smaller, the same phenomenon and particularly second year mortality rates have been demonstrated in developed countries such as England and Wales, and this applies to all the social classes (5). Women having their third or later delivery in Tientsin, China, have more than four times as many miscarriages and early infant deaths as women having their first or second births.

One reason for the high fertility observed is that, in some cultures, the status of a woman is considerably enhanced by the number of her children, especially boys. Due to the high infant mortality rates and the experience or expectation of infant or child death by many families, many are born in the hope that a few will survive.

Birth Intervals

Not only parity but also short intervals between births may cause dangers to the newly born child or his siblings. In many developing countries, lactational amenorrhoea and sexual abstinence supported by many taboos, customs and superstitions, is the commonest form of child spacing practiced. It may enable families to achieve a spacing of 24 to 33 months or more between births (6, 7). Full breast feeding prolongs the period of postpartum amenorrhoea longer than does partial breast feeding. The introduction of any supplementary feeding to the suckling infant therefore shortens the period of amenorrhea. Because of the adaption of bottle or artificial feeding, this period is shortened. The effect is most marked in the urban than in the rural areas. The death of an infant is also recognized as a major influence in reducing birth intervals due to the termination of lactational amenorrhoea.

Studies in the Punjab have demonstrated that the shorter the preceding interval between birth, the higher the infant mortality rate of newborns (8). Following the birth of a child after a short interval, the preceding child may develop kwashiorkor due to early cessation of breastfeeding. The phenomenon was first noticed by Williams in Ghana in 1938 and is now widely recognized. A similar study in the U.S.A. (9) demonstrated a definite improvement in the survival of the index child as the preceding birth to conception interval is prolonged from 4 months to 3 years or more.

Mother's Age

Babies born of mothers under the age of 21 or over 35 are subject to higher mortality and morbidity. More data, particularly from South America, Canada and the U.S.A. indicate clearly that neonatal mortality is higher for babies born to mothers under the age of 20 than for all other mothers in the community. The same is true of infant deaths whereby it is higher for those born to mothers less than 20 years than for all the mothers. In this maternal age group, prematurity and low birth weight are probably the most important causes of high neonatal and infant mortality with congenital defects, mental and physical handicaps, including epilepsy, cerebral palsy, blindness and deafness (10).

Studies from England and Wales show that fetal deaths during the last two months of pregnancy and during the first week of life is high if the mother is less than 20 years and above 30 (11). The breakdown of customs or other traditional mechanisms which affect adolescent sexuality has given rise to an increase in premarital sex and early pregnancy. This tendency is accentuated by the migration of population from the rural to the urban areas and their exposure to foreign customs through the communication media.

Apart from the dangers to the adolescent mother and her offspring, the social consequences are enormous. The adolescent mother may have to leave school or work, her prospects for future marriage reduced and both mother and

child may face social and legal discrimination. For these
reasons, the United Nations Population Conference Study on
the interrelationship of the status of women and family
planning concluded that "the benefits of family planning
are important, not only for regulating the number and
spacing of children, but also in enabling girls and young
women to avoid pregnancy" (12). In the United States,
one-half of the decline in infant mortality from 1960 to
1970 is attributed to the increasing concentration of
births among women of more favorable age and family size
(13). An added danger to babies of mothers over the age
of 30 is the high probability of congenital malformation;
Down's Syndrome is a typical example.

Large Families

High parity and close child spacing give rise to
large families which contribute to an increased mortality
and morbidity due to overcrowding and poor hygienic conditions. There is increase in the transmission of infection
and shortage of household goods and food for each member
of the family leading to an increased incidence of gastroenteritis and common respiratory infections. In Africa,
Morley and his co-workers showed that after the seventh
parity, there was a marked increase in the chances of malnutrition in the children of the family (14). Similar
studies in Bangkok (15), India (16) and Columbia (17) have
demonstrated the same phenomenon in large families.

The quality of maternal care may be diluted where
there are many children. Studies in many countries have
indicated that children from larger families tend to have
lower intelligence quotients than those with fewer siblings, and within the same family, the higher the birth
order, the lower the IQ (18, 19). In Britain, heights and
weights of children were found to be inversely proportional to family size. This association was present in upper
and lower working classes to the extent that at age 5
years, the difference between the first and third child
was around 10.2 cm or 4 inches (20, 21).

ROLE OF HEALTH SERVICES AND FAMILY PLANNING

There are few studies which have shown a reduction in
child mortality and morbidity as a result of available
family planning services. The Danfa Project in Ghana
demonstrated that when family planning services were combined with comprehensive health care programs and health
education, substantial reduction in fertility and birth

Table 1.   Changes in Observed Birth Rates (BR) and
            General Fertility Rates (GFR).

		1971 to 1972	1976 to 1977
Family Planning plus			
Comp. High School plus	BR	42.8	32.9
Health Education	GFR	226	178
Family Planning plus	BR	44.7	44.6
Health Education	GFR	235	235
Family Planning	BR	51.2	54.2
	GFR	241	283

Source: Danfa Project Final Report (22).

rates were achieved as compared with the rates when family planning services alone were provided. No difference was however found in child survival rates or in the percentage of children who fell below 80 percent of the standard weight for age between children born before contracepting intervals as compared to those born before non-contracepting intervals (22).

In many developing countries, due to high perinatal infant and child mortality rates, attempts to introduce family planning service, or to induce the members of the community to use them when available have proved difficult. It is believed that if parents perceive that their children will survive due to efficient child care services, they will take steps to reduce the size of their families. In Narangwal, an attempt made between 1971 and 1973 by the Johns Hopkins' Group to demonstrate the "child survival hypothesis", and came to the conclusion that "the measurable child replacement effect operates through the parents' subconscious expectation of child death" (23). Parents do not seem consciously to link child mortality with high fertility. However, when the project came to an end after three years of service activity, analysis of their data, which included attitudes and beliefs, showed definite evidence supporting a shift in subconscious awareness of child survival and its relation with variables associated with the use of family planning in those areas where family planning, women services and child care services were introduced (24). The group recognized that the child survival hypothesis would probably have a built in lag of at least 5 years, while parents became aware of declining mortality and improved health in children.

Table 2.   Relationship Between Number of Child Deaths
            and Number of Children Ever Born in Ebendo,
            1974.

Deaths/ age of mother	Number of women	Median of children ever born	Median of children alive	Death in percent of total births
15 - 29				
No deaths	78	2.1	2.1	0
death	17	3.4	2.4	29.4
2-7 deaths	24	5.2	2.6	50.0
39 - 49				
No deaths	55	4.7	4.7	0
1 death	41	5.7	4.7	17.5
2-7 deaths	103	8.0	5.0	37.7

Source: Mott (25)

        A 1974 study by Mott in Ebendo village, Nigeria,
where he examined the number of children a woman ever had
by age of mother and number of deaths, helped to draw the
conclusion that in this community, the women compensate by
having additional children almost exactly equal the number
of deaths they have had (25).   Table 2 show that for the
15 to 29 year old women, the range of the number of children currently alive is 2.1 to 2.6, while the range of
children ever born is wide, i.e., 2.5 to 5.2.   This find-
finding is even more dramatic in the older women (30 to 49
years) who show the wide range, from 4.7 to 8, for the
number of children ever born and the number currently
alive is almost stable at about 5 per woman.   Moreover,
deaths expressed as a percentage of total births increase
sharply as one moves from the women who have had no deaths
to those who have had several deaths, and these additional
deaths are compensated for exactly in terms of additional
births.   The conclusion drawn was that the Ebendo women
react rationally to actual mortality events within their
frame of reference and that if infant and child mortality
could be reduced, there might well be a compensating one
associated with a corresponding decline in completed
family size.

        In Imesi-Ile, Nigeria surviving children and the me-
dian number of additional births desired were studied in
two villages, one with an efficient under five clinic
(26).   There is a suggestion that mothers perceiving that

Table 3.   Surviving Children and Median Number of
             Additional Births Desired by 253 Imesi-Ile
             and Oke-Imesi mothers (1967)

Surviving Children	Imesi-Ile with Under 5 Clinic	Oke-Imesi Control
1	5.9	10.9
2	6.3	8.5
3	4.6	6.8
4	3.6	3.6

Source: Cunningham (26)

their children are surviving, have began to realize the
need to reduce their fertility.

    In our Lagos clinic, where maternal, child and family
planning services are provided in a target area, preliminary analysis of our data indicate a trend whereby between
December 1976 and December 1977, the percentage of mothers
who were "not ready for another baby" increased and the
percentage of those who were "ready" decreased. In October 1977, our maternity services were taken over by the
local government. Figures from April 1978 showed that the
percentage of those who were "not ready for another baby"
remained the same and those "ready" increased. It may be
a subconscious response of members of the community to un-
certainties surrounding the maternity service during this
period. Due in a large part to the widespread availability of contraceptives in Costa Rica, the impact of declines
in high risk pregnancies on infant mortality has been reported. Between 1960 and 1977, births of fifth and higher
order, and births among older women decreased sharply
(27). During the same period, the infant mortality rate
fell by almost 60 percent. An estimated one-fifth of this
decline is due to changes in child-bearing patterns.

CONCLUSION

    The case for an integrated maternal and child service
with family planning is clear. Fear that integration may
lead to a neglect of family planning services has led many
to separate them and sought cooperation between the services. But integration means the application of family
planning to all the activities in a health service system,
and must therefore be integrated at the planning during
implementation and into the training programs. The

purpose for family planning must be seen clearly, by the members of the community, to be aimed at improving their health and that of the children and not to reduce population, particularly in areas where mortalities are high. A reduction in fertility and thus population, will follow as an added dividend.

REFERENCES

1. Bamisaiye A, de Sweemer C, Ransome-Kuti O (1978): Developing a clinic strategy appropriate to community family planning needs and practice: An experience in Lagos, Nigeria. Studies in Family Planning, 9:44.
2. Mott LF (1976): Some aspects of health care in rural Nigeria. Studies in Family Planning, 7:109.
3. Speed DE (1971): Population crisis in Central Africa: Rwanda and Burundi. In: Health and Diseases in Africa. The community approach. LC Gould, Editor. Proceedings of the East African Medical Research Council Scientific Conference, Nairobi, Kenya, 1970. East Africa Literature Bureau, p. 243, Kampala.
4. Maine D (1978): Family planning. Its impact on the health of women and children. Center for Population and Family Health, Columbia University.
5. Morris JN, Heady JA (1955): Social and biological factors in infant mortality: Objects and methods. Lancet, 1:393.
6. Baimisaiye A (1978): Personal communication.
7. Martins W, Morley D, Woodland M (1967): Interval between births in a Nigerian village. J Trop Pediat, 10:82.
8. Gordon JE, Wyon JB, Ascoli W (1967): The second year death rate in less developed countries. Am J Med Sci, 254:357.
9. Yerushalmy J (1945): On the interval between successive births and its effect on the survival of infants. An indirect method of study. Human Biology, 17:65.
10. Hunt WB (1976): Adolescent fertility - risk and consequences. Population Reports Series J, No. 10.
11. Adelstein AM, Davies IMM, Weatherall JAC (1980): Perinatal and infant mortality. Social and biological factors 1975-77. Studies on medical and population subject No. 41. Her Majesty's Stationery Office, London.
12. WHO (1975): Pregnancy and abortion in adolescents. Report of a WHO meeting in Geneva June 24-28·, 1974. WHO Technical Report Series, No. 583, p. 27.

13. Wright NH (1975): Family planning and infant mortality rate decline in the United States. <u>Am J Epidemiol</u>, 101:182.
14. Morley DC, Bicknell J, Woodland M (1968): Factors influencing the growth and nutritional status of infant and young children in a Nigerian village. <u>Trans R Soc Trop Med Hyg</u>, 63:164.
15. Wray JD (1971): Population pressure on families. Family size and child spacing. In: <u>Rapid Population Growth. Consequences and Policy Implications</u>. Volume 2, The Johns Hopkins Press, Baltimore.
16. Copolan C, Visweswara Rao K (1969): Nutrition and family size. <u>J Nutr Diet</u>, 6:258.
17. Wray JD (1971): Population pressure on families. Family size and child spacing. <u>Reports on Population/Family Planning</u>, No. 9.
18. Nortman D (1974): Parental age as a factor in pregnancy outcome and child development. <u>Reports on Population/Family Planning</u>, No. 16, p. 52.
19. Wray JD, Aguirre A (1968): Protein calorie malnutrition in Candelaria, Columbia. Prevalence, social and demographic factors. <u>J Trop Pediat</u>, 15:76.
20. Douglas JWB, Simpson HR (1964): In: <u>Pediatric Priorities in Developing Countries</u>, D. Morley, Editor. Butterworths, London, 1973.
21. Scott JA (1962): Intelligence, physique and family size. <u>Brit J Prev Soc Med</u>, 16:165.
22. University of Ghana Medical Schools and UCLA School of Public Health (1979): <u>The Danfa Project</u>, Final Report.
23. Taylor CE, Takulia HS (1980): Integration of health and family planning in village sub-centers. <u>Report on the Fifth Narangwal Conference</u>, November 1970. Rural Health Research Center, Narangwal.
24. Narangwal Population Study (1975): Integrated health and family planning services. Rural Health Research Center, Narangwal.
25. Mott FL (1974): The dynamics of demographic change in a Nigerian village. <u>Human Resources Research Unit Monograph</u>, No. 2, University of Lagos, Lagos.
26. Cunningham N (1971): <u>Report to the US AID Conference on the use of weight charts</u>. Washington.
27. Sosa Jara D (1979): <u>Family planning</u>. Its impact on the health of women and children. Center for Population and Family Health, Deborah Maine, Editor, Columbia University.

SOCIO-ECONOMIC, CULTURAL AND PSYCHOLOGICAL ACCEPTABILITY OF FERTILITY CONTROL FOR PROTECTING THE LIFE AND HEALTH OF MOTHER AND INFANT

P. Senanayake

Medical Director
International Planned Parenthood Federation
London, United Kingdom

INTRODUCTION

The study of motivation in human reproductive behavior is of central importance in any attempt to understand fertility patterns and in the design and implementation of family planning services. A great many factors are involved in determining a couple's desired family size, and their preferences for the timing and spacing of births. These include cultural, social, economic and psychological factors. With a better understanding of such issues, fertility regulation methods and the service system through which they are provided can be made consonant with the knowledge, cultural values, beliefs and behavior of the consumer.

The central theme of this conference is the health of the mother and her child. I will look therefore primarily at socio-economic, cultural and psychological acceptability of fertility control for protecting the life and health of mother and infant. As the health benefits of family planning are the subject of other papers at this session, this paper will focus on issues related to acceptability. For a moment, however, let us digress, and look at the attitudes and values in general that affect reproductive behavior. These fall into two basic groups - favorable and unfavorable [Table 1]. Effective participation in a family planning program necessitates three decisions on the part of the couples or individuals who become acceptors. First, there must be a willingness or motivation to avoid pregnancy. The second decision concerns the

Table 1.   Attitudes and Values Affecting Reproductive
            Behaviour.

Favourable to birth control	Unfavourable to birth-control efforts
Valuing self and others as persons	Sense of inferiority and inequality (immaturity, minority status, etc.)
Education (more than minimal)	Minimal education, fear and superstitions about interfering with natural forces
Knowledge about parental and familial responsibilities	Ignorance about sexuality and family life
Partners on equal footing	Male dominance over women
Extrafamilial role opportunities for both partners	Emphasis on large families and the mothering and housewife roles
Availability of contraception and health care and social supports	High infant mortality and morbidity, dearth of human services
Ready access to abortion and voluntary sterilization	Anti-abortion attitudes and laws
Day care centers for infants and young children	Absence of communal child-care services
Children an economic liability	Children an asset as workers and earners
Pension systems	Dependency on children in old age
Decline in sense of national destiny following famine, epidemic, defeat in war	Nationalism, chauvinism, post-victory climate
Active concerns with communal planning - future is valued and human mastery over nature believed possible	Value orientation emphasizing the present; mysticism; belief in nature's dominance over man's fate

selection of a technique for pregnancy prevention. The
third decision becomes necessary once a technique is
selected, and requires a commitment on the part of the
acceptor to carry out the necessary steps to make the
program effective.

     In this paper, it is assumed that there is a willing-
ness to avoid or postpone a pregnancy for protecting the
life and health of the woman and her child. The success

of technological innovation and service programs ultimately depends on their acceptability to consumers. In the
areas of family planning, consumers consist not only of
couples who wish to space or avoid a birth, but the policy
makers, administrators and program personnel responsible
for providing methods and services. Consumer acceptability is a quality which makes these fertility regulation
methods, and the systems through which they are provided,
attractive and satisfactory.

Defining acceptability in this context is difficult.
The World Health Organization stated in 1973 that: "Acceptability refers to the degree to which a method or any
one of its attributes is perceived by potential users to
be consonant with their well being". Because acceptors
and consumers vary, acceptability is clearly a subjective
evaluation, and may differ according to the source, context and timing of the evaluation. Rates of acceptance
and continuation of specific methods do not necessarily
reflect their acceptability - for example, methods and
services attractive to particular users may not be easily
available. Also, the biases of clinic personnel for or
against particular methods may influence which of these
are used.

FAMILY PLANNING AND MAJOR LOGISTICAL PROBLEMS

Family planning is a relatively new area of health
care all over the world, and its very newness gives rise
to many questions, only some of which can be answered with
our present knowledge. In the field of family planning,
it is difficult to transfer experience from one setting to
another, not only because of strong cultural connotations,
and the great variation in administrative and political
structures, but also because family planning requires an
individual and local approach to the provision of services. Furthermore, family planning has, in particular,
to reach a very large segment of the population - i.e. all
couples of reproductive age, roughly a third of the total
population. This presents major logistical problems.

User Perspective

Contraceptive service programs need to become more
and better oriented to the perceptions of individuals who
are potential or current users of contraceptives. We need
to respond to their perceived needs, wants and problems.
The assessment of risks and benefits on contraceptive use
is important. Although there are mortality risks asso-

ciated with pregnancy, it is unlikely that many women
think of their own pregnancies as life threatening.
Further, it is unlikely that the individual woman chooses
contraceptives in preference to a pregnancy because the
former is less life threatening. Yet how often do we hear
of administrators and professionals discussing these issues as being the most crucial factors in the acceptance
of fertility regulation? The perceived needs, wants and
problems of the individual must be assessed and the programs must be geared to meeting these needs for a family
planning program to be successful.

        Socio-economic acceptabilty. The success of any
program ultimately depends on the acceptability not only
of the concept of family planning, but of the various methods offered. Socio-economic acceptability for the user
is determined chiefly by the perceived benefits of low
fertility. In many societies, there is strong economic
pressure to have many children, to provide security for
the future, and help for manual labor in the meantime. In
polygamous societies, the status of a wife is, to a large
extent, dependent on her ability to produce children.
These factors obviously discourage women from accepting
family planning, but, of course, it can be argued that
gaining control of fertility is a major step towards
raising the status of women. If the health rationale for
family planning is accepted, then in socio-economic terms,
a method for giving birth to fewer but healthier children
becomes more attractive.

        Psychological factors influencing acceptability.
Acceptability of fertilty control are deep-seated, but
people can be reassured if their apprehensions are understood, and their fears allayed. Again, securing the
involvement of community leaders is helpful, so that
contraceptive methods offered are suitable for specific
groups, as, for example, the IUD project in Bali, which
was successful for many reasons, one of which was that
there are male Traditional Birth Attendants (TBAs), so
that the insertion of the IUD by male doctors did not
constitute an embarrassing ordeal for potential acceptors.
Again, if the health rationale is accepted, then psychological factors encouraging high fertility, such as the need
to produce children to prove the virility of a husband, or
to quieten a mother-in-law, can be placed in the context
of the risks of rampant fertility.

        Cultural acceptability of fertility control. Cul-
tural acceptability is by definition difficult to overcome, as it is derived from time-honored traditions and

practices which have gone unquestioned for generations.
Aside from cultures where survival of a tribe makes high
fertility important, there are other pressures, such as
the necessity in India, for example, to be survived by a
son, and therefore to produce as many children as seems
necessary to ensure that at least one son survives into
healthy adulthood. Aside from necessities such as these,
there are more specifically religious factors which
encourage high fertility, or at least make family planning
more difficult to establish. Many religions prohibit premarital sex, and therefore early marriage is encouraged,
which results in longer periods of exposure to pregnancy.
However, if the help of religious leaders is secured, as
happened in the Bali program, this problem can be
minimized, if not overcome.

     Other major influences. Another major influence on
the acceptability of fertility control is the way contraception is handled as an issue in the media, and the
tendency of bad experiences to become widely known far
quicker than beneficial ones. The inescapable fact that
denials never have the impact of the original statement is
unfortunate, but reassurance of individuals can help in
this respect.

Barriers

     Illiteracy, religion, culture and the long suffering
mother-in-law have all been collectively or individually
blamed for the so-called resistance to fertility control.
It is accepted that these factors, along with traditional
social norms (need for sons, children to provide social
security, etc.) are partially responsible for creating a
bottleneck, but these are not insurmountable.

     Psychological barriers. Tradition and illiteracy
are recognized as obstacles in bringing about any social
change. However, fears, anxieties, apprehension and
suspicion act as hurdles in family planning acceptance.
Aside from factors touched upon earlier which inhibit
psychological acceptance of fertility control, there are
real fears which need to be taken into account. Fear of
insecurity is a major factor, due primarily to high infant
mortality rates and limited social security arrangements.
There is also a fear of bodily injury, since no method is
100 percent safe. Anxieties about the effects of contraceptives on sexual activity - the link between condoms and
decreased sex drive, and hirsutism in women on hormonal
contraception present further barriers to acceptability.
Other prevalent fears include fear of group inquiry -

differential acceptance by various religious and socio-
economic groups, and moral fears, due to increased
permissiveness (1).

Political barriers. A fundamental requirement for
a successful family planning program is the individual
family and the community at large. In Africa, for examp-
ple, while 18 out of 51 governments have some involvement
in family planning, only 14 have a family planning program
(2). If a country has no family planning program, what
opportunity is there for the rural population to obtain
information and supplies (3)?

There are still some countries in the developed
world where there continues to be major restriction on
access to all types of fertility control. The family
planning workers in these areas find themselves fighting
battles not dissimilar to those fought by Margaret Sanger,
Marie Stopes and others. In Spain, the penal code drawn
up under Franco banned the dissemination, public display
or offer for sale of anything intended to avert pregnancy.
As the country moves towards democracy, following the
death of Franco, the law has been changed, but abortion
remains illegal, and a growing number of Spanish women are
travelling to England each year to seek a safe termination
of pregnancy.

In the Republic of Ireland, the 1980 Health Act
(Family Planning) has made contraceptives available on
prescription. However, both doctors and pharmacists are
able to refuse to supply contraceptives as conscientious
objectors, and, as this Act has outlawed the sale of
contraceptives through other channels, it has not made
family planning more accessible.

Administrative barriers. Family planning programs
are often designed at international or national level.
Those responsible for the program draw up targets, and the
people are motivated to accept the methods chosen for
them. The interest of the providers of the services seem
to play a much more important part than the needs of consumers. Family planning services are often designed with
the convenience of providers in mind, without due consideration for the needs of consumers. Service outlets are
located far from the people who they are meant to serve.
Opening hours clash with other commitments, and people are
asked intimate questions within full hearing of other
attendants. Furthermore, in many countries, all too often
the greatest share of the program is devoted to the urban
areas. Even if rural couples wish to plan their families,

they have to travel long distances for their supplies.

Sometimes well-meaning "outside" agencies can provide barriers to acceptance of fertility controls. One such example is vividly described by Potts: "To 'help' Laos, an international agency built a single clinic in one village. It happens to express all the physical and social limitations of this type of approach; second only in size to the school and larger than the temple, it was the only building in the village with its own water supply and sewage and without doubt the most expensively constructed building in the area. Heavily built of red hardwood, it stood out aggressively beside the flimsy but charming houses raised on stilts with thatched roofs. Even from the road it was possible to see the culturally inappropriate posters which lined the veranda and depicted the anatomical details of a midline section of the male and female pelvis. To complete the picture, it was surrounded by a barbed wire fence and only opened for a few hours each week. Technically, nothing was ever required of that clinic which could not have been performed on the immaculately kept bamboo floor of any house in the village" (4).

Instead of working backwards, taking into account views of potential consumers and asking common-sense questions, most family planning programs are heavily over-engineered. The poliical wrappings cost much more than their technical contents.

Medical barriers. Contraceptive services have traditionally been in the hands of the medical personnel. This immediately means that contraceptive services can be adequately handled only in locations where doctors are easily available, and in most developing countries, this means the large cities.

The doctor/population ratio in most rural areas of the developing world is as low as 1 per 20 or 30 thousand. It is almost impossible for a doctor in this situation to cope with the disease problems of his community, let alone practise preventive medicine. Many rural women in developing countries deliver babies at home usually attended only by an older female member of her family or by a traditional birth attendant. She may have borne 8 or 10 children, but very likely would never have been subject to a vaginal examination. If this same woman wanted to obtain some oral contraceptives, she would very likely have to have a vaginal examination, blood pressure check and a detailed health record. It is not surprising that many rural women are ill at ease in doctor or health personnel-dominated family planning clinics.

"Choice of methods" barriers. To many health administrators, family planning services are synonymous with
IUD pogrammes, pill programs, condom programs or a combination of these. This does not, in reality, make a family
planning program. An ideal program should make available
through appropriate channels, all methods of fertility
regulation, from indigenous methods of contraception to
early abortion and elective sterilization. If this
definition is applied, it is seen that, even in countries
which have a commitment to family planning, programs are
not comprehensive.

It is obvious that what is acceptable to one couple
may be totally unsuitable for another, and this is why the
so-called "cafeteria" approach has emerged.

India has had a national family planning program
since 1952, but even after about 30 years of existence,
oral contraceptives are still only used to a limited extent. It is believed that the average rural woman is too
ignorant to be asked to take the pill correctly, and that
it is dangerous to dispense them without medical supervision. This myth has already been exploded in many rural
areas in developing countries, including some rural areas
in India, for example, the Howrah project (5).

Method-related barriers. During most of human
evolution, lactation was the sole factor governing the
spacing of conceptions. Today, in traditional societies,
it remains the prime factor, but can be supplemented by
varying periods of abstinence, the practice of coitus
interruptus and sometimes abortion.

In the past 20 years or so, the world has seen the
emergence of "modern" methods of contraception - the pill,
IUDs, injectables, etc. Contraceptive choice does not necessarily reflect the method preference of the individual
who uses it. Actual choice involves a compromise between
the partners explicitly and implicitly, within the context
of cultural pattern of dominance and division of responsibility in the given society's culture and situation.

Continuation and discontinuation of contraceptive
practice is a topic attracting much research. Typically,
a number of socio-demographic characteristics of users are
linked to duration and use. Often, a few service variables such as distance to clinic, service provider, and
waiting time at clinic, are included. Discontinuation,

broadly speaking, could be due to medical reasons, dis-
satisfaction and desired pregnancy.

Women's attitudes to contraceptive methods vary tre-
mendously. In a pilot study conducted in Australia (6),
the adjectives "unnatural", "tense", "messy", "frighten-
ing", "unsafe", and "repulsive" were chosen frequently by
women to describe contraceptives, while "immoral",
"sinful", and "ill-health" were not used.

Availability (logistical) barriers. Availability
is an important factor which will ultimately determine the
effectiveness of the family planning program. The initial
number of acceptors depends on the motivation, publicity,
support from local leadership and widespread availability
of commodities. However, the continued use of contraceptives will depend on knowledge of proper use and
availability. The necessity for maintaining adequate
stocks and supplies cannot be overemphasized. The case of
the Howrah CBD project is a sad example: - "Due to various
bureaucratic procedures, a large shipment of pills was
unduly delayed, and this proved to be a most serious and
costly setback. The opening of several new depots had to
be postponed, even though the community was all geared to
start. The depot holders were reluctant to recruit new
acceptors due to the uncertainty of supplies. The entire
momentum was halted, and even though the pills were available shortly afterwards, it took some time to resume the
original pace."

SOME SOLUTIONS

Community Participation

Many a program has been known to fail because the
contraceptive method or its delivery system has not been
acceptable to the community. It is essential to determine
what the people want, and not impose what is supposedly
good for them. By involving the community right from the
start, it is possible to counteract any opposition that
could arise from local practitioners and community leaders. If these leaders are involved at the inception of a
project, then many socio-economic and psychological factors affecting an individual's fears concerning fertility
control will be allayed, as cultural traditions will be
shared and understood by the organizers of the program,
and the idea of family planning will become more acceptable. A Ministry of Health Official of the Philippines
once said "Consider people not merely as targets or num-

bers to be accounted for, but as people who have feelings,
emotions that can be hurt, and who have reasons for doing
almost anything they do". Contraceptive service programs
can be integrated into the broader aspects of women's
lives, for example in the Korean Mothers' Clubs program or
in income generating schemes.

Government Commitment

Developing nations have moved from public apathy or
antagonism towards family planning, to government policies
and national programs in less than 20 years. Until 1956,
the Thai government offered bonuses for large families;
the Prime Minister said he wanted 100 million people, and
the Ministry of Health had a Wedding Promotion Committee.
Today, Thailand has a population policy; the government
spent US $3.4 million on family planning in 1978 (7); the
Prime Minister frequently endorses the need for small
families, and the population, now at 45 million (8), is
growing more slowly than previously. These changes, which
have their parallel throughout Asia, parts of Africa and
in an increasing number of Latin American countries, have
occurred at a relatively earlier stage in the demographic
transition than did the evolution of public approval and
assistance to fertility regulation in the West (4).

Availability and Choice

Even though the "perfect" fertility regulation method
is still not with us, and many of us believe it never will
be, we do have a wide range of methods to choose from. It
is generally accepted that, even in countries with a government commitment to family planning, it is still rare to
find ready access to all these methods of fertility control. No one method of fertility regulation is suitable
for all couples at all times. A wide range of choices
will be more likely than a narrower one to fill perceived
needs and wants, and to solve perceived problems. Such
availability and choice would also make switching from one
contraceptive to a different one easier.

Today, biomedical research efforts are aimed at
improving the currently avaiable methods of fertility regulation and developing new ones. Many important factors
play a part in deciding the method most suited to the
individual. For example, the way a fertility regulation
method is administered to the human body plays a role in
its acceptability, both to potential users, and to service
personnel. For example, potential users may prefer an
injected contraceptive, as it may be perceived as more

effective and safer than a pill in some socio-cultural
settings. On the other hand, clinic workers may prefer
methods which require the fewest demands on scarce staff
time and facilities. For example, contraceptives inserted
into the uterus normally have higher requirements for
skills, equipment and time than do orally ingested
methods.

Service Providers

     Methods of distribution are as important as the
physiological side effects of the method. The interaction
between consumers and providers of family planning
services is one of the most important aspects of program
success. The providers - doctors, nurses, midwives,
villagers - must not only be knowledgable about fertility
regulation methods and willng to make them available, but
must understand and be sensitive to the beliefs, customs
and cultural values of clients.

     When oral contraceptives were first introduced, it
was reasonable to limit these physiologically powerful and
relatively poorly understood drugs to medical prescriptions. With the passage of time, however, a large
amount of data has become available. The rare potentially
serious side-effects that may occur, are not made any less
frequent by medical examination. If the need for a medical prescription for oral contraceptives is recommended,
then large groups of rural women in developing countries,
in addition to other women in the so-called developed
countries where legislation demands such prescriptions,
would have very limited access to the pill.

     In order to meet the shortage of medical personnel
which has already inhibited surgical methods of family
planning in developing countries, nurse-surgeons are being
taught female sterilization using minilaparotomy. Pilot
schemes have been successfully implemented in Thailand and
Bangladesh, and these personnel are providing a service to
a population that would normally have been denied this
service.

SOME EXAMPLES

Japan

     Japan is a country of paradoxes. It is illegal to
prescribe the Pill for contraception, but abortion is
readily available; it has the highest use of the rhythm

method in the world, but has no significant number of
Roman Catholics in the population; three-quarters of all
family planning users adopt the condom, yet male sterilization is rare. The IUD, which was partly a Japanese
invention, was only made legal in 1974.

Contraceptive practice in Japan has increased from 20
percent in 1950 to 60 percent currently using some form of
contraception in 1975. The same socio-economic pressures,
the same urban and rural differentials and the same effects of education and income apply in Japan as they do in
Britain and the United States. However, the range of
methods used is different. Over 75 percent of contraceptive users in Japan are condom users, whereas, in Sweden
and Great Britain, less than a third rely on the condom.
This is the highest single use of one method in any country, and exceeds the popularity of the pill in Europe and
the United States.

The positive reasons for the success of the condom
have included aggressive, imaginative and comprehensive
marketing, where the Japanese Family Planning Association
(JFPA) has made an outstanding contribution. The JFPA saw
the need to enter the community rather than wait for
people to seek out its services. It created mobile teams
which sold condoms on a door-to-door basis. Of course, a
great many users buy condoms directly, often from the
pharmacy and cosmetic stores, which remain the main condom
outlets, and account for 60 percent of the total trade.

The packaging of the condom is imaginative, sophisticated and designed to appeal to a highly diverse and
segmented market. In the case of condoms sold to women,
the packages simulate non-contraceptive domestic items,
such as sweets, boxes of biscuits or cigarette cartons.
JFPA made constructive use of local midwives who were
becoming increasingly unemployed because of the declining
birth rate, but who proved to be appropriate condom sales
ladies.

China

Changes which have affected a few million people in
isolated areas of Asia seem to have extended to hundreds
of millions in the People's Republic of China. At first
sight, the Chinese program appears to be unique, but on
closer examination does not turn out to be as unusual as
is sometimes believed.

First and foremost, the Chinese effort involves a

realistic availability of all possible methods of family
planning. Condoms and oral contraceptives are available
at household level and involve the barefoot doctor. China
is the only developing country to manufacture oral contraceptives from plant raw materials. Abortion is available
and widely used.

The Chinese do not call their activities family
planning, but "birth planning". In some areas, "group
planning" has evolved. This is a unique system: almost
as fascinating for the reactions it arouses among Western
observers, as for its intrinsic interest. Briefly, the
larger units of Chinese administration, such as the municipality, determine the optimum birth rate for a locality.
This is then translated at the commune level to actual
numbers of births possible. All the fertile couples in a
production brigade together select who will have children
over the next year or more. There may even be a chart
displayed in a public place, setting the target number of
pregnancies.

To the Western mind, the system seems illiberal,
threatening and incomprehensible, but group birth planning
is worth studying. It assumes that couples have total
control over fertility - which indeed they do, as early
abortion is available. Human beings are asked to plan
children with regard to community needs as well as family
needs, in the same way that they plan to use their resources to build a bridge or temple. There is no coercion
in the sense that a woman who accidentally gets pregnant
is forced to seek abortion, but there are strong social
pressures.

Strangely less rational and perhaps even less
desirable patterns of social conformity are found in other
cultures: millions of healthy young men have lost their
lives in brutal war. Is it odd for millions of young
Chinese women whose parents knew the reality of starvation
to agree not to have babies indiscriminately? (4)

Proposed Model

In order to better illustrate some of the interrelationships between the three main groups involved (the
user, the service provider and the policy maker), and the
influences which bear upon the individuals who make up
these groups, a "model" can be drawn up. This "model" is
an extension of one used previously in describing the use
of fertility regulating services, but has been modified to
include a description of the social, familial and psycho-

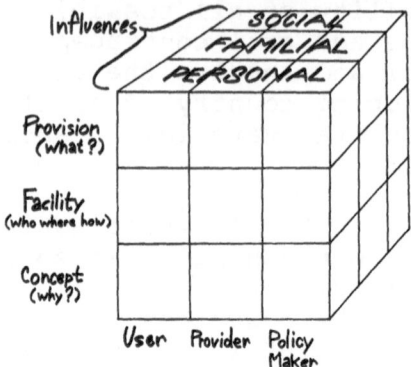

Figure 1.   A conceptual model showing inter-relationships
            among three main groups involved.

logical pressures bearing upon the individuals involved.

        The model demonstrates the perceptual viewpont of the
user, the service provider and the policy maker, as the
three interact and are influenced by each other. The view
of each individual is shaped by three basic levels of
concern, with each level becoming more narrowly focused at
each step. The broadest level relates to the general
question "why is there an interest in this topic at all?"
The second level assumes that interest in the subject matter is justified. At this level, the questions relate to
"who and from what source can further information be provided?" The final, most specific level again assumes that
the previous two levels have been dealt with, and concerns
itself entirely with the content of the information to be
provided. It is evident that each of these levels may be
seen differently, according to which of the three groups
the individual belongs. The view of the policy maker in
relation to each of the three levels is likely to be very
different from that of the user.

        But each of the perceptual positions is being taken
by an individual who as an individual is being influenced by social pressures of various kinds, by his or her
own familial ties and perceived obligations and expecta-
tions, and by psychological pressures resulting from
personal experiences, training and socialization. It is
not just the user who is influenced by peer group and
family pressure; the service provider and the policy
maker also experience and respond to such influences.

        The advantage of such a model is that it may be used
to demonstrate more clearly gaps in existing knowledge and

possible strategies of action which have not previously
been considered. It provides an indication of the source
of influence bearing on each of the individuals involved,
and at the same time indicates the degree of specificity
that is being considered and avoids unequal comparisons.
It should be kept in mind that irrespective of the issue
being specifically examined, pressure is being continually
exerted within the total framework of the model. The model is a dynamic one, with each component part influencing
the others. Many important factors are brought into play
before the right contraceptive can be given to the right
person at the right time, in the right place.

CONCLUSION

It is reasonable to argue that the family planning
programs in the Third World may have been too optimistic
in assuming that they alone can rapidly bring fertility
down to replacement level. However, failure should be
examined in relation to demand versus supply. Many family
planning programs, as has been pointed out earlier, use a
"target group" approach, ignore questions of cultural
suitability, and are heavily over-doctored.

The success of voluntary family planning depends on
human decisions. The spread of information, the provision
of services, the acceptance and continued use of methods
of fertility regulation all depend on individuals, couples, groups and societies. Phychological, social and
cultural aspects need to be considered in formulating government policies that enable family planning communication
and education programs to fit particular audiences, in
order to allow services to be adjusted to meet the needs
of clients, and to ensure that new methods are culturally
appropriate.

REFERENCES

1. Potts M, Bhiwandiwala P (1974): Birth control: an
    international assessment. MTP Press Ltd., Lancaster,
    England.
2. International Planned Parenthood Federation (1979):
    Family Planning in Five Continents. IPPF, London.
3. Senanayake P (1977): Family spacing and limitation.
    In Royal Society discussion proceedings. Technologies
    for rural health. Royal Society, London.
4. Potts M, Selman P (1979): Society and fertility.
    MacDonald and Evans Ltd, Plymouth, England.

5. International Planned Parenthood Federation (1979):
    People, IPPF, London, 6:3,
6. Wood C, Leeton J, Downing B, Mahews J, Williams L
    (1970): Emotional attitudes to contraceptive methods.
    In: Contraception 2:2.
7. Nortman DL, Hofstatter E (1980): Population and
    family planning programmes: a compendium of data
    through 1978 - 10th ed. Population Council, New
    York.
8. United Nations (1980): World population situation in
    1979. UN, New York.

FUTURE PROSPECTS OF FAMILY PLANNING PROGRAMS

S. Surjaningrat

Minister of Health and Chairman of the
National Family Planning Coordinating Board
Jakarta, Indonesia

INTRODUCTION

In the post World War II era, there has been an increased conciousness of the relation of population factors to a number of major world problems. Population growth and other aspects of population also have an important bearing on social change and economic growth, especially in the less developed nations. Although much attention has been focused on the relationship of high fertility and population growth rates to economic development, many other facets of population are also important.

The estimated population of the world in mid 1975, a year after the conclusion of the World Population Conference at Bucharest, was about 4.0 billion. Five years later in 1980, the estimated population of the world is just over 4.4 billion. In other words, the human species has increased by a total of about 400 million or, approximately 80 million per year over five years. We are continuing to grow at a rate of 1.8 percent per year according to current medium-variant estimates. The population of less developed countries increases at rates of 2 to 3 percent annually while the more developed countries grow at about 0.7 percent annually.

It is therefore obvious that global concern should be focused on the less developed countries where population problems are so closely related to unsolved development difficulties. There is a dangerous gap between the less developed countries and the more developed ones. Indeed

we are all concerned about this widening gap in socio-
economic conditions between developed and developing
countries in the world today. We are now entering the new
decade of the 80's where human sufferings are still
prevalent around the world. Developing countries are
struggling to improve the life of their people through
many efforts but constraints have still to be overcome in
establishing the New World Social and Economic Order as
recommended during the Second World Population Conference
in Bucharest in 1974.

It was the historic post-war fall in mortality, especially in infant mortality, that created the potential
for a drastically increased rate of population growth.
This situation forced developing countries to deal actively with the persistent high level of fertility which did
not fall immediately as mortality fell. The increasing
number of poor people and the unfavorable new age distribution were consuming most of the resources and gains from
economic development of these countries.   Therefore vigorous measures were essential and the control of fertility
through family planning programs became a necessary
element of the development effort itself.

We know that macro-level analysis of the relationships between socio-economic development and fertility
have identified various social and economic changes that
are highly correlated with fertility declines at the national level. Also, socio-economic status has been found
to be inversely related to fertility, using such indices
as educational level, occupation and income. Also of some
importance are the economic utility of children, female
labor-force participation and family structure. It is
clear therefore that development is not an alternative to
family planning but rather a companion to it, and that of
course is the way most developing countries, including
Indonesia has been proceeding. In addition however, the
benefits of family planning to individual families can be
appreciated from an immediate point of view such as reducing the suffering of mothers from childbearing, providing
better quality of food and education, enabling mothers to
work outside the house and participate in development
activities.

CHARACTERISTICS AND NEEDS OF FAMILY PLANNING PROGRAMS

Our experience in conducting an intensive fertility
control program has led us to an understanding that family
planning cannot be expected to arise spontaneously from

socio-economic development efforts. Members of individual
families and communities must view fertility reduction on
their own terms and interests. Their appreciation of a
small family has to develop through links to basic needs
such as education, food, housing and income. Modern aspirations have to be created and this must be carefully
approached, for inspite of our awareness to the importance
of modern aspirations in accelerating the process of acceptance of small family norm, we have to be aware that
not all forms of modern innovation are acceptable to the
cultural standards of many developing countries. They may
have to be adapted appropriately with a definite selective
process. Therefore, we in the developing countries must
be able to identify which among the forms of modernization
achieved in developed countries are useful to our effort
to improve the quality of life without negatively affecting our cultural standards.

Contraceptive Acceptance

However, in other areas we should be able to take
advantage of the latest developments in science and
technology and in so doing accelerate our development
processes. In particular, achievements in recent years
have improved the efficiency and effectiveness of the
management of family planning programs. Developments in
contraceptive technology and reproductive biology constitute one of the important backbones of family planning,
and here we are continuously challenged by the need for
more effective, more practical and safe contraceptive
devices or drugs. Besides the historic breakthrough of
modern contraceptive technology, recent research has led
to the testing and use of several new fertility control
methods. Some are refinements of present methods; others
are based on application of fundamental research. These
include medicated IUDs, new form of copper IUDs, improved
injectable contraceptives, and the five year implant.
Other new methods are now at a very advanced stage of
testing including clinical trials with human subjects.
Some others are still at very early stages of development.

With any contraceptive method, community acceptance
remains very important. In countries where the delivery
of contraceptives has reached the grassroot level, as with
our case in Indonesia, management problems arise in
maintaining continuity of use due to the logistics of oral
contraceptive pills. To date the number of "current
users" in our program has reached a total of more than 7
million couples, most of whom use the oral pill. The
management of the program would have been easier if there

were equally attractive contraceptive methods available
that involved less resupply.

    To approach this problem, a strategy was developed
for the regular provison of oral pills through distribution points accessible to rural couples. In this context,
the effort is to gradually shift the responsibility for
the distribution of pills and condoms from the program
infrastructure to community institutions such as women
organizations, mothers' club, acceptors clubs, village
committees, and the like at the village level which
function on a voluntary basis. Institutions like those
mentioned are encouraged by the government to gradually
assume the responsibility for coordination of community
participation in various development projects. Those
institutions also serve as a forum for the meeting of
minds between the community members and local government
workers. This forum can effectively be used for introduction of various innovations and for adjustment and
adaptation of various development inputs to the local
needs and conditions.

    This kind of approach is not unique to Indonesia
since similar methods are also applied in other countries.
The development of primary health care in rural areas is a
good example of this kind of approach. In family planning
program implementation, the role of village institutions
is vital to success, since they not only reinforce continuous use of contraceptives among their members but are
also very effective in recruiting new acceptors and in
motivating couples to use the most effective device.

Institutionalization

    These village mechanisms are gaining an increasing
degree of recognition due to their success in transforming
development plans and messages into action. Although it
is rather easy to demonstrate their success, a substantial
amount of effort and dedicated work was needed on the part
of the program to get this mechanism operational. In the
Indonesian family planning program, the strategy focuses
on the establishment of "acceptor groups" in every village
in the country, especially so in more advanced areas.
This phase was labelled the "institutionalization phase"
in which success depended upon the level of motivation of
both the community and program personnel. Once the institutions were established, we were faced with the problem
of maintaining their functions over a period of time. To
ensure this, new innovations and other kind of inputs had
to be introduced. The need for continued functioning of

these institutions is based on the following reasons:

(a) An effective family planning program needs
continuous use of contraceptives among the accepting
couples. The impact on the fertility level depends upon
the number of couple-years-of-protection.

(b) Through frequent and regular meetings among
members and through the introduction of various development inputs into these groups, the traditional values,
norms and attitude related to reproduction are expected to
change gradually towards new forms.

Internalization

It is in this institutionalization phase that we in
developing coutries are trying to operationally integrate
the family planning elements with those of other development programs. Such efforts to integrate family planning
with nutrition, with income-generating activities, and
other community incentive schemes, has been successfully
done in many developing countries. These programs, though
labelled as beyond family planning, is becoming part and
parcel of the family planning program. In fact the program
is trying to reach the next phase termed "internalization
phase" once institutionalization is established. In this
phase of "internalization", we expect that the desire for
a small family will become part of the basic human
outlook.

YOUTH PROGRAMS

To cite other programs beyond family planning activities being developed, is the population education program
which was initiated in most developing countries in the
mid 70s. It covered only those attending the intermediate
level of education, but is at present being expanded to be
included in the university curriculum as a "population
science".

Moreover, approaches to organizations of young women,
university students, religious groups and other non-
governmental organizations are being made to deal with the
young generation of the nation. Youth has a unique
position in the context of family planning and population
programs for development. Adolescents represent those who
are potential eligible couples for family planning in the
course of the present and the next decades, and they also
represent those who will be the leaders and managers of

various development programs in the country. It is for
these reasons that special programs have to be developed
to make them fully aware of the present population problems we are facing and to comprehend the various efforts
we are making to cope with these problems. Through various orientation courses, we are trying to make them
understand the nature of the interrelationships between
demographic variables and development variables, and to
involve them in discussions of feasible alternative
approaches to influence those interrelationships. By
bringing them into a wider scope of orientation to see
population on one side and development on the other as
systems that interact, we will help them to comprehend the
importance of the role of lower fertility and of other
demographic variables as conducive to development itself.

Our motivation program is also tring to encourage the
young generation, especially those in the villages, to
postpone their marriages. We are working to make them
aware of the existing marriage law which sets the minimum
age for marriage at 16 year for women and 19 years for
men.

Another approach which still has to be developed concerns the incentive and disincentive systems which can be
introduced through formal policies governing salary
schemes, public housing rules, school enrollment regulations and the like. It is part of our responsibility to
prepare the necessary documents on all these subjects, to
be used as a basis for the formulation of a comprehensive
and integrated national population policy, which is badly
needed in Indonesia at the present.

These are examples of the characteristics and needs
at various levels of the family planning program
development. Many of you have probably shared similar
experiences in the implementation of a nationwide family
planning program. Many ideas have to be developed in the
course of a few years during the early period, and crea-
tive extensions are necessary in the later years to relate
the work to other sectors. People can equally benefit
from other sectoral development programs, and in time
people become convinced that planning the family is a prerequisite of a better life. Therefore, we are convinced
that family planning is part and parcel of the overall
socio-economic development.

In addition, we have to be aware that while one objective of family planning is the reduction of fertility,
the broader objective is a state where demographic

characteristics and behavior are conducive to the overall improvement of life. The ultimate goal is to improve the quality of all aspects of life of the people which merges with the hope of all development programs in evey country in the world.

CONCLUSION

(a) The very nature of all efforts in family planning in developing countries is education.

(b) Family planning programs should be integrated in other development programs acceptable to the local people in the rural areas.

(c) Family planning programs reaching grassroot levels need an effective program infrastructure and community participation.

(d) Developments in contraceptive technology and reproductive biology constitute one of the important backbones of family planning.

REFERENCES

The Population Council (1981): Family planning in the 1980's, challenges and opportunities. Recommendations of the International Conference on Family Planning in the 1980's in Jakarta, Indonesia. In: Studies in Family Planning, 12, No. 6/7, New York.

Population Reference Bureau (1977): Indonesia's family-planning story: success and challenge. In: Population Bulletin 32:6, Washington.

United Nations (1979): National experience in the formulation and implementation of population policy, 1960-1976, Indonesia. UN, New York.

Clinton JJ et al, Editors (1980): East Asia Review 1978-79. In: Studies in Family Planning, 11:11, The Population Council, New York.

United Nations (1979): The world population situation. In: 1977 Concise Report, United Nations, New York.

Rich W (1973): Smaller families through social and economic progress. Monograph Series No. 7, Overseas Development Council, Washington.

SOCIAL BENEFITS OF FAMILY PLANNING

M. B. Concepcion

Dean, Population Institute
University of the Philippines
Manila, Philippines

INTRODUCTION

Throughout the world, women marry, have children, watch their children grow, marry, and form families of their own. By the end of the eighties, an estimated one billion or so young people in the Third World will be entering the age groups, 15 to 29 years. Their decisions concerning marriage and family formation and their knowledge about the benefits of a smaller family size and of birth spacing will influence future population growth rates and ensure health and welfare of families.

The results of nationally representative, internationally comparable, fertility surveys conducted under the aegis of the World Fertility Survey (WFS) in some 54 countries since 1974 indicate a high level of contraceptive awareness in the countries surveyed in Asia and in Latin America. Women in these regions are most familiar with the latest methods and have taken the pill at one time. The gap between knowledge and action is evident with the majority of women still unprotected from the risk of pregnancy. Current contraceptive use rose with each additional child and with advancing age in Asia and the Pacific but peaked at about four children and at about age 35 in Latin America and the Caribbean.

Current users identified in these surveys tended to be concentrated among the more highly educated urbanites. A sizeable portion of the fecund women interviewed had never resorted to family planning nor intended to do so in the future despite their acquaintance with a wide variety of contraceptive measures. Inconsistencies in contracep-

tive behavior and desired family size were prominent among
the older, less educated village inhabitants who had borne
more than five children, were either newlyweds or had
already been married over 20 years.

This article deals with some of the social benefits
that families would derive from planning the number and
spacing of their children.

SOCIAL BENEFITS TO FAMILIES

In the seventies, changing patterns of social and
economic development and the possibility of timing and
spacing of children have had an important impact on family
structure and functioning. The changes influence not only
women's and men's economic and social roles but also child
bearing and child rearing patterns and family health as
well.

The changing social situation has influenced family
life styles and the role of women in society. The changes
in the structure and life style of the family seem to indicate the emergence of a new type of family, of new types
of relationship between men and women and between parents
and children. Modified patterns of child-bearing and
child rearing have led to increasing involvement of women
in economic life, reduction of female dependency on their
families for economic and pscyhological support and
increased freedom of movement.

A breakdown of the extended family system such as
that occurring in the suburban areas of many developing
countries, threatens the social and physical well-being of
the people, particularly the children, owing to continued
high death rates and the absence of a functioning system
of nuclear families with adequate organized support. For
example, in the least developed countries where life expectancy at birth is about 40 years, some two-fifths of
the population aged 20 years have only one parent left
alive and about 8 percent have lost both parents. In
other words, every other 20-year old in the least economically developed populations is either a full or partial
orphan. At the mortality level of developed countries
where the corresponding life expectancy at birth is about
70 years, fewer than one in fifty will be complete orphans
and only a further tenth will have lost one parent. This
implies that nine out of ten 20-year olds in the industrialized nations will have both parents still living.

In countries characterized by high fertility, many women have several pregnancies very early in their child-bearing years and continue to bear children up to the time of menopause. Extremely young mothers, mothers at the peak of child-bearing, mothers with closely spaced pregnancies - all are high parity risks. Except in the most favored socio-economic groups, evidence suggests that a short interval between pregnancies depletes the mother's capacity to give her baby a good start. She also carries a higher risk for her own health and safety, especially if she has had several pregnancies very early in her child-bearing years. Under such circumstances fetal loss is higher, infant survival is lower, and malnutrition and some impairment of growth and development are found among the surviving children.

Mothers not only fall prey to illnesses associated with pregnancy and childbearing but they are also more vulnerable to other more general health hazards. They bear the burden of child care frequently under unfavorable conditions. More often than not, such mothers have fewer opportunities to avail themselves of any existing health services.

High parity or closely spaced pregnancies or both lead to greater risk of early pregnancy interruptions and of prematurity. Where breast-feeding is the only chance of child survival, early birth of another infant curtails the benefits from the mother's lactation and predisposes the child to kwashiorkor or other types of malnutrition.

In the following paragraphs, studies supporting the social benefits described in the previous section will be briefly cited.

Lower Incidence of Infant and Child Mortality

In less developed countries, infant and child mortality is much lower in small families than in large ones. In a survey of eleven Punjab villages during 1955- 1958 (14), 116 infants out of 1000 babies born to families with only two children died before their first birthday. By way of contrast, the infant mortality rate was 206 in families in which the mother had given birth to seven or more living children. The difference in mortality rates was even greater for children between 1 and 2 years of age: 15 child deaths per 1000 for two-child families as against 95 per 1000 for the children in families of seven or more live births. The same proportionate differences in mortality rates between children of small and large families

were found in New York City, although the levels of
mortality were much lower (2, 3).

The effect of birth spacing on infant and child
mortality in low-income families are dramatically illustrated by data from the same Punjab villages cited above.
From 1955 to 1958, 196 out of 1000 children born between 3
and 4 years after a previous birth, died before reaching
age two years. The corresponding rate was 137 among
children born after an interval of more than 4 years. But
when the birth interval was less than a year, the
mortality rate rose alarmingly to 310.

Reduced Morbidity.

In low income countries, the high mortality rates
among children in large families and in families with
close birth intervals, are in part due to malnutrition.
The greater the number of children, the greater is the
likelihood of malnutrition among impoverished families.
Studies of pre-school children in Colombia (12) showed
that only 32 percent of children in families with only one
pre-school child were seriously malnourished as compared
to 51 percent of the children in families in which there
were 5 or more children of pre-school age. In Thailand
(1969), 42 percent of children from families with no more
than 3 children were malnourished, 16 points less than
that reported for children coming from families with 4 or
more children.

Among the children examined in the Thai study, four
out of ten of those in families without a younger sibling
were malnourished; the comparable figure for those whose
next youngest sibling was born within 2 years was 7 out of
ten. In rural Colombia, the prevalence of malnutrition
declined appreciably only among children who were over 3
years of age at the birth of the next child.

Faster Physical Development.

Since growth is related to nutrition, it would be
expected that the height and weight of children in small
families would be greater on the average than in large
families. Even in high-income countries the children of
poor families are taller and heavier at any given age when
there are fewer children in the family. Scott (10) collected data in 1959 on height and weight of 2169 London
day school students 11.25 years old which showed that
children from one-child families were about 3 percent
taller and 17 to 18 percent heavier than children from

families with five or more children.

The difference in physical growth between children of small and large families studied in Great Britain (4) seemed to affect mainly the poorer social classes. In the upper and lower manual working classes children in small families were, on the average, 3 to 4 percent taller than those in large families at 7 and 11 years of age, and 1.4 to 2.8 percent taller at 15 years.

Greater Intellectual and Educational Performance

The number of children in the family are associated not only with physical size but also with linguistic skills, intelligence and educational performance. To some extent, these elements are interrelated. For example, heavier children mature earlier, and early maturers do better in school than late maturers. Experiments show that the apathy associated with malnutrition is highly correlated with such psychological elements as lack of ambition, low self-discipline, low mental alertness, and inability to concentrate.

Both physical growth and the greater cultural nurturing associated with small families appear to affect intelligence. In the sample of British day school children cited above, intelligence increased with height and decreased with family size. The average verbal reasoning scores of children over 135 centimeters tall in families of one or two children surpassed those of children of the same height in families of four or more by 5 to 7.5 percent. The difference for children of the same age but less than 135 centimeters tall between small and large families average about 7 percent.

In studies of Scottish children the average I.Q. of only children was 113, that of children with five or more siblings was 91. In France, only children between the ages of 6 and 12 had an average mental age 1 to 2 years higher than children with eight or more siblings (6).

That the difference in children of small and large families persists in adult life is indicated by the average scores of army recruits on tests of different types in Great Britain (11). In the tests that measured general, verbal, and special mechanical intelligence, the scores of recruits from small families exceeded those from families with five or more children by 11 to 16 percent. The difference increased with larger family size. On the other hand the difference in results of physical ability tests was much smaller by about 5 percent.

Better Parental Health

There is some evidence that family size takes its toll on parents too. Hare and Shaw (5) studied fifty-five British families divided according to the number of children under 16 years of age. They observed that both physical and mental ill-health in parents increased with family size, more marked among mothers than among fathers.

In a study of the relationship between parity and the incidence of diabetes in England, Pyke (9) compared the number of women in each parity group among the diabetics with that of a control population. He found a dramatic and highly significant increase in diabetes with increasing parity of the women.

Repeated pregnancies followed by prolonged lactation periods will produce sustained needs for high quality protein in the diet. In the many parts of the world where these needs are poorly met, the result is what Jellife (7) has termed the "maternal depletion syndrome". This process may contribute to low birth weight of their infants, to poor performance in lactation and, ultimately to the premature aging and early death often seen among women in developing regions.

Indirect evidence concerning this condition is provided by Wright (13) who studied maternal mortality figures by age group for Thailand in 1971. He found that maternal death rates rose from 154 deaths per 100,000 births among women in their twenties to a grim 474 per 100,000 among women in their forties.

Clearly, general health would improve markedly if family planning measures were more widely available and more widely used - to reduce early and late pregnancies, to place a reasonable limit on family size, and to keep a healthy interval between births. Examining data from around the world, Dorothy Norman (8) has calculated the health benefits for women that would result if births in the risky early and later periods of female fertility were eliminated. She reported that if women had births only in the age interval from 20 to 34, maternal mortality would be reduced by 19 percent in Mexico, Thailand, Venezuela, and the United States; by 23 percent in Colombia and France; and by 25 percent in the Philippines. As it is, more than a third of the world's births each year are to mothers younger than 20 or older than 34 - mothers outside their safest child-bearing years.

CONCLUSION

Majority of the health problems of developing countries stem from malnutrition, infectious diseases and unregulated fertility. These factors usually go hand in hand with poverty, handicapping social conditions and the absence of health services. Alleviating these conditions therefore, would bring benefits to the families and the communities to which they belong.

In the regulation of fertility through family planning, the families derive social benefits such as:

(a)   A woman and her family are able to maximize their nutritional resources, a crucial factor in family health especially where the majority of people live in poverty.

(b)   Confining childbearing to the best years of the woman's reproductive life preserves the woman's health and lengthens her life expectancy.

(c)   The fewer the dependent children the less the strain on the family economy as a greater part of income can be diverted into savings which are eventually channelled into investment.

(d)   A woman who has access to family planning can take advantage of educational and employment opportunities and participate more actively in community life.

(e)   Woman's absolute dependency on their families for economic and psychological support is lessened, their freedom of movement is increased, the realization of ambitions and of social, economic and psychological needs is facilitated.

REFERENCES

1.   A Health and Demographic Survey of Bang Pa-In,
         Bangkok. Community Health Care Program,
         Ramathibodi Hospital Faculty of Medicine, 1969.
2.   Chase, HC (1961): The relationship of certain
         biologic and socio-economic factors to fetal,
         infant and early childhood mortality. I.
         Father's occupation, parental age and infant's

birth rank. New York State Department of Health, Albany, New York.

3. Chase HC (1962): The relationship of certain biologic and socio-economic factors to fetal, infant and early childood mortality. II. Father's occupation, infant's birth weight, and mother's age. New York State Department of Health, Albany, New York.

4. Douglas, JWB and Simpson HR (1964): Height in relation to puberty, family size and social class. A Longitudinal Study. Milbank Mem Fund Quart, 40:20-35.

5. Hare EH and Shaw GK (1965): A study in family health. I. Health in relation to family size. Brit J Psychiat, 3:461-466.

6. Hunt JM (1961): In: Intelligence and Experience, The Ronald Press Co., New York.

7. Jelliffe DB (1966): The assessment of the nutritional status of the community. World Health Organization Monograph Series No. 53, Geneva.

8. Nortman D (1974): Parental age as a factor in pregnancy outcome and child development. Reports on Population/Family Planning.

9. Pyke DA (1956): Parity and the incidence of diabetes. Lancet, 1:818-820.

10. Scott JA (1962): Intelligence, physique and family size. Brit J Prev Soc Med, 165-173.

11. Vernon PE (1951): Recent investigations of intelligence and its measurements. Eugen Rev, 43:125-137.

12. Wray JD and Aguirre A (1969): Protein-calorie malnutrition in Candelaria, Colombia. I. Prevalence, social and demographic factors. J Trop Pediat, 15:76-98.

13. Wright NH (1975): Thailand: estimates of the potential impact of family planning on maternal and infant mortality. J Med Ass Thailand.

14. Wyon JB and Gordon JE (1962): A long-term prospective-type field study of population dynamics in the Punjab, India. In: Research in Family Planning, CV Kiser, Editor, Princeton University Press, Princeton, 17-32.

HEALTH CONSEQUENCES OF UNPLANNED PREGNANCIES

VERSUS CONTRACEPTION

R. W. Rochat

Department of Health and Human Services
United States Public Health Service
Centers for Disease Control
Atlanta, Georgia, USA

INTRODUCTION

Virtually everyone considers at least once in his or her life the health consequences of childbearing or family planning. Many still view the addition of each child as an inevitable gift of God or an act of fate. Others have learned that they may plan both the number and the timing of the births of their children. To the extent that conception and childbearing are viewed as controllable events, it is useful to examine the consequences of different strategies of control.

The safety of childbearing, of terminating unplanned pregnancies, and of using contraception are important in selecting preferred strategies. Epidemiologic data on mortality risks are better defined than on morbidity. Epidemiologic data on non-contraceptive health benefits of contraception, particularly oral contraceptives, are less well known but extremely important in affecting individual health. We have made great strides in recent years in lowering maternal mortality and improving the safety of family planning methods (1-6). We know how to prevent over 90 percent of all deaths related to reproduction.

PREGNANCY-RELATED MORTALITY (7-12)

For pregnancy-related mortality in 1977, the data from 66 countries were used to estimate that about 427,000 women died as a result of pregnancy or its sequelae (Table 1).

Table 1. Estimated Maternal Mortality - the World and
          Each Region, 1977.

	Number Countries[1]	Number Countries With Data[2]	Percent Population in Countries With Data	Births[3] (in millions)	Maternal Deaths[2] (in 1,000s)	Mortality Rate[4]
World	160	66	42.1	122.5	426.6	348
Africa	52	5	21.2	19.0	19.5	103
Asia	43	13	44.7	74.4	388.4	522
North America	2	2	100.0	3.6	0.4	11
Latin America	31	19	56.1	12.1	14.4	119
Europe	27	25	99.4	7.2	2.3	32
USSR	1	0	0	4.7	1.5	32
Oceania	6	2	77.7	0.5	0.1	12

[1]All United Nations members and all geopolitical units with a population larger than 200,000.

[2]Sources: World Health Statistics Annual Report, Vol. 1, Geneva 1977; 1975 Demographic Yearbook, United Nations, New York 1976; Bose A, et al: Population in India's Development, 1947-2000, Vikas, Delhi 1974; Chen L, et al: Maternal mortality in rural Bangladesh, Stud Fam Plann 5(11):334-341, 1974; Government of Afghanistan, National Demographic and Family Guidance Survey of the Settled Population of Afghanistan, Vol. 1, 1975 (all death data for years between 1965 and 1975).

[3]1977 World Population Data Sheet, Population Reference Bureau, Washington, D.C.

[4]Per 100,000 live births.

Data were available from only 13 of 43 Asian countries representing less than half the population of Asia.
Nevertheless, based on these limited data, it is estimated
that 388,000 women in Asia died that year from pregnancy.
This represents about 1 in every 200 women who becomes
pregnant.

        Data on maternal mortality and its causes are absent
or under-reported for virtually all nations, including the
United States. Unless all pregnant women receive pregnancy and delivery care from hospitals, one might expect that
hospital data will be biased with respect to causes of
maternal mortality. In the United States, it has been
determined that from 1974 to 1978, over 25 percent of
maternal deaths were not reported on death certificates
such that they can be properly classified in national
statistics as pregnancy related. Except for voluntarily

Table 2.   Reported Maternal and Abortion-Related Deaths,
           by Type of Health Facility, Bangladesh,
           1978-1979.

	Total	Maternal	Abortion	Percentage From Abortion
Overall	1,933	1,435	498	25.8
Non-Hospital Facilities	1,154	857	297	25.7
Population Control-Family Planning Clinics	790	571	219	27.7
Thana Health Complexes	298	239	59	19.8
Maternal/Child Welfare- Maternal/Child Health Clinics	57	39	18	31.6
Other	9	8	1	11.1
Hospitals	779	578	201	25.8
Medical School	423	313	110	26.0
Subdivision	152	108	44	29.0
District	159	136	23	14.5
Other	45	21	24	53.3

terminated pregnancies, information is lacking on whether
pregnancy-associated deaths result from planned or
unplanned pregnancies.

HEALTH CONSEQUENCES OF ABORTION

        Determination of health risks of pregnancy and
childbearing in countries without vital statistics
requires innovative epidemiologic methods. A recent
nationwide survey in Bangladesh offers some data on
pregnancy-related deaths known to health workers. One-
fourth of pregnancy-related deaths were attributed each to
the termination of unplanned pregnancies by induced
abortion, to obstructed labor, to hemorrhage, and to other
causes. Sixty percent of the 1933 pregnancy-related
deaths were reported from non-hospital facilities, chiefly
freestanding family planning clinics. Both clinics and
hospitals reported about one-fourth of the deaths were
attributed to traditional methods of abortion (Table 2).
About 80 percent of the reports of abortion-related deaths

were subsequently verified through visits to villages of
the deceased. Overall, Measham estimated that 7800 women
died from abortion complications in Bangladesh in 1978.
Most of these abortions were performed by traditional
birth attendants inserting sticks and tree roots into the
cervix.

While abortion is the most dramatic, widely
recognized and highly controversial outcome of unplanned
pregnancy, it is not the only possile consequence.
Studies in Sweden and Czechoslovakia have examined the
health and social consequences of children born to women
who were denied abortion. The most recent report from the
prospective study in Czechoslovakia showed that the emotional and physical health of these children is adversely
affected. The study matched 110 boys and 110 girls born
to women twice denied abortion for the same pregnancy with
220 children born to women who had not requested pregnancy
termination. Both the children and the mothers were
matched for appropriate epidemiologic risk factors and
subsequently studied by members of a research team who did
not know which child belonged to what group. Despite the
fact that the two groups did not differ in intelligence
test results, the school performance of the children in
the study group was significantly poorer than the control
group, and the study group had a higher incidence of
illness and hospitalization. This research suggests that
giving birth to children following explicitly unwanted
pregnancies may lead to adverse emotional and health
consequences detectable 17 to 18 years later.

SURGICAL STERILIZATION

Most studies on abortion in Asia suggest that women
in this region who obtain abortion are usually married,
have several children, and presumably do not wish to have
further children. The most effective way of preventing
these abortions is to make safe methods of surgical steril-
ilization widely available. Westoff recently reported
that the high rate of sterilization in Korea from 1977 to
1978 averted an average 0.84 pregnancies per woman, but
that 64 percent of the averted pregnancies would have been
terminated by induced abortion had the sterilization not
been done. Thus, surgical sterilization in Korea
contributes more to preventing abortion than to lowering
fertility.

Because of its high effectiveness in preventing
unplanned pregnancy, surgical sterilization has become one

Table 3. Results of Eight Preliminary and Published
          Studies on Sterilization Death Rates

Study (Chief Investigator)	Years	Procedure	Number	Deaths	Rate[1]
International (AVS) (Aubert)	1973-1979	Tubectomy	255,812	15	5.9
International (IFRP) (Bhiwandiwala)	1971-1979	Tubectomy			
		Interval	24,037	1	5.1
		Postabortion	5,577	4	75.1
		Postdelivery	10,726	5	76.8
Rural Thailand (Chaturachinda)	1974-1977	Laparoscope	5,632	4	71.0
Bangladesh (Grimes)	1979-1980	Tubectomy	108,875	21	19.3
Bangladesh (Rosenberg)	1979-1980	Tubectomy	5,042	5	99.2
Korea (Ory)	Late '70's	Tubectomy	260,000	10	2.6
Colombia (Trias)	1973-1980	Laparoscope	93,098	2	2.1
		Minilaparotomy	92,073	2	2.2
United States (Peterson)	1977-1978	Tubectomy	414,500	15	3.6

[1]Per 100,000 procedures

of the most popular methods of contraception in the world
(13-16). Epidemiologic studies of its short and long-term
complications have only recently been initiated. At the
invitation of the governments of Bangladesh and Korea, we
have participated in the evaluation of sterilization mortality and morbidity in these countries. Sterilization-
associated deaths were defined as the death of a patient
from any cause occurring within 42 days of tubectomy or
vasectomy. Sterilization-attributable death is a death
resulting from the complications of the operation itself
or from a chain of events initiated by the operation.
Despite the lack of common definitions among studies and
the small numbers in each study, the mortality rate has
ranged from 2.1 and 99.2 deaths per 100,000 procedures
(Table 3). The higher death rates are associated with
either concurrent pregnancy termination or small numbers
of cases. Deaths are undoubtedly under-reported in some
of these studies.

     The single most common cause of mortality in the
United States, Korea and Bangladesh is related to the use

of local and general anesthesia. The use of excessive
amounts of drugs intended for local anesthesia can cause
general anesthesia. Infection and hemorrhage were two
other common causes of fatal complications.

Mortality is such a rarely occurring event that the
Center for Disease Control has established an international registry for sterilization-associated deaths. In
collaboration with other international agencies and individual physicians, we collected case reports on over 100
sterilization-associated deaths.

ORAL CONTRACEPTION

Oral contraception is one of the most commonly used
methods of contraception in the world (17-19). Numerous
clinical and epidemiologic studies have been conducted to
determine the noncontraceptive health effects of oral
contraception on humans. The benefits and risks of oral
contraception have been fairly well defined for selected
populations in the United Kingdom and the United States.

Oral contraception has its most harmful effect
through cardiovascular diseases, especially for women age
30 and older who smoke. The three most important diseases
affected by oral contraception are myocardial infarction,
thrombotic stroke, and subarachnoid hemorrhage. While
oral contraception is asociated with a small but meaningful increase in risk of myocardial infarction for
otherwise healthy women, its greatest risk is incurred by
women who smoke cigarettes, particularly those who are age
30 or older.

In the United States, fewer than 10 percent of oral
contraceptive users are 30 and older and smoke. Ory (17,
18) estimates that about three-fourths of heart attacks
that occur in oral contraceptive users in the United
States could be eliminated if those who are over 30 stop
both smoking and using oral contraceptives. Similar
preventive measures appear to be appropriate to prevent
thrombotic and hemorrhagic strokes.

Oral contraception is associated with eight known
major noncontraceptive benefits. It has been repeatedly
shown to reduce the incidence of benign breast diseases by
50 to 75 percent. This effect has been shown in 11 different studies conducted by different investigators. The
protection is greater the longer oral contraception is
used, and there is a strong association with greater

Table 4.   Estimates of Lifetime Mortality Risk Associated
           With Reproduction and Fertility Control for
           Hypothetical Cohorts of 20,000 Women in the
           United States.

Abortion for Contraceptive Failure	Deaths[2] Yes	No	Relative Ratio[3] Yes	No
Contraceptive Method				
Oral Contraception (smoker)	674	661	112	110
No Contraception	149	320	25	53
Oral Contraception (non-smoker)	123	126	21	21
IUD	96	109	16	18
Condom	24	79	4.0	13
Postpartum Sterilization	7	6	1.2	1.0

[1]Maternal mortality is 11.6 deaths per 100,000 live births.
Infant mortality is 19.7 for males and 13.6 for females per 1,000 live
births. Mean postpartum anovulation is 2 months.

[2]Per hypothetical cohort, 20,000 women using this method from age 15 to
49.

[3]Compared to women who choose surgical sterilization after the birth of
the second child.

amounts of progestin in the oral contraceptive.

Functional cysts of the ovary are either suppressed
or prevented by oral contraception. In addition, oral
contraception reduces the incidence of iron deficiency
anemia by 45 percent. More recently, oral contraception
has been shown to reduce the risk of developing pelvic
inflammatory disease by 50 percent as compared with
non-users of contraception. Oral contraceptives also
provide protection against ectopic pregnancy, probably
because they protect from pelvic inflammatory disease.
Less persuasive evidence currently exists that oral
contraceptives may protect against rheumatoid arthritis,
endometrial and ovarian cancer.

Ory et al at the Center for Disease Control are
currently conducting a large-scale, multi-center study on
the possible relationship between steroid hormones,
including oral contraceptives, and cancer of the breast,
ovaries and endometrium. We should have some preliminary
results within the next 12 months.

OTHER CONTRACEPTIVE PROCEDURES

The intrauterine device which has contributed so greatly to the reduction of fertility in South Korea, Taiwan, Chile and China has also had relatively limited epidemiologic study outside the United States States and United Kingdom. Several studies have shown an increased risk for pelvic inflammatory disease among IUD wearers (20, 21).

Injectable contraceptives such as depo-medroxy-progesterone (DMPA) are used in over 80 countries (22-23). DMPA is not currently approved as a contraceptive in the United States by the Food and Drug Admnistration. Its status for use as contraception is currently being reviewed by an expert panel. No epidemiologic study has demonstrated any serious adverse health effect from using DMPA, but the studies which have been conducted in the United States have been limited by the number of users. Preliminary data from our studies in Atlanta have shown no detectable increased risk of either endometrial cancer or overall mortality among DMPA users.

SELECTION OF SAFEST STRATEGY

Given the empirical data on mortality risks due to pregnancy and different methods of contraception, how can one determine the safest strategy? The analysis is complicated by the varying use of breast feeding and abortion, the different age at which women marry, the number of children they want, and the age at which they choose to stop childbearing. Tietze has used a simple graphic model to show that the safest strategy for women in the United States is a highly safe, relatively ineffective method of contraception with abortion for contraceptive failure.

The same principles in a probabilistic computer model to determine the relative risks of alternative strategies cumulated over the reproductive life span of a woman were used. To illustrate the maximum effect of cumulated risk, a hypothetical cohort of 20,000 women who marry at age 15, use either no contraception or use oral contraceptives, IUDs, condoms, or postpartum sterilization was examined (Table 4). Each woman may or may not choose abortion for contraceptive failure. She does not breast feed her infants, but infant mortality is low. She wants only two children. Using effectiveness and mortality risk data from the United States, the safest strategy is surgi-

Table 5. Pregnancies and Their Outcomes for Hypothetical
          Cohorts of 20,000 Women in the United States.

No Abortion	None	Condom (10% Failure)	Intrauterine Device (4% Failure)	Oral Contraception (2% Failure)	Postpartum Sterilization
Conceptions	362,030	109,880	73,140	59,625	45,150
Live Births	304,750	93,985	61,840	52,170	40,290
Spontaneous Abortions	55,800	15,480	9,340	7,260	4,790
Ectopic Pregnancies	1,460	416	1,970	194	69
Infant Deaths	5,010	1,579	1,010	877	651

Abortion For Contraceptive Failure					
Conceptions	516,630	129,820	81,110	63,780	
Live Births	40,510	40,730	40,500	40,530	
Spontaneous Abortions	61,280	14,795	8,920	7,000	
Induced Abortions	413,110	74,080	30,110	16,075	
Ectopic Pregnancies	1,720	418	1,590	178	
Infant Deaths	662	666	645	677	

cal contraception after the second child. The next safest
is to use condoms with abortion for contraceptive failure.
Condoms alone, the IUD, oral contraceptives for women who
do not smoke, or the use of abortion alone fall within a
twofold range (13 to 25) in relative risks. Using no
contraception has 53 times greater risk of death than the
safest strategy. Even more dangerous, however, is the use
of oral contraceptives by women who smoke; this combination is over 100 times more dangerous than the simple
strategy of surgical contraception after completing one's
family.

        Decisions on choices among these different strate-
gies are based on many factors other than mortality risks.
The computer model permits one to examine the consequences
of pregnancy outcomes and infant mortality, of choosing
methods with different effectiveness levels, and using or
not using abortions for contraceptive failure. If this
hypothetical cohort of 20,000 American women used no method of contraception, they would have 362,000 conceptions,
an average of 18.1 each and, by implication, an average of

15.2 children (Table 5). This high fertility is achieved
by early and sustained childbearing without breast feeding
or any family planning method. This cohort would have
1450 ectopic pregnancies and, among the children born,
5010 would die as infants. Using the least effective
contraceptive method (condoms), reduces the number of
births to an average of 4.7 each and the number of infant
deaths to 2579 or, 68 percent fewer infant deaths than for
those who used no contraception. Clearly the number of
infant deaths is directly related to the effectiveness of
fertility control strategy. Without any other change in
health care, highly effective family planning prevents 85
percent of all infant deaths as compared to maximum levels
of childbearing.

        This model has not yet incorporated benefits of oral
contraceptives. The reduced risks of pelvic inflammatory
diseases, ectopic pregnancies,anemia, and breast and ovarian disease make oral contraceptives even safer than
shown in this model.

CONCLUSIONS

        (a) The wide difference in maternal mortality in
different populations makes it clear that we currently
know how to prevent over 90 percent of the half million
deaths resulting each year from pregnancy.

        (b) Any method of family planning which prevents
pregnancy also prevents infant deaths. Highly effective
contraception prevents 85 percent of the infant deaths
associated with no contraception.

        (c) The safest contraceptive strategy for women is
voluntary surgical contraception.

        (d) Cigarette smoking combined with oral contra-
ception is the most dangerous family planning strategy.

        (e) Unexpectedly, epidemiologic studies have shown
that oral contraceptives in the United States have important non-contraceptive health benefits in preventing
pelvic inflammatory disease, ectopic pregnancy and anemia.

        (f) The epidemiologic risks of pregnancy and family
planning in developing countries need to be periodically
measured to determine our success in achieving healthy
reproduction.

(g) Couples the world over are choosing a new path in planning pregnancies effectively. Epidemiologic studies provide a rational information base in considering different family planning strategies. To implement informed decisions requires that minimal pregnancy and family planning services be readily accessible to those who need them.

REFERENCES

General

1. Hatcher RA, Stewart GK, Stewart F et al (1981): Contraceptive Technology 1980-1981, Irvington Pub., New York.
2. Kaminetzky HA, Ingelman-Sundbert A (eds.) (1979): Proceeding of an international symposium: A reappraisal of fertility control risks and benefits. Int J Gynaecol Obstet, 16:447-578.
3. Moghissi KS (1979): Controversies in Contraception. Williams and Wilkins, Baltimore.
4. Rochat RW, Ory HW, Schulz KF (1978): Methods for measuring safety and health hazards of presently available fertility regulating agents in the developing world. Singapore J Obstet Gynec, 9:1-15.
5. Sciarra JJ, Zatuchni GI, Speidel JJ (eds) (1978): Risks, benefits and controversies in fertility control. Harper and Row, Hagerstown, Md.
6. Suchindran CM< Rochat RW, Krasowski RS, Leeds (1980): FERTMORT, a computer model to study mortality risks of different birth control strategies. In: Modeling and Simulation, Vol. II, Part 4, Social Economics, Proceeding of the Eleventh Annual Pittsburgh Conference on Modeling and Simulation, 1421-1428, University of Pittsburg, Pittsburg.

Pregnancy-Related Mortality

7. David HP, Matejcek (1981): Children born to women denied abortion. An update. Fam Plann Perspect, 13:32-39.
8. Liskin LS (1980): Complications of abortion in developing countries. Population Reports Series F, No. 7, Pregnancy Termination, Johns Hopkins University.
9. Rochat RW (1981): Maternal mortality in the United States of America. World Health Statistics, 34:2-13.

10. Rochat RW, Jabeen S, Rosenberg MJ, Measham AR, Khan
    AR, Obaidullah M, Gould P (1981): Maternal and
    abortion related deaths in Bangladesh, 1978-1979.
    Int J Gynaecol Obstet, 19:155-164.
11. Rochat RW, Rubin GL, Selik R et al (1981): Changing
    the definition of maternal mortality. A new look
    at the postpartum interval. Lancet I:831.
12. Westoff CF (1980): Abortions averted by sterilization
    in Korea, 1977-1978. Fam Plann Perspect,
    6:60-64.

Sterilization

13. Auber JM, Lubell I, Schima M (1980): Mortality risk
    associated with female sterilization. Int J
    Gynaecol Obstet, 18:406-410.
14. Chaturachinda K (1980): The use of the laparoscope in
    rural Thailand. Int J Gynaecol Obstet,
    18:414-419.
15. Grimes DA, Peterson HB, Rosenberg MJ et al (1981):
    Sterilization-attributable deaths in Bangladesh.
    Int J Gynaecol Obstet (in press).
16. Rosenberg MJ, Rochat RW, Akbar J (1981):
    Sterilization in Bangladesh. Mortality, morbidity
    and risk factors. Presented at American Public
    Health Association, October 1981, Los Angeles.

Oral Contraception

17. Ory HW (1981): Maximizing the non-contraceptive
    benefits of oral contraceptive use. Presented at
    Leuven, Belgium, September 25, 1981.
18. Ory HW, Rosenfield A, Landman L (1981): The pill at
    20. An Assessment. Fam Plann Perspect,
    12:278-283.
19. Petitti DB, Wingerd J, Pellegrin F, Ramcharan S
    (1979): Risk of vascular disease in women:
    Smoking, oral contraceptives, non-contraceptive
    estrogens, and other factors. JAMA,
    243:1150-1154.

IUDS

20. Burkman RT and The Women's Health Study (1976):
    Association between intrauterine device and pelvic
    inflammatory disease. Obstet Gynecol,
    57:269-275.
21. Cates W, Ory HW, Rochat RW, Tyler CW (1976): The
    intrauterine device and deaths from spontaneous
    abortion. N Engl J Med, 295:1155-1159.

Injectables

22. Greenspan AR, Hatcher RA, Moore M, Rosenberg MJ, Ory HW (1980): The association of depo-medroxy-progesterone acetate and breast cancer. Contraception, 21:563-570.
23. Gold RB, Willson PD (1981): Depo-provera: new developments in a decade-old controversy. Fam Plann Perspect, 13:35-39.

Natural Family Planning

24. Wade ME, McCarthy P, Braunstein GD et al (1981): A randomized prospective study of the use-effectiveness of natural family planning. Am J Obstet Gynec, 141:368-376.

SYSTEMIC CONTRACEPTION AT PRIMARY HEALTH CARE LEVEL

AND WHO SHOULD APPLY THEM

R. A. Apelo

Professor of Obstetrics and Gynecology, College
of Medicine, University of the Philippines and
the National Family Planning Office
Manila, Philippines

INTRODUCTION

The term "systemic contraception" in this paper
refers only to that induced by oral pills and by long-
acting progestin injectables because they are the ones
more commonly available in most countries. Other
contraceptives which make use of steroids for contraception control like vaginal rings, the implants (both the
biodegradable and non-biodegradable), the nasal sprays and
the male pills are still investigated and therefore are
not included in the discussion.

At present, 80 million women are using the oral pills
while around 100 million have used them at one time or
another. On the other hand there are 10 million users of
the injectables today. The pills have reached women all
over the world through many ways such as hospitals,
clinics, drug stores or community supply points (food
shops or retail stores). The pills have been dispensed by
doctors, midwives, other health personnel and even by lay
volunteers. The question of who can safely dispense the
pills has been raised repeatedly. Some physicians would
not want to dispense the pills until after a thorough
physical and laboratory examination. At the other
extreme, some programs allow the pills to be freely given
by lay people without any safe- guards. At one time there
was even a suggestion of dispensing pills in vending
machines. Clearly these practices and considerations are
influenced by each country's resources and the extent of

need for population control measures.

Presently, when governments are concerned with total
coverage of the population to be able to provide health
care for all, the question of who should dispense these
contraceptives again arises. This is a natural sequela
since some of the basic principles in primary health care
relate to the multisectoral approach, i.e. the participation of communities and the maximum use of existing resources. In order to answer the question, it is necessary
to reassess the advantages and disadvantages offered by
the pills and the injectables.

CONTRACEPTIVE PILLS AND PLAN OF ACTION

The pills have been in use for 20 years. There is no
doubt that its use has helped millions of women contracept
successfully. Aside from its role as ovulatory suppres-
sant, the pills have beneficial effects such as regulation
of menstruation, prevention of dysmenorrhea, maintenance
of body iron, protection from breast cysts and ovarian
tumors.

There are certain risks involved with the use of
pills. Considered to be the most serious is the risk of
circulatory system disease. Retrospective and prospective
studies on the incidence of cardiac failure, thromboembolism and myocardial infarction among pill users have been
conducted in the United States and Great Britain. The
findings show that British women who were aged 35 to 40
years old and were pill users had a death rate of 13.8 per
100,000 per year against 5.5 per 100,000 per year among
non-pill users in the same age group. This incidence increased to 39.5 per 100,000 per year among pill users who
smoked. Although Goldzicher and Dozier raised questions
on the statistical validilty of these case control
studies, findings of prospective studies being currently
published support these earlier reports.

Some studies suggest that 5 or more years of use may
lead to an increased risk of heart attacks. Whether this
is due to the pill itself or to concurrent risk factors is
not clear because of the difficulty of interpreting study
results especially since heart attacks are recognized to
be quite infrequent among women. At this point, it is
appropriate to recall that Pincus, the pill discoverer,
said that the pills were never intended for long term use.

Hypertension, or a substantial elevation of blood

pressure, has been noted among oral contraceptive users:
In most instances, the blood pressure returns to normal
levels within 6 months of contraceptive discontinuance.

Some investigators consider diabetes as a contraindi-
cation to pill use as the latter may cause an increase in
insulin requirement. Others recommend that the oral
contraceptives can be suitably and safely given to
diabetics, which incidentally is the recommendation of the
British Diabetic Association.

There have been reports on the development of benign
hepatic nodules among long term users of oral contraceptives. However, this has not created as much controversy
as the risk of cardiovascular disease because of the
rarity of liver tumors and the difficulty of reaching an
agreement on the nomenclature of hepatic tumors and on
their histopathologic interpretation.

As to the relation between oral contraceptives and
cancer of the reproductive system, an epidemiologic case
control study is presently being conducted by the World
Health Organization with its collaborating research
centers in different countries. Previous studies have not
shown any definitive relationship. Researchers like Stern
and associates observed that pills may promote progression
to carcinoma in situ of already existing cervical
dysplasia. However, Boyce and associates analyzed a large
series of women with cervical carcinoma in situ and an
equal number of matched controls without the disease. No
significant difference was found among pill users in both
groups. At present, there is no statistically significant
evidence of a causal relationship between pill use and
cancer of the cervix.

Less cause of concern are side effects whch are
relatively minor such as headache, urticaria, weight gain,
nausea, vomiting and irregular bleeding. A cause and
effect relationship for these side effects has not been
establised except that bleeding occurred among users of
combined pills containing noresthisterone, and nausea and
vomiting among those taking preparations containing
norgestrel.

Another consideration which may be important to women
suffering from endemic diseases who need prolonged and
specific therapy is the possibility of drug to drug interaction. While many studies have been undertaken, only two
drugs have so far been established to affect the
metabolism of the combined pill leading to decreased

effectivness.   They are rifampicin and ampicillin.

Suggested Plan of Action

     The controversy regarding the validity of research
methodology and interpretation of results will probably
continue. Meanwhile, there are a growing number of women
who need the pills and must be heeded. However, in so
doing, the following precautions should be taken so that
potential risks could be reduced:

(a) Restriction of pill use among women over 35 years,
     and heavy smokers.
(b) Limitation of pill use to not more than five years.
(c) Consideration of the following absolute contraindica-
     contraindications: history of thromboembolism or
     cardiovascular accident; impaired liver function;
     malignancies of the reproductive system including the
     breast; and pregnancy;
(d) Consideration of the following relative contraindi-
     cations: hypertension; jaundice; and diabetes.

     A medical checklist, though not as comprehensive as
suggested above, has been introduced in the Philippine
Population Program for use by full time outreach lay-
workers. However, its use is limited because the initial
prescription is still being provided by trained nurses and
midwives stationed at health centers. Only resupplies are
available through field workers, barrio supply points, rural health units, government hospitals and various private
agencies. Some form of control of distribution exists in
government health stations, but no such restriction exists
in the drug stores because pills can be bought over the
counter.

     The need for a wider acceptance of the pills is
recognized but they should be administered discriminately.
Full time outreach workers who are mostly lay persons
should be reoriented in the use of the checklist and be
allowed to provide both the initial and succeeding
supplies of the pills. While these workers are employed
by the Commission of Population, the Ministry of Health
has piloted the Sarikaya approach which is the utilization
of indigenous volunteer leaders who have been chosen by
the community to act as "extension communicators" in
health and family planning. They conduct home visitations
and organize informal gatherings to influence their peer
to adopt proper health and family planning practice. In
effect, this is primary health care in a limited scale.

Sarikaya is a contraction of two Filipino words, "sariling kakayahan" or self-reliance. They too can dispense pills if properly trained in the use of the check list. With this approach, a few women who are in need of pills might be denied its use because of the existence of conditions included in the checklist, but this is to their advantage.

Injectables and Plan of Action

Unfortunately, this simple, effective, and reversible method of conception control is not allowed in the Philippines inspite of its proven acceptability and safety as evidenced by the result of local studies conducted in different parts of the country for the past 13 years. Filipino women prefer to use injectables even if they experience prolonged periods of amenorrhea.

The long-acting progestin injectables have less metabolic effects than the combined pills. The injectables do not affect lactation. Studies in humans here and abroad have yielded favorable results. However, governmental approval for its use has been withheld possibly because of the published adverse reaction of beagle dogs and monkeys to medroxy- progesterone. The Task Force on Injectables of the World Health Organizatin has concluded that the beagle dog is not an appropriate animal model and that the finding of two endometrial cancers and 10 endometrial atrophies among 12 rhesus monkeys that were given 50 times the human dose level is irrelevant.

All the above reactions occurred in animal models. In more than 10 million women who have used the injectables, not a single death has been established that can be attributed to the drug. Despite this favorable outcome, the WHO Task Force and other expert committees continue to remain alert for adverse effects. It is my opinion there is no longer any reason to withhold its use. It is unlikely that new methods will be forthcoming in the near future. There will only be improvements on the existing ones - the pills, the injectables, the IUDs, and sterilization.

The administration of injectable contraceptive is a type of service delivery suitable to this country of 7000 islands. Injections can be administered by nurses and midwives at the community level. Filipinos, by culture, welcome injections as it is considered to be superior to oral medication in terms of effectiveness.

CONCLUSION

Lay volunteers who are appropriately trained in the use of a medical checklist may be deployed to distribute pills at the community level. However, the checklist must be updated continuously to include new precautions. Low dose combination contraceptive pills should be made available for initial users. An effective referral system must be established or strengthened for back-up support.

Injectable contraceptives should be included in the population program. Nurses and midwives should be allowed to give the injection.

REFERENCES

Apelo R et al (1974): Acceptability of injectable contraception in the Philippines. IPPF Medical Bulletin, (April).

Apelo R, dela Cruz J (1973): Depoprovera, an effective contraceptive agent. J Phil Med Assoc, 49:179-196.

Back DJ, Breckenridge AM (1978): Drug interactions with oral contraceptive. IPPF Medical Bulletin, 12(4).

Back DJ, Breckenridge AM et al (1980): The effect of rifampicin and the pharmacokinetics of ethinyl estradiol in women. Contraception, 21(2).

Back DJ et al (1979): Drug - drug interactions, studies with oral contraceptive steriod. In: Drug Assessment, Criteria and Method, Elsevier/Northhill Biomedical Press, pp. 185-206.

Boyce JG, Lu T, Nelson JH Jr, Fruchter RG (1977): Oral contraceptives and cervical carcinoma. Am J Obstet Gyn, 128:761-766.

Briggs M (1978): Rationale of dosages and ratios of oral contraceptive steroids in combined products. Meeting of the Steering Committee, Task Force on Oral Contraceptives, World Health Organization, Singapore.

Edmunson HA, Henderson B, Benton B (1976): Liver cell adenomas associated with use of oral contraceptives. New Eng J Med 294:470-472.

Egren R, Strutevart FM (1976): Potencies of oral contraceptives. Am J Obstet Gyn 125:(8).

Fraser I, Weisberg E (1981): A comprehensive review of injectable contraception with special emphasis on depot medroxyprogesterone acetate. Med J Australia 1:(1).

Goldzieher JW, Dozier TS (1973): Oral contraceptive and thromboembolism. A reassessment. Am J Obstet Gyn, 123:878-914.

Kay CR (1980): The happiness pill. <u>J Royal Col Gen</u>
     <u>Pract</u>, (Jan).
Mann JL, Doll T, Thorogood M, Vessey MP, Waters WE (1976):
     Risk factors for myocardial infarction in young
     women. <u>Brit J Prev Soc Med</u>, 30:94-100.
Nora AH, Nora JJ (1978): Maternal exposure to exogenous
     progestogen/estrogen as a potential cause of birth
     defects. <u>Advances in Planned Parenthood</u>,
     12:156-169.
Population Report (1979): Oral contraceptives - Update on
     usage, safety and side effects. <u>Population Report</u>,
     A(5).
World Health Organizatin (1979): The effect of female sex
     hormones on fetal development and infant health. <u>Re-</u>
     <u>port of the WHO Scientific Group</u>, (December).
Ministry of Health, Philippines (1980): <u>Sarikaya</u>
     <u>Manual</u>. National Family Planning Office.
Shapiro S et al (1979): Oral contraceptive use in
     relation to myocardial infarction. <u>Lancet</u>, (April).
Poller L (1978): Oral contraceptives, blood clotting and
     thrombosis. <u>Brit Med Bull</u>, 34:151-156.
Report (1978): The Special Advisory Committee on
     Reproductive Physiology report to the Health
     Protection Branch. (March)
Royal College of General Practitioners (1974): <u>Oral</u>
     <u>contraception and health</u>. An interim report from the
     Oral Contraception Study of the Royal College of
     General Practitioners. Pitman, New York.
Royal College of General Practitioners (1977): Oral
     contraceptive study. Mortality among oral
     contraceptive users. <u>Lancet</u>, 2:727-731.
Steel JM, Duncan LPJ (1978): The effect of oral
     contraceptive on insulin requirements in diabetes.
     <u>Brit J Family Planning</u>, 3:77.
Stern EB (1977): Steriod contraceptive use and cervical
     dysplasia. Increased risk of progression. <u>Science</u>,
     196:1460-1462.
Vessey MP, Mann JI (1978): Female sex hormones and
     thrombosis. <u>Brit Med Bull</u>, 34:157-162.
Vessey MP, Kay Clifford R, Wingrave S (!979): Oral
     contraceptives and diabetes mellitus. <u>Brit Med J</u>,
     (Jan).
WHO (1977): Multinational comparative clnical evaluation
of two long acting injectable contraceptive steriods:
norethisterone enanthate and medroxyprogesterone acetate.
<u>Conception</u>, 15:(15).

INTRAUTERINE DEVICE INSERTION AT THE PRIMARY HEALTH CARE LEVEL: WHO SHOULD APPLY THEM?

I. Kamal

Professor of Obstetrics and Gynecology
Faculty of Medicine
Cairo, Egypt

INTRODUCTION

The intrauterine device (IUD) is an effective, in-expensive method of conception control that is bound to a single decision and intervention for years. Because of the socio-cultural status in our countries, this contra-ceptive modality should rank first among other methods of family planning.

However, the method requires manpower and a degree of clinical training and skill which creates a problem in countries where physician to population ratio is low. The question then arises: who should apply the IUD at the primary health care level, physician or non-phsycian? To what extent is the attendant who inserts the device, responsible for the occurence of side effects and complications?

SKILLS NECESSARY IN INSERTION OF IUD

Presented below are a selection of hysterograms, demonstrating and answering the following questions on intra-uterine contraception.

(a) How is a device retained in the uterus?
(b) Why do most IUD users remain asypmtomatic?
(c) What are the causes of bleeding, pain and expulsion?
(d) How is perforation produced?
(e) Why do unwanted pregnancies sometimes occur with the IUD in situ?

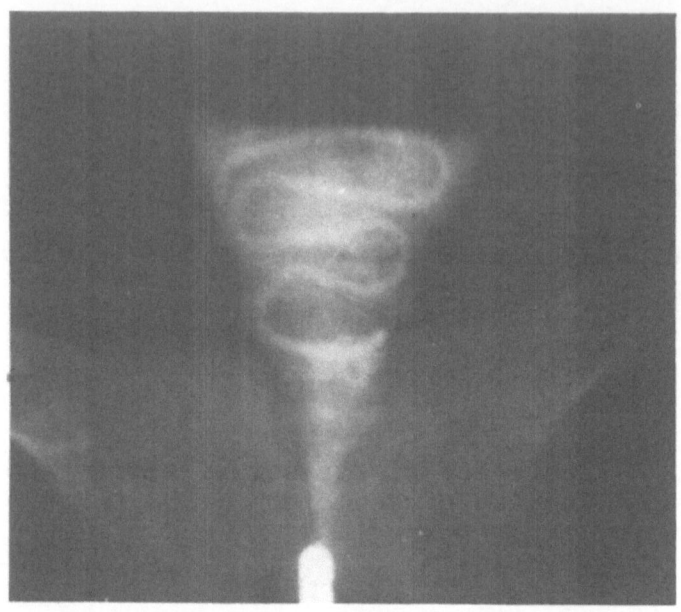

Figure 1.   A hysterogram of a Lippes Loop user that
             remained asymptomatic for years since inser-
             tion. It demonstrates a triangular uterine
             cavity with a closed isthmus. In the cavity
             the loop is oriented in the frontal plane oc-
             cupying virtually its entire space. The base
             of the loop is totally covering the fundus and
             its edges fit snugly against the lateral
             walls. On theoretical consideration, the
             loop is retained by the two convergent side
             walls of the uterus and the closed isthmus.

     For a device to be retained and the woman remain
asmptomatic, the IUD should conform harmoniously with the
uterine cavity (Fig. 1). This could be achieved by the
choice of a proper device and the use of an appropriate
technique of insertion. "Individual fitting" is impossible for programatic efforts, but certain devices approach
this ideal more than others. The inert Lippes loop 30 mm
C, as regards shape, size and its multidirectional
pliability, approaches this ideal in 80 percent of cases.

     Disparity in size and/or shape between the uterine
cavity and the device (Fig. 2) unleashes fundal hypertonia
and myometrial irritation, which in turn excite uterine

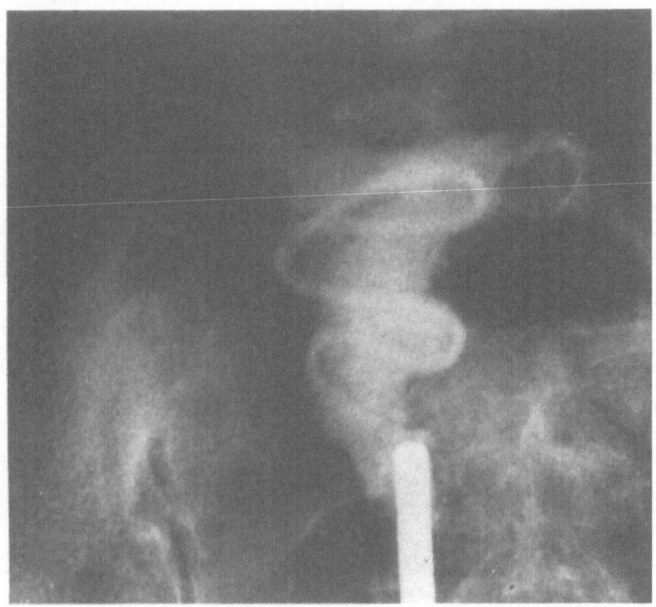

Figure 2. Bleeding and pain are directly linked to a dis-
harmonious fit relationship between the uterine
cavity and the device. This hyperactive uterus
shows contractions in the alleys of the loop;
symptoms included colic and bleeding for two
days since insertion. The loop was expelled
the morning after hysterography. If it were
not expelled, it should have been removed,
otherwise bleeding and pain would have
persisted.

contractions that trigger the entire battery of side
effects: bleeding, pain, expulsion and pregnancy.

The observation in Fig. 2 has been noted in severe or
moderate cases of pain and bleeding (10 to 12% of cases).
The only therapy of choice is the removal of the device
which in the final analysis is considered an iatrogenic
form of trauma. The device should not be left too long or
else the woman is bound to lose much blood with a resultant severe anemia. However, an alternative may be the
reinsertion of a different device as to shape and size
(Fig. 3).

Perforation at the time of insertion is a traumatic
event. It can be entirely prevented if gentle manipula-

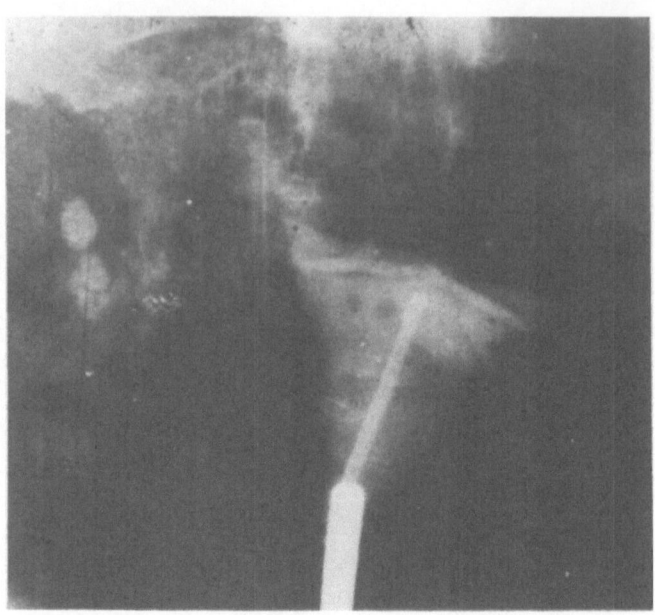

Figure 3.   The copper "T" is smaller than the Lippes
             loop; because of its structural characteris-
             tic of a square double beam, it has two free
             tips to anchor itself into the walls of the
             uterus. Fixation helps retention and this
             minimizes traumatic bleeding.

tions are used and a proper insertion technique is
followed. Proper IUD insertion technique includes five
precautions:

(a)   the use of tenaculum to pull on the cervix and to
      straighthen the angle of flexion.
(b)   the use of uterine sound to estimate the length and
      direction of the canal.
(c)   dilatation of the cervix to facilitate insertion.
(d)   introduction of the insertion tube with the device
      up to the fundus.
(e)   the use of tube withdrawal instead of plunger push
      technique.

COMPLICATIONS

     Congenital anomalies, malposition of the uterus and
soft myometrium after labor or abortion are the three most
important predisposing factors to perforation (Fig. 4, 5).

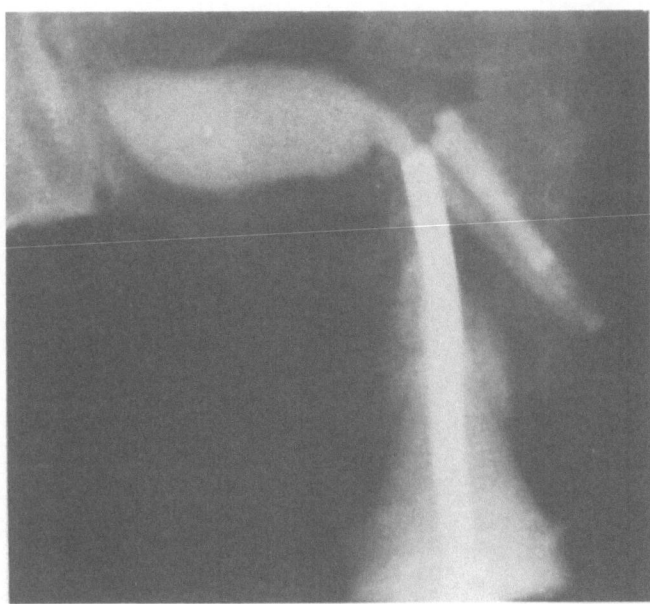

Figure 4.   A hysterogram demonstrating a long cervical
             canal, an acute dextro-lateral flexion of the
             body of uterus and a Lippes loop in the
             vesico-uterine pouch of the peritonium.
             Gentle manipulations and a proper technique of
             insertion would have prevented this
             perforation.

For optimal contraceptive protection, the IUD should virtually completely occupy the cavity, and therefore must be
very near the fundus. Because of a lack in optimal fit,
some areas of the uterine cavity is left unprotected which
may invite pregnancy. This was found to be due to three
reasons: congenital anomalies, disorientation of the
device, and empty uterus.

     Congenital anomalies such as a bicornuate uterus have
been shown to give rise to unexpected pregnancy following
insertion of a single IUD (Figs. 6 and 7). The observations indicate that no matter what improvement is made in
an IUD design, the morphological factors in the population
will render a 100 percent protection rate almost
impossible (3 to 5/100 woman years).

     Disorientation of the IUD occurs in uterine cavities
which are larger than the device. Such disorientation
increases the risk of pregnancy for both the inert and the

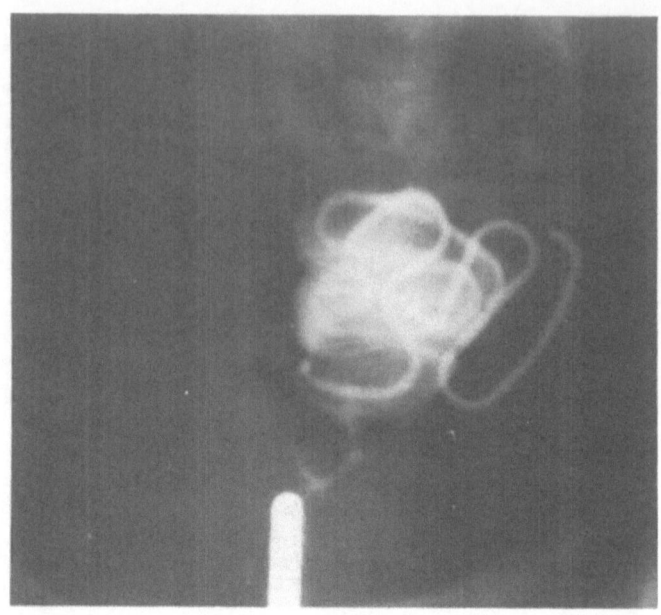

Figure 5.   A hysterogram demonstrating two Lippes loop,
             one inside and another outside the uterus.
             The primary insertion was immediately post-
             partum. Three months later, the woman con-
             sulted her physician because she could not
             feel the thread. Another loop was inserted on
             the assumption that the first was expelled. A
             month after the second insertion the woman
             complained of unexplained bleeding. Double
             contrast hysterography revealed the loop that
             was missing.

copper-carrying devices (Fig. 8 and 9).

     An empty uterus or a uterine cavity devoid of an IUD
is subject to the usual pregnancy rate. Post-insertion
emptiness of the uterus results either from unnoticed
expulsion or perforation (Fig. 10 and 11).

PHYSICIANS AND NON-PHYSICIANS

     The above pictorial presentations of case records
demonstrate that apart from perforation, IUD side effects
(bleeding, pain, expulsion and pregnancy) are due to disparity in size or shape between the uterine cavity and the
device. Accordingly, the attendant who inserts the device

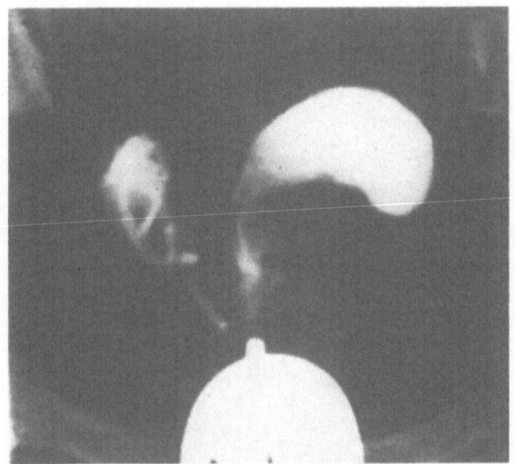

Figure 6.   A hysterogram demonstrating a bicornuate
             uterus, the right horn holding the Lippes loop
             and in the left horn which is unprotected,
             pregnancy is in progress.

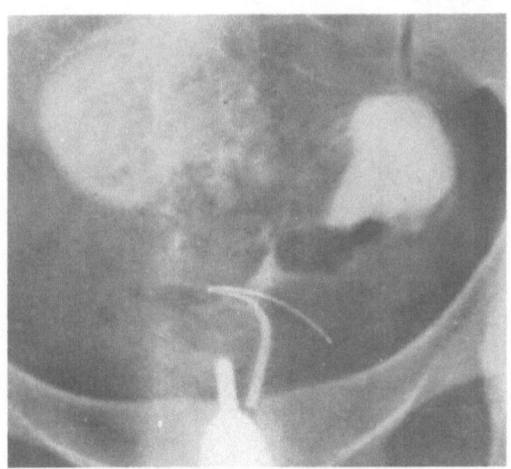

Figure 7.   Failure to recognize the existence of a bicor-
             nuate uterus can make insertion and correct
             positioning of an IUD difficult. Here a Cu'7'
             is located low in the uterus. The septum be-
             tween the two horns had prevented proper
             orientation of the device. Pregnancy is in
             progress in one of the unprotected areas
             above.

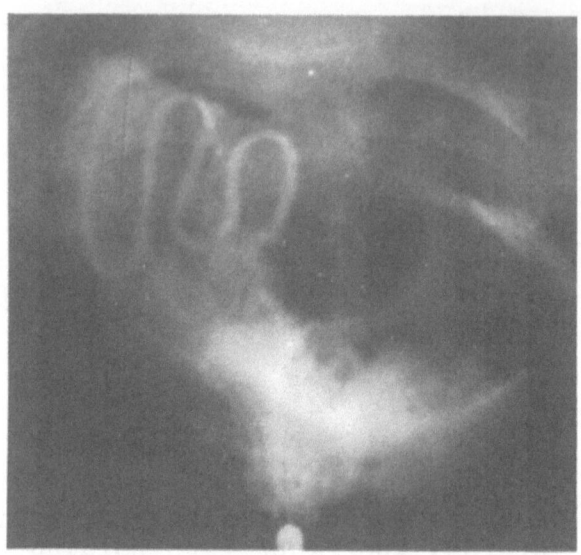

Figure 8.   A Lippes loop disoriented and laterally
             rotated, providing incomplete fundal coverage
             and cavity occupation that allowed pregnancy
             to occur.

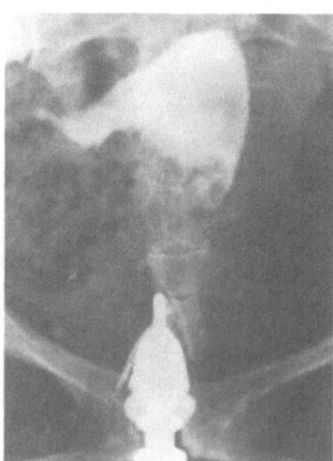

Figure 9.   Two Lippes loops expelled before a Cu'T' (a
             less risky expulsion device) was fitted.
             Because of the large uterine cavity, the Cu'T'
             came to be anchored low in the uterus leaving
             a large unprotected area above, that invited
             pregnancy.

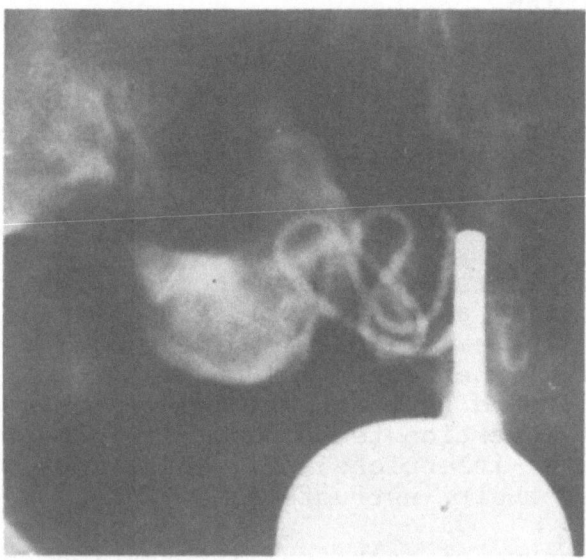

Figure 10.   A referral case of perforation of a Lippes
loop with pregnancy in progress in the empty
uterus.

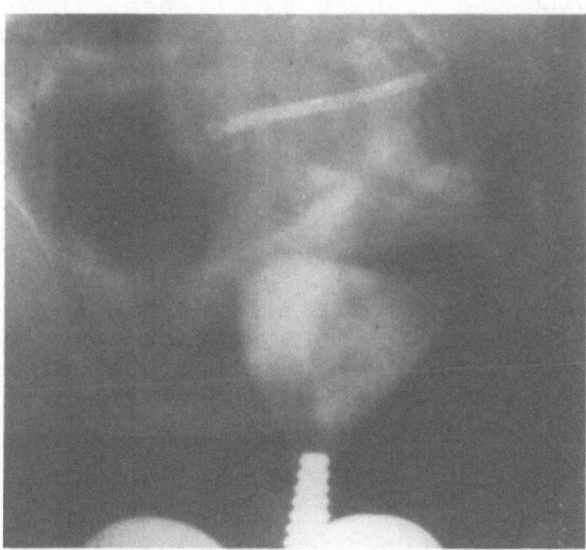

Figure 11.   A referral case of pregnancy secondary to a
Cu'T' perforation. The case was not diagnosed
until after evacuation when a double contrast
hysterogram was made.

should not always be blamed, whether he is a physician or a non-physician.

In developing countries where physician shortage is a problem, non-physicians usually provide primary health care for the rural inhabitants. The traditional midwife has the tasks of delivery and the care of mothers and children which place her in a position to be a trusted provider of family planning and contraception.

Non-physicians from local communities, after special training courses under medical supervision, can in a short period, be of great help to family planning programs including IUD insertion. The major part of their training should be devoted to practical demonstrations, including the correct insertion technique. Trainees are allowed a few supervised-insertions; solo insertions will only be permitted by their instructors.

As a source of technical information, a properly designed training manual incorporating check lists and management instructions would be an asset to the trainees. A mobile team which includes a physician should periodically monitor family planning centers to answer questions and deal with difficult cases and problems.

Following the Iranian experience, it was concluded in one of the WHO Conferences that a rural midwife can, after a short training course in the technique, insert IUDs as safely and effectively as a physician.

CONCLUSION

Does it matter then who should apply the IUD at the primary health care level: physician or non-physician? Non-physicians are usually more strategically located in rural areas. They have more contact with rural women and can offer more time for counseling. Their continuous availability in the area can be of great help to promote any family planning program.

MOBILE FACILITIES FOR VASECTOMY-

A RATIONAL APPROACH FOR A DEVELOPING COUNTRY

A. Nirapathpongporn and M. Viravaidya

Population and Community Development
Association (PDA)
Bangkok, Thailand

INTRODUCTION

Medical service delivery in developing countries is facing problems and limitations mainly due to the shortage and maldistribution of medical manpower. A broad range of services are available to the population in urban communities, but the majority of people living in the rural areas are not being adequately served by the existing resources. A ratio of one physician for every 100,000 rural population makes it difficult, if not impossible, to deliver good quality medical care to each individual.

To remedy this situation in many countries, paramedics have been trained and allowed to carry out the diagnosis and treatment of simple ailments and some surgical operations (1, 2). Village volunteers have been used for community-based distribution (CBD) of contraceptives in some countries (3). These village distributors, together with other paramedics, have helped recruit a great number of acceptors of pills, IUDs, injectable contraceptives and even sterilization without notable increase in the rate of complications. Furthermore, these village volunteers can be trained to be auxillary health workers to serve the people in their villages (4). The policy of using non-physicians for distribution and prescription of the temporary effective methods of contraception will make these methods more widely available at the primary health care level in most countries.

While great advances have been made in the avail-

ability of temporary contraceptive methods, much less progress has been made in the area of sterilization. Once a
couple has achieved its desired family size, they will
need permanent effective contraception. Unlike the temporary methods, surgical contraceptive is more sophisticated
and requires well-trained personnel and expensive instruments to provide the services. It is also associated with
higher risks and complications.

With limited numbers of physicians having a broad
range or responsibility for many aspects of health service
delivery superimposed on the geographical and cultural
barriers existing in some countries, a question can be
raised as to whether voluntary surgical contraception
services may be made available to meet the demand at the
primary health care level.

APPROACHES TO SOLVE THE PROBLEMS

The delivery of voluntary surgical contraceptive
services at the primary health care level may be brought
about by a variety of alternative approaches. The following are some of the issues involved in the service
delivery system:

Vasectomy vs Tubal Ligation.

Vasectomy and/or tubal ligation can be provided at
the primary health care level. It is well accepted that
vasectomy is relatively more convenient and economical to
perform and is associated with fewer complications than
tubal ligation. Although it appears that the acceptance
of vasectomy is more difficult due to traditional male
resistance, it is possible that with extensive and appropriate motivational strategies, this attitude can be
changed and acceptor recruitment can be achieved.

Paramedics Performing Sterilization.

Because of the shortage of physicians, especially in
rural areas, paramedical personnel working at the primary
health center can be trained to provide sterilization services. It has been demonstrated that this can be carried
out with satisfactory results in many countries (1, 2). A
great number of paramedics have to be trained and equipped
in order to expand the service throughout the country.
This will be quite an expensive program unless it is
limited to certain areas. The training of these paramedics may not be feasible in some countries with limited

budgets and personnel who can conduct such training.

Physician in Clinic-based Service and Mobile Units.

The physcian in the provincial or district hospital may be encouraged to provide sterilization services in both clinic-based and local mobile outreach programs. It has been demonstrated that this approach is quite effective (5). However, due to the scarcity of doctors in rural areas and the fact that most are already overburdened with other responsibilities, the local mobile service team can not be deployed frequently enough from their hospital base to provide service at the primary health center. This approach, if selected for widespread service, is also expensive because equipment for sterilization and facilities for the mobile team must be provided.

Centrally Controlled Mobile Service.

A mobile team specially trained to provide sterilization services in rural areas can be combined with an existing community-based family planning infrastructure to maximize the effect of mobile service delivery at the primary health care level. Ths mobile team can be deployed daily from a centrally or regionally situated logistical staging center.

In this program, a one day orientation and training of the family planning volunteers in the villages will be carried out by the motivation team. After the training, the motivation and acceptor recruitment activities by these volunteers will be coordinated with the mobile service team which will visit their villages two weeks after the orientation.

With all the facilities in the self-contained mobile vans, the mobile teams are deployed from the center for periodic sterilization service of about one week in each target area. Good management of mobile team activities and cooperation with local health offcials are key factors in the success of the program. The mobile team may be deployed in the following manner:

(a) Centrally controlled mobile service. In this arrangement, one or more self-contained mobile vans will be deployed from the central office to the target areas, providing services in one area after another until all the target areas have been visited. Second and third round service may be scheduled if necessary.

(b) Regional center with mobile satellite. One or more self-contained mobile vans will be deployed from regional centers to target areas within the operational radius for one day round trips.

This mobile service approach offers some advantages over other alternatives in that it does not require too many doctors and the equipment used for sterilization need not be duplicated and distributed throughout the country. It also covers a wide operational area at the primary health care level. Theoretically, the service provided by this mobile team should have a lower failure rate and minimal complications because the procedures are performed by well-trained physicians. The use of this mobile team service program in Thailand by the Population and Community Development Association (PDA) will demonstrate this operational approach. The Population and Community Development Association is a registered, tax-exempt, non-profit organization engaged in service delivery in family planning, parasite control, sanitation, general health and community development at the village level and some urban communi- ties in close collaboration with government agencies.

COMMUNITY-BASED VOLUNTARY STERILIZATION PROJECT

The Population and Community Development Association has had special interest in providing sterilization ser-vices since its inception in 1974. A good number of male and female sterilizations have been performed at two sta-tionary urban clinics each year. From July 1980 through April 1981, a special campaign called "The Community-Based Voluntary Sterilization Project" was launched to supplement the government sterilization program, especially in the rural areas where services are needed most. Self-contained vasectomy buses travelled throughout rural Thailand; simultaneously, new urban acceptors were channeled to PDA's urban clinics using a variety of innovative promotion strategies.

Under this project, sterilization services were delivered to both rural and urban communities. Two mobile vasectomy teams were deployed from the PDA Bangkok office to rural areas where the government's vasectomy program has not provided adequate service. Forty-eight (48) of 158 districts already serving as operational areas in the Community-Based Family Planing Services (CBFPS) rural program with an infrastructure of contraceptive volunteer distributors in the villages were chosen as the target

areas for this project. Two stationary clinics in Bangkok
served as referral centers for acceptors in urban areas
for vasectomy and tubal ligation procedures. The planing, selection of target areas, and implementation of this
project was done with the complete approval of and under
the direct supervision of the Ministry of Public Health.
Good cooperation with government officials at the Ministry, provincial and local levels was a key factor toward
the success of the program.

In the rural component, a one-day orientation and
training on voluntary surgical contraception was organized
by the project's staff for 3360 village volunteers in the
48 districts. After the orientation period, village volunteers carried out motivation and recruitment activities
for vasectomy acceptors in their villages. Vasectomy
service was provided by the mobile team which visited
their respective villages two weeks after the training.
Female acceptors were referred to the nearest government
health facility for tubal ligation.

In the urban areas, a similar training was organized
for 500 volunteer distributors who after training, referred both male and female acceptors for the service to
Bangkok clinics. Occasional mobile van forays to mass
gatherings in Bangkok for vasectomy service was also
included in the urban program activities.

An extensive motivation campaign using mass media
and every possible promotional strategy was carried out
throughout all project areas. Two mobile vans were self-
contained with operating tables and facilities for 50
vasectomy procedures and were air-conditioned. Necessary
equipment for medical emergency management was also
included. Each mobile team consisted of 5 staff members:
one physician, one nurse, one nurse assistant, one cleaner
and one driver. Vasectomy and tubal ligation were performed by qualified physicians specially trained for this
purpose.

Vasectomy was performed through a single median
scrotal incision by standard method, i.e., removing one
piece of the vas deferens about one centimeter long from
each side and tying both sectioned ends with nonabsorbable
suture. The skin was closed with one plain catgut stitch.
After the procedure, a specimen of seminal fluid was obtained at 3 months time or after 15 ejaculations for sperm
analysis.

Minilaparotomy or laparoscopic approaches were used

Table 1.   Percentage of Sterilization Acceptors
By Type in Urban Areas.

| | Sterilization Type | | |
	Vasectomy	Female Sterilization	Total
Acceptors over nine months	79.1 (2020)	20.9 (535)	100.0 (2555)

in female sterilization. Whenever possible, the fallopian
tubes were occluded using the Falope Ring technique.
Post-operative follow-up of all acceptors was made by regular visits of the vounteers and their supervisors. If
any complaint or complication associated with the procedure arose, the district supervisors and local health
officials helped manage it themselves or referred to appropriate medical facilities. However, the mobile service
team providing the service in a particular area usually
remained in that area for about one week before departing
to the next nearby district. If immediate serious post-
operative complications occurred, the physician from the
mobile team was usually within reach to solve the problem.

RESULTS

The Urban Component.

     Through two standing clinics in Bangkok and
occasional mobile van forays to mass gatherings, the urban
sections of the PDA project recruited 2020 male and 535
female sterilization acceptors over nine months for an
average of 213 cases per month (Table 1). The male-to-
female ratio of nearly 4:1 is highly unusual even for
Bangkok, whose hospitals have generally averaged seven
females for one male procedure (5).

     By far, most referrals for female sterilization were
through PDA project staff (40 percent) followed by women
who were already predisposed to accept but simply needed
the guidance as to source of service (34 percent self-
referred). All other promotional channels were
insignificant for the women (Table 2).

     The men however, represent a broad range of referral
sources, from those who referred themselves to those who

Table 2. Percentage Referral Sources by
          Sterilization Type in Urban Areas.

| Referral Source | Sterilization Type | | Total |
	Vasectomy	Female Sterlization	
Self-Referred	21.3	34.2	24.0
Friend and Previous Acceptors	19.3	7.1	16.7
PDA Staff/Distributor	12.8	40.0	18.5
Government Official	3.6	6.7	4.2
Mass Media	16.0	0.2	12.7
Ad Van	14.0	0.4	11.2
Commercial Co./Factory	3.3	4.5	3.5
Others	9.1	6.0	8.5
No Answer	0.6	0.9	0.7
Total	100.0	100.0	100.0
	(2020)	(535)	(2555)

were referred by friends or acceptors, the mass media,
ad van, project staff and other sources. These findings
have clear implications for optimizing sterilization
promotion budgets. Women, already easily predisposed to
new acceptance, require the least expenditures. Some
staff outreach is significant but the emphasis should be
on announcements of source and time of service. The men
on the other hand, emerge from a variety of motivational
dispositions that respond to different kinds of promotion. Eliminating any one of these motivational channels
might cause a significant reduction in the number of
acceptors.

The Rural Component.

     PDA village agents and their district supervisors
joined in a case recruitment effort that helped produce an
average of over 20 vasectomy acceptors per operating day
in the nine months of mobile visits. A total of a remarkable 4481 cases of vasectomy were recruited, mostly in
the North followed by the North-east and Central Regions.
However, the overall number of acceptors in the rural program for only 5 days of services in each target district
is comparable to or has exceeded the total government's
statistics in the same operational area in either the year
1979 or 1980 (Table 3).

Table 3.   Vasectomy Acceptors by Region.*

Region	No. of Districts	No. of Acceptors CBVSP 5 Days	Annual Government Vasectomy Acceptors		
			1978	1979	1980
North	15	2202	1221	1193	1022
Central	12	960	1449	775	874
Northeast	21	1319	2602	1647	1314
TOTAL	48	4481	5332	3615	3210

*A comparison of 5 days of services in each of the 48 districts (August 1980 - March 1981) of the Community-Based Voluntary Sterilization Project (CBVSP) with the Annual Government Statistics.

Finally, referral success for vasectomy bus acceptors is largely dependent on PDA village distrbutors in all three regions where approximately 40 percent of acceptors were motivated by these community agents (Table 4). Government health centers play as important a role in referral only in the Central region while local administrative officials, the project's ad van, and self-referral are secondary sources in the North and Northeast.

DISCUSSION

The Community-Based Voluntary Sterilization Project (CBVSP) implemented by the Population and Community Development Association (PDA) was designed to meet the need for voluntary sterilization in both rural and Bangkok urban areas and to supplement the activities of the government's mobile voluntary sterilization project by deploying mobile teams to those districts that are not presently being adequately served by the government teams. This was accomplished by tapping into CBVFPS's already established infrastructure in 48 of 158 operational districts. With extensive motivation programs and effective service delivery system of the mobile teams and stationary clinics, the project has recruited a good number of sterilization acceptors. In 1980, the National Family Planning Program (NFPP) recruited 31,105 new acceptors of vasectomy (which includes that portion of the PDA total performed during the calendar year).

Table 4. Referral Sources of Vasectomy Acceptors in
Percent by Region

Referral Source	% of Acceptors by Region			
	North	Central	North-east	Average
Distributors	43.0	38.1	42.7	41.9
Gov't Health Center	17.8	35.1	17.1	21.3
Govt Official	10.2	2.7	12.8	9.4
PDA Staff	3.8	3,3	5,9	4.3
Ad Van	10.0	5.9	3.6	7.3
Mass Media	6.9	11.6	0.8	6.1
Friend/Previous Acceptor	4.4	0.6	2.8	3.1
Self Referred	1.6	2.2	13.6	5.2
Other	2.0	0.4	0.2	1.1
No Answer	0.3	—	0.5	0.3
TOTAL	100.0	100.0	100.0	100.0
	(2202)	(960)	(1319)	(4481)

The combined PDA total over nine months of 4481
rural procedures and 2020 urban procedures (or 6501 cases)
re- presents an astounding 21 percent of the 1980 national
total. Clearly, this potential contribution to acceptance
of the most cost-effective of contraceptive methods cannot
be ignored.

Despite the traditional male resistance to sterilization, it is notable that the acceptors of vasectomy in
the urban program outnumber the female acceptors by 4:1.
This is in contrast to the general figure of the national
program where female to male ratio is 5:1.

In previous years, Bangkok has traditionally contributed approximately 15 percent to the NFPP achievement
of sterilization recruitment. In nine months, two clinics
and a vasectomy bus have contributed 10 percent to this
Bangkok sub-total. Over the coming five-year plan period,
the equivalent of this project's urban efforts would generate 17,033 acceptors or roughly 2 percent of the
projected national requirement (6). With over 800 NFPP
sterilization service outlets, the PDA project's three
urban outlets would seem to have the potential to contribute a disproportionately large amount to this total.
Demonstration to the potential acceptors of the easy,
trouble-free and relatively painless vasectomy procedure

plus prompt and effective service by qualified physicians in this projects has been one of the most effective motivational strategies of the male acceptors.

In rural areas, the number of vasectomy acceptors recruited by CBVSP during 5 days of services in each rural district is significantly higher in most cases than the annual record of that district, especially in 1979 and 1980. This confirms the effectiveness of the mobile service in the rural areas.

The demographic and new family planning acceptor requirements of the next two five-year plan periods make it not a question of whether large numbers of couple can be recruited. Disregarding the traditional caveats of male resistance to vasectomy and saturation of contraceptive services in Bangkok, the PDA has shown that widespread and demographically significant acceptance of sterilization is within the grasp of any outreach program. Different media and promotional approaches were used according to the social setting and some would appear on the surface to be more cost-effective than others in Bangkok. For the rural sector, reliance on the existing network of distributors and local health and administrative personnel is more than adequate to generate enough acceptance to justify the cost of operating the mobile unit.

In this project, a centrally controlled mobile vasectomy service strategy, i.e., deploying the mobile vans from the Bangkok central office to the target area was employed. The organization and management of the mobile team are under the direct responsibility of the Bangkok headquarter. Cooperation with local health officials is arranged prior to the visit of the mobile team. With the same personnel moving from one district to another, the vasectomy services given are relatively uniform as far as the quality of service and result of the operation are concerned. Revisit to the target area can be made at appropriate times. Campaign efforts for motivation usually result in greater numbers of acceptor recruited in shorter periods of time.

According to one study (7), operating the mobile service delivery in the manner described above is the most cost-effective of all other programs in Thailand. Mobile tubal ligation service can be arranged in similar fashion but it is difficult to justify providing such service at primary health care level in the presence of a much more cost effective and more convenient procedure for vasectomy.

While speakers at a recent regional seminar on "Expansion of Sterilization Service" in Thailand repeatedly complained of traditional male resistance to vasectomy, this project has shown that men do indeed accept the service if the providers go a bit out of their way.

CONCLUSION

Voluntary Surgical Contraception may not be adequately and conveniently provided by the personnel at the pimary health care level because of shortage and maldistribution of medical manpower in most developing countries. However, mobile vasectomy service is possible and is an appropriate approach to solving this problem. Deploying a mobile team from a center to provide periodic services to one target area for about one week before moving to another is much more effective than distributing the equipment and personnel throughout the country. By providing orientation and some training for local family planning volunteers a few weeks prior to the visit of the mobile service team, recruitment of vasectomy acceptors can be carried out without too many difficulties.

The success of the mobile service depends on good management and local cooperation. Intensive motivation efforts aimed at potential clients by local village family planning volunteers greatly increases acceptance. The Community-Based Voluntary Sterilization Project in Thailand has demonstrated this approach to be appropriate and highly effective.

REFERENCES

1.   McDaniel EB (1978): The use of operating theatre nurses as surgeons in the performance of minilaparotomy female interval sterilization, compared to the performance of the same operation by a physician-surgeon. A pilot study paper presented at the Joint IGCC/IPPF Workshop on the Policies and Programmes for the Utilization of Non-Physicians in the Delivery of Family Planning Services, Thailand, December 13-15.
2.   Chowdhury S and Chowdhury Z (1975): Tubectomy by paraprofessional surgeons in rural Bangladesh. Lancet 567-69.
3.   Foreit RJ, et al (1978): Community-based and commercial contraceptive distribution: An inventory and appraisal. In: Population Report

Family Planning Programmes, Series J, No. 19.
4.   Viravaidya M (1980): Non physician in family
     planning and family health in Thailand. In:
     Proceedings of a conference - The Nonphysician
     and Family Health in Sub-Sahara Africa,
     Pathfinder Fund, Boston.
5.   Ministry of Public Health (1980): Monthly report,
     National Family Planning Programme 1976-1980.
     Thailand.
6.   National Social Economic Development Board (1982):
     National 5th Five-year Plan (1982-1986).
     Thailand.
7.   Bennet T: Personal communication.

PROSPECTS FOR A FUTURE FAMILY PLANNING PROGRAM-

WHAT CONTRACEPTIVE TECHNIQUES ARE FEASIBLE AT THE

PRIMARY HEALTH CARE LEVEL AND WHO SHOULD APPLY THEM:

BARRIER METHODS

H. Furuya

Professor of Obstetrics and Gynecology
Juntendo University School of Medicine
Tokyo, Japan

INTRODUCTION

As one aspect of national health policy, it was
decided to popularize family planning among the Japanese
people in 1952. This policy was adapted soon after the
end of the Second World War at a time when the nation was
attempting to overcome postwar chaos and poverty.
However, this movement actually got underway in 1955,
therefore maternal health conditions had become worse.
Table 1 shows a comparison between the 1952 and 1979
statistics. The figures in 1952 on birth rate, death rate
and maternal death rate are high compared to more recent
rates.

Since contraceptive techniques had not become popular
in Japan at that time, some women who did not want to bear
children had no choice but to undergo induced abortions;
this was their only way to achieve birth control. These
abortions were performed by licensed doctors in accordance
with the law. Table 2 shows the numbers of induced abortions according to statistics of the Ministry of Health
and Welfare. There is a reduction in the number of
induced abortions (for all ages) from 50.3 per 1000 women
population in 1955 to 19.6 in 1980. The government was
aware of these conditions and wanted to minimize the
number of induced abortions to protect the health of both

Table 1.   Summary of Vital Statistics in Japan

Vital Statistics (per 1000 population)	1952	1979
Live Birth Rates	23.4	14.2
Death Rates	8.9	6.0
National Increase Rate	14.4	8.3
Infant Mortality Rate	49.4	7.9
Maternal Death Rate (per 10,000 live births)	17.0	2.2

Table 2.   Induced Abortions by Age of Women (1955-1980)
(Rates per 1000 women population)

Age in Years	less than 20	20 to 24	25 to 29	30 to 34	35 to 39	40 to 44	45 to 49	Total
1955	3.4	43.1	80.8	95.1	80.5	41.8	5.8	50.3
1975	3.1	24.7	34.3	38.3	29.2	13.9	1.5	22.1
1980	4.8	23.3	29.3	33.1	26.7	12.0	1.3	19.6

the mother and child. It was decided that the concept of family planning and the basic methods of contraception had to be disseminated among the public as an alternative to abortion.

FAMILY PLANNING WORKER SYSTEM AND CONTRACEPTIVE METHODS

As part of the health policy, the Japanese government decided to enact a law to establish the family planning worker (FPW) system. This law alloted government funds to cover the costs of training the FPW, of teaching materials required to instruct and guide the public concerning family planning, of contraceptives and their distribution throughout the country.

The first qualification to become an FPW is to have a license as a midwife, a public health nurse, or a clinical nurse. Persons with these qualifications are trained in accordance with the specified curriculum; the period of training is 33 hours for midwives and 63 hours for public health and clinical nurses. The government provides persons who had been trained by

Table 3.   Percentage of Live Births by Hospital Staff
            and Midwives (Urban and Rural, 1950-1979.

Birth Attendants	1959	1960	1970	1979
Hospital Staff				
Total	4.6	50.1	96.1	99.4
Urban	11.3	63.6	97.6	99.6
Rural	1.1	27.0	91.2	98.9
Midwife				
Total	90.1	56.1	15.0	5.6
Urban	88.8	46.9	11.9	4.7
Rural	90.8	71.9	24.9	8.5

this curriculum with an FPW certificate.

The FPW and other paramedical personnel are active in spreading family planning throughout Japan. In addition to their routine work, this group establishs family planning programs which gradually started to achieve important results. In 1950, many midwives who were involved in maternal care and care of the newborn babies practiced everywhere in Japan under their own responsibility. They were licensed midwives who underwent a specified education and practical training and passed a government examination. These women formed close personal relations and strong bonds of trust with the local people, especially mothers. This was so because up to about 30 years ago, most of the births in Japan were undertaken with the aid of local midwives; very few were performed in hospitals or by physicians (Table 3). Under the conditions prevailing at the time, the occupation of midwife was usually passed from one generation to the next in a family. There were many cases where both mother and daughters used the same midwife. Therefore, the midwives knew local families intimately and were often popular and trusted.

In 1955, the contraceptive methods officially permitted by the government included condoms, diaphragms, intravaginal tablets and jellies, and the rhythm method. The use of contraceptive materials such as rings and IUDs were not approved; the pill had not been developed. The IUD was not approved until after 1974. The role of instructing the Japanese people concerning contraceptive techniques naturally fell more to the FPW than to the physicians.

Table 4.   Percentage of Use of Contraceptive Methods
            and Materials in Japan (1959 and 1979).*

Year	Con-dom	Diaph-ragm	Tab-let	Jelly	Rhythm	With-drawal	IUD	Pill	Sterili-zation
1950	35.6	7.8	_	15.4	27.4	12.7	_	_	_
1979	81.1	1.1	2.3	5.2	23.1	1.9	8.3	3.2	4.0

*Using the Multiple Answer Method.

Among these four types of contraceptives, condoms
were used by 35.6 percent of the people surveyed in 1950
and 81.1 percent in 1979. They are by far the most
popular type of contraceptives and continue to be so at
present. The rates of use of diaphragms, tablets and
jellies are much lower than that for condoms and these
rates have been reduced recently (Table 4). The Ogino
rhythm method is used but mostly together with condoms.
The rate of use in 1979 was 23.1 percent, which is the
next highest rate after that of condoms alone. However,
for ordinary women, it is difficult to understand Ogino's
method and its correct application so that if this method
is used alone, it has the great disadvantage of unsuccessful contraception resulting in pregnancy. This appears to
be one of the reasons why this method is not widely used.

There are many reasons why condoms are still used at
a high rate in Japan, but the major reason is because the
FPW distributed condoms to each family at the time when
contraception was first popularized in Japan. The FPW
would assemble the housewives living in their region and
form groups. The contraceptives would then be supplied to
each family through the leader of the group. The main
contraceptive distributed in this way were condoms. This
distribution method was highly effective and contraception, using condoms, rapidly spread throughout Japan. At
present, condoms are not only distributed by FPW but are
also sold by many local pharmacies and supermarkets. They
can also be purchased from sales people who visit each
household.

Contraception using condoms is the traditional method
and is known to have a higher rate of failure than methods
using the pill or IUD. The rates for the pill and IUD in
1979 was 3.2 percent and 8.3 percent respectively.
Therefore, condoms can not be said to be the best method
of contraception. However, the use of the pill and the

Table 5.   Reasons for Contraception in Japan (1975).*

Reasons	Percentage
1. Preserve maternal health	46.2
2. Restrict number of children in order to give better education	41.9
3. Difficult living due to small income	17.5
4. Enjoy pleasant life	13.7
5. Other reasons, or no answer	12.7
6. Follow what others are doing	4.9
7. Dislike for children	2.8
8. Lessen division of property in the family	0.9
9. Prevent hereditary disease	0.9

*(Survey Result wherein two reasons were selected)

IUD requires a visit to a doctor's clinic; the use of such methods will probably increase gradually in Japan.

CONCLUSION

According to the statistics of the Ministry of Health and Welfare, induced abortions reached a peak in 1955, but with the spread of contraceptive techniques, the number of live births dropped drastically and significant changes were found in the rate of birth order. This situation caused a sharp decrease in family size.

Since births are almost always now performed by doctors or in hospitals, there has been a sharp decrease in the number of midwives: 55,356 in 1955 to 26,493 in 1978, or a total decrease of 34,863. Most of the midwives who practise independently have become quite old. Almost all of the midwives now work in doctor's clinics, hospitals, maternity clinics or other medical facilities. This suggests that changes are underway to improve maternal health care, which used to be undertaken by midwives working closely with each local family, to meet the new needs of families in the futures. Table 5 shows a recent statistics on the main reasons for contraception of couples. Majority of the couples practise contraception mainly to preserve maternal health and give better education to children if the number of children was restricted. From these results, we can make a fairly good guess at the recent direction of family planning in Japan.

REFERENCES

(Available by correspondence with H. Furuya)

REVERSIBLE METHODS OF FIMBRIAL ENCLOSURE

L. E. Laufe

Medical Director
International Fertility Research Program
Research Triangle Park, North Carolina, U.S.A.

INTRODUCTION

In December of 1977, the Program for Applied Research on Fertility Regulation (PARFR), held a workshop in San Francisco on the reversal of sterilization. Included in the program was a section of new potentially reversible techniques for sterilization of women. Included were presentations on tubal plugs placed either in the ostia, hysteroscopically (1), or through the fimbria at laparotomy (2). Droegemueller outlined his approach of placing the tubal fimbria in teflon stockings, and then burying them inside the broad ligament by a modified Aldridge procedure (3). The author reviewed and presented the concept of a fimbrial enclosure or fimbrial cap which could provide a reversible technique of female sterilization via minilaparotomy (4). The application of this approach to the developing country setting was emphasized.

One of the most interesting presentations at this seminar was the report of El Kady et al (5), who had performed the procedure in 35 women, using hoods made from the middle fingers of disposable medical gloves and tying them in place with a No. 0 black silk purse string suture. At the time of the workshop, no woman had requested reversal as yet. The authors commented that "Reversibility will not only increase the acceptability of sterilization in a population that includes more than 700 million Moslems - persons with a strong bias against sterilization - but it will also offer a most welcome advantage to people worldwide".

The potentially high acceptability of a reversible technique has been confirmed by Shain in a study of Texas women (6). Perhaps most impressive is the November 1979 State Department cable from New Delhi which reports the government of India's request for collaborative research programs (7). Included in the priority list of four areas of assistance is a request for a reversible method of female sterilization.

HISTORY

As reported in 1977, the concept of using a fimbrial hood was tested on five rabbits at Battelle, Columbus in 1971 at the suggestion of John Marco (8). Although the reversibility of this technique was demonstrated, little enthusiasm was expressed as the medical community pursued improved technologies of permanent sterilization to meet the worldwide demand. The critical role of the laparoscope in providing these services and attracting both physicians and patients to sterilization programs cannot be denied. By the mid-1970s the advantages of minilap to meet the rural needs were becoming apparent and many nations with limited medical resources adopted complete minilap programs. During these years of attempting to train personnel and establish service programs, numerous requests for a reversible technique were made from the field, and the concept of a fimbrial enclosure applied and removed by minilap was pursued. Despite anecdotal reports of adhesions, failure and disappointments, there was nothing in the literature by the critics.

The availability of better materials, fabrication techniques, device preparation, and fixation made the development of the fimbrial enclosure a reality. The preliminary work was performed at the University of Leuven in cooperation with the International Fertility Research Program (IRFP). Original attempts to develop the technique in rabbits included a variety of empirically developed devices and fixation techniques which gave proper direction to a delivery and surgical technique and the development of candidate devices. Three years ago, with a pilot project grant from PARFR, the research activity began.

RABBIT STUDIES

White New Zealand rabbits, five months of age and not of proven fertility, were used. The animals were

obtained from the official Belgian breeding station at the
University of Ghent. Animals were quarantined for one
month prior to surgery. Candidate materials chosen were
silastic and PTFE (commercial Gorotex, a teflon polymer
employed by Droegemueller in his studies).

The original silastic prostheses were designed empirically and proved to be too large. Accurate in vivo
dimensions were obtained and appropriate sized devices
were fabricated as follows: Teflon mandrels of appropriate dimensions were made. These were dipped into liquid
medical-grade silastic and dried. The devices were then
cured at 200 degrees centigrade for 45 minutes. The
devices were removed from the mandrels by soaking them in
tetrohydrofuran and redrying them in the inflated position
which allowed them to shrink to their original sizes. After drying they were placed in ethyl alcohol for shipping.

Two silastic devices were developed - one 0.002
inches thick and another 0.006 inches thick, depending on
the number of times the mandrel was dipped. The former
devices were pliable and the latter were rigid. Both were
semipermeable. A third device was made of the teflon
material; this material, due to its thinness, proved to
be difficult to work with and could not be made into the
specific sizes of the silastic ones. The teflon devices
were larger than the silastic hoods.

A special telescoping, double-barreled forceps was
developed for the implantation of the devices. The design
is similar to that used for delivery of the Falope ring.
The neck of the device was stretched over the inner barrel, then the device was inverted into the barrel. It was
placed over the fimbria by flushing or sucking the fimbria
into the devices and then pushing the collar over the
distal tube. The devices were soaked in 0.02 percent
chlorohexidine for ten minutes prior to placement.

A variety of fixation techniques using interrupted,
inert 11-0 sutures were tried. Due to the necessity of
dissecting the mesotubarium of each tube, the first animals were done with only two sutures per cap per side. As
experience grew and this technique proved unsatisfactory
for holding the devices in place, a 6-suture technique was
employed and finally a continuous suture technique was
evaluated. All surgical procedures were carried out under
the operating microscope using a magnification of anywhere
from 5 to 20 power.

Four animals had teflon devices placed bilaterally.

The neck of these devices had been reinforced with liquid
silastic, which proved to be too rigid and made anchoring
difficult. The devices, due to their size, had a tendency
to collapse with folds which invited excessive peritoneal
overgrowth. Six devices remained in place, but all pro-
voked adhesions. Further experiments with these devices
were abandoned.

The rigid 0.006 inch devices proved to be too heavy.
They were difficult to anchor and the few that were placed
became detached almost immediately after placement and
dropped into the pelvis. This was confirmed by repeated
laparoscopic examinations. The thin silastic 0.002 inch
devices proved to be the most rewarding to work with.
Thirty-three enclosures were placed in 17 rabbits using a
2-stitch technique. One animal was used for morphologic
studies, using the uncapped horn as a control. Only six
caps remained in place in six different animals. One cap
remained in situ eight months, four for ten months and
one for twelve months. These animals periodically underwent laparoscopy and for these six devices there was no
infection or indications of hydrosalpinx or adhesions.

In this group, 27 caps became detached from the
fimbria. All these events occurred within two months by
laparoscopic examination. Twenty-four detachments were
complete, and three were partial, allowing at least 50
percent of the fimbria to be freed from the prosthesis.
These observations led to the conclusion that two sutures
were inadequate for fixation. The active motility of the
tube and mesotubarium where the sutures were placed
afforded easy opportunity for detachment. One tube in
this group did develop infection as evidenced by mild
adhesions of the fimbria to the meso and ovary.

Twenty thin enclosures were placed in ten rabbits
using a 6-stitch technique for fixation. Seven rabbits
were challenged for pregnancy but only two ovulated. In
these two animals, three caps were in place. In the unprotected horn there were two implants, and that ovary had
four corpora lutea. For the three caps which remained in
place, each had two challenges for pregnancy at six week
intervals. On the first challenge there were six corpora
lutea in two ovaries and three in the other. On the
second challenge, there were five corpora lutea in two
ovaries and three in the other. In this limited group,
where the enclosures remained in place and ovulation was
confirmed, there were no pregnancies. Five additional
rabbits have recently had enclosures placed using a
continuous suture technique of 10-0 nylon. One device

became detached. In the other four rabbits fixation was successful and after removal of the enclosures at three months, six of the eight uterine horns had implants for a reversal rate of 75 percent. The other animal did not ovulate but tubal morphology was normal.

Histologic Changes

Scanning electron microscopy (SEM) on biopsies were obtained at different intervals from the animals whose caps became detached and from the six tubes where they remained in situ. Multiple biopsies through eight months of cap placement and examination under various magnifications revealed no fimbrial damage to either the secretory or ciliated cells. Two SEM photos from the rabbit used for a control at 2100 magnification taken at 6-1/2 months reveal no difference in the fimbria biopsied from the control and the cap sides. Additional SEM studies at 3-1/2 through 12 months following prosthesis placement confirm that the 0.002 inch silastic hood can remain in situ for long periods without provoking morphologic alterations.

Rabbit Results

The results of these studies can be summarized. A biocompatible device has been developed for the rabbits. A simple instrumental delivery system of placing the cap over the fimbria appears to be applicable to humans. Fixation techniques of the cap to the tube must be improved. When displacement occurs, it is usually early, occurring within the first two months following cap place- ment. The devices become covered with a thin layer of peritoneum and usually a single mesentery-carrying blood supply develops. The devices were easily removed by a circular incision over their neck and transecting the mesentery. The fimbria are not adherent to the interior of the hood. Extensive SEM studies up through one year of placement revealed no damage to the epithelium of the fim- bria. With this information at hand and again under the sponsorship of PARFR, a primate study was initiated at the University of Texas at San Antonio with Dr. Carlton Eddy employing the 0.002 inch device.

PRIMATE STUDIES

Studies with the nonhuman primate have been under- taken to further define and validate the effectiveness and reversibility of fimbrial enclosures as a female steril- ization technique in a species more closely related

anatomically, physiologically and endocrinologically to
the human. Two types of experiments are underway, one to
determine fertility effects and one to document device-
induced changes in fimbrial morphology.

Twenty female Rhesus monkeys were fitted bilaterally
with silastic fimbrial enclosures. The devices remained
in place for nine months. The animals were bred to males
of proven fertility during the periovulatory period of
each endocrinologically documented ovulatory menstrual
cycle. At the end of nine months the devices were
removed.

A second group of five animals were used to monitor
the effects of the devices on tubal morphology. The induction of pelvic adhesions, hyrosalpinx and anovulation
were monitored laparoscopically at weekly intervals. Fimbrial biopsy was performed following removal of individual
devices at monthly intervals from one to nine months post
placement. Biopsy specimens were examined by light and
scanning electron microscopy for changes in the fimbrial
mucosa. To date there are no morphologic alterations in
the fimbria.

Placement of Devices

The fimbrial-ovarian relationship of the Rhesus monkey was determined in order to define how best to fit and
anchor the devices with minimal disruption of normal anatomy. In the Rhesus, the oviduct is relatively straight
with the ampulla forming a loop at its anterior end. The
tubal infundibulum is funnel shaped and terminates in a
well-developed fimbria of roughly lenticular shape with a
centrally located ostium. Medially, the fimbria is continuous with, and supported by, the mesotubarium superious.
Laterally, the fimbria is directly attached to the upper
pole of the ovary via the fimbria ovarica. Measurement of
fimbriae performed in vivo and using excised tracts
indicated the necessity to fabricate devices in a range of
sizes to accomodate normal variation between subjects.
The mesotubarium superious was severed adjacent to the
fimbria following hemostatic bipolar microcauterization.
Mobilization of the fimbria was completed by similarly
severing the fimbria ovarica. A fimbrial cap of proper
dimension was then fitted. Several anchoring sutures of
9-0 monofilament were placed around the perimeter of the
device. Exposed fimbrial folds were gently pushed into
the device and anchored in place with additional sutures.
This process was repeated until the entire fimbria was
encapsulated. Each device was anchored around its entire

perimeter with six to eight interrupted sutures. The
thickness of approximately one millimeter of the device
was included to prevent the suture from tearing through.
Similarly, sutures were anchored where possible to the
mesosalpinx and the base of the ovary through the ovarian
cortex for greatest strength. Other sutures were placed
in the tubal mesenteris.

Fertility Studies

Monkeys were housed individually and checked daily
for vaginal bleeding in order to determine menstrual
cyclicity. Blood samples were drawn daily by femoral
puncture from Day 8 and assayed for total plasma estrogen.
Following detection of the pre-ovulatory estrogen peak,
the female was placed with a male of proven fertility for
72 hours for breeding. The occurrence of pregnancy was
determined by monitoring peripheral plasma progesterone at
weekly intervals and urinary macaque chorionic gonodo-
tropin on Days 19 to 22 postmating. Animals were mated
during all ovulatory menstrual cycles during the initial
nine-month period of the study. At the end of nine
months, animals underwent a second laparotomy and the
fimbrial devices were removed. The animals with devices
successfully fixed underwent a second nime-month period of
mating without devices. A total of 90 matings has been
accomplished. Twelve subjects became pregnant within six
months after fimbrial enclosures. Diagnostic laparo-
scopies were performed and revealed displacement of the
devices in each of these animals. One animal died due to
chronic nephritis confirmed by a veterinary pathologist.
It was the pathologist's finding that this condition was
pre-existent, chronic, and did not result from an ascending infections induced by placement of the fimbrial
devices.

Morphology Studies

Morphologic studies are underway. The initial
devices fitted were found to have a high detachment rate
despite placement of six to eight interrupted 9-0 monofilament nylon sutures at regular intervals along the entire
circumference of the device's base. Detachment invariably
occurred within two months of placement and appeared to be
the result of at least two mechanisms: inclusions within
each suture of insufficient tissue to properly anchor the
device , and tying the suture too tightly, resulting in
necrotizing tissue, ischemia, slough and subsequent loss
of anchorage. Due to the need of replacing animals in
which devices spontaneously dislodged, no fimbrial biop-

sies have been examined as of yet. The silastic material
used to fabricate the devices has shown remarkable inert-
ness and freedom from tissue reactivity. The presence of
fimbrial caps does not appear at this time to produce
extensive adhesions. Adhesions, when present, have been
minor and tend to form a band around the base of the
device or, less frequently, a peritoneal covering.

Based on weekly laparoscopic observation following
placement of devices, a well-defined pattern of healing
may be described. During the first several weeks, the
tissue to which the base of the device is sutured is
transformed into a band of tissue undergoing adjustment
either to the mechanical presence of the device, if
sutures are well-placed and tied, or undergoing necrotic
changes if excessive tightness produced ischemia. In the
former case, this band of tissue appears to form a cuff
and remains otherwise intact. In the latter case, extensive healing and remodelling occurs following sloughing.
At this time, adhesions may begin to form between the raw
area at the base of the device and any adjacent areas
which are deperitonized, either by the dissection required
to free the fimbria from its ovarian and uterine connec-
tions prior to placement of the device, or through
iatrogenically-induced abrasions of abdominal or pelvic
viscera. Adhesions, if and when they form, appear to be
restricted to this area, leaving the bulk of the device
free of adhesions. With increasing time, adhesions become
better organized but generally remain string-like. If
sloughing of tissue is extensive, anchorage of the device
is compromised. The formation of adhesions may place the
device under tension, leading to further compromise and
eventual displacement, either partial or complete. By two
months postplacement, devices are either displaced or in
position with an apparently steady state reached. Presence of devices has in no way compromised menstrual
cyclicity or the occurrence of ovulation. Furthermore, in
no case have adhesions been observed to form between the
device or the ovulatory stigma or corpus hemorrhagicum.
One tube has been observed to develop a mild hydrosalpinx
which first became evident three weeks postplacement. In
the ensuing two months it did not worsen nor regress. The
ampulla is approximately 30 percent larger in diameter.
The device has remained adhesion-free.

DISCUSSION

The concept of using fimbrial enclosure as a means
of reversible female sterilization is based upon preven-

tion of ovum pick-up and interaction between the male and female gametes. Implicit is the requirement that such a device be easy to attach to the fimbria, remain in place throughout the desired period of sterilization, demonstrate marked efficacy in preventing pregnancy, and be reversible.

Ease of Attachment

Access to the fimbria in both rabbits and monkeys in the present studies has been obtained via laparotomy and has not presented any difficulty. In view of the fact that minilaparotomy and colpotomy are widely used clinically for tubal sterilization by fimbriectomy or tubal interruption, these approaches would obviate the need for laparotomy and would thus make sterilization by fimbrial enclosure suitable as an outpatient technique. In both the rabbit and monkey, the fimbria are supported by two mesenteries, the fimbria ovarica and the mesotubarium superious. Placement of the device requires transection of both mesenteries in order to mobilize the fimbria. Since the latter mesentery is absent in women, the placement technique is simplified. Because of the relatively small size of the internal genitalia of the rabbit and monkey and the preliminary nature of both studies, an operating microscope together with micro-suture has been used to attach fimbrial caps. Because of the greater size of the human ovary and fimbria, a microscopic technique using relatively large, inert sutures would probably be suitable clinically.

Retention of Devices

Premature detachment of devices has been experienced in both studies. Improved fixation will, therefore, have to be evolved prior to clinical use. At this time it appears from both studies that detachment is the result of insufficient numbers of sutures to anchor the device. It would appear that sufficient sutures consistent with avoiding devitilization of tissue will assure permanent retention of devices.

Efficacy

When retained, fimbrial enclosures appear to be highly successful in preventing pregnancy. Although efficacy studies are only half complete in the primate, results to date are highly promising. Animals continue to experience normal menstrual cycles, the majority of which appear to be ovulatory. The pregnancies that have occurred were clearly the result of fimbrial enclosure detachment.

Reversibility

Reversibility, or more accurately, its potential, is of major clinical importance since this aspect of the sterilization technique will have great recruitment value among women in the developing world, particularly those with Moslem populations.

In the rabbits, removal of devices has proved simple since the fimbriae do not adhere to the interior of the device and the devices themselves tend to form adhesions. The peritoneal envelope that forms around devices in this species is easily removed by incising it and severing the cord-like vascular mesentery.

In the primate, fimbrial devices appear to be essentially devoid of reactivity. Adhesions, when present, are invariably thin and involve only the base of the device and adjacent tubal and ovarian tissue. Peritonealization of devices has not been a consistent observation. In the limited experience to date, removal of the devices has essentially entailed cutting each individual suture and removing the device. The importance of reattaching the severed fimbrial mesenteries, particularly the fimbria ovarica, does not appear to be necessary since the pregnancies that have occurred were established without surgical restoration of the normal fimbrial/ovarian anatomy. We are therefore encouraged to anticipate reversibility of the device-induced sterilization with removal of devices and little, if no, restorative surgery.

CONCLUSION

The silastic fimbrial devices being used appear to elicit no foreign body reaction in either species, nor do they create excessive adhesions. In the primate, by whatever mechanism, fimbrial enclosure appears to be effective. Currently, we are investigating the continuous suture technique for fixation in the primate and exploring the use of surgical staples in rabbits. Once a standard technique of fixation is developed, human trials are planned both in the United States and internationally.

REFERENCES

1. Hosseinian AH, Lucero S, Zaneveld LJD (1978):
    Hystero- scopically delivered tubal lugs. In:
    Reversal of Sterilization, Sciarra JJ, Zatuchni
    GI, Speidel JJ
    (eds), Harper & Row, Hagerstown, Maryland, pp.
    220-223.
2. Meeker DI (1978): A tubal occlusive device in mon-
    keys. In: Reversal of Sterilization, Sciarra
    JJ, Zatuchni GI, Speidel JJ (eds), Harper & Row,
    Hagerstown,Maryland, pp. 226-231.
3. Droegemueller W, Chvapil M, Christian CD (1978):
    Modern modified Aldridge procedure. In: Reversal
    of Sterilization, Sciarra JJ, Zatuchni GI, Speidel
    JJ (eds), Harper & Row, Hagerstown, Maryland, pp.
    224-225.
4. Laufe LE (1978): The fimbrial prosthesis. In: Re-
    versal of Sterilization, Sciarra JJ, Zatuchni GI,
    Speidel JJ (eds), Harper & Row, pp. 220-223.
5. El Kady AA, Sami G, Laurence KA, Badawi S (1978): The
    tubal hood: a potentially reversible sterilization
    technique. In: Reversal of Sterilization,
    Sciarra JJ, Zatuchni GI, Speidel JJ (eds), Harper &
    Row, Hagerstown, Maryland, pp. 232-240.
6. Shain R (1979): Acceptability of reversible versus
    permanent tubal sterilization. An analysis of
    preliminary data. Fetility & Sterility, 31:13.
7. Department of State Cable (1979): No. R291209Z,
    November.
8. Laufe FE, Hassler C, Lower BR (1972): A laboratory
    prototype for reversible female sterilization. In:
    Female Sterilization. Prognosis for Simplified
    Outpatient Procedures., GW Duncan, RD Falb, JJ
    Speidel, editors. Academic Press, New York, 65-71.

ACKNOWLEDGEMENT

Presented in part at the PARFR International Workshop in
Mexico City, February 1980 by Leonard E. Laufe, Carlton
Eddy, Ivo Brosens and Willy Boeckx.

PREVENTION AND CURE OF PREVALENT INFECTIONS

IN THE MOTHER AND THE NEWBORN

W. H. Foege

Assistant Surgeon General
Director, Center for Disease Control
Department of Health and Human Services,
Atlanta, Georgia, U. S. A.

INTRODUCTION

In the global village of the late 20th century, there is no problem we share with more conviction, no priority more universally accepted, than the health and future of the world's children. For therein lies the health and the future of civilization. We are fortunate in one way. Problems in this area have been reasonably well defined, and their preventability is well established. It is a matter of applying what we know how to do, to what we know is wrong in the areas of maternal and child health in developed and developing nations of the world. It is a matter of emphasis on sanitation, availability of pure water and food, immunization, and health education.

Almost all the diseases killing children in developing nations today, are preventable and are often the same ones which killed children in the developed nations at the turn of the century. Life expectancy in India for example, estimated in 1970 to 75 to be 49.5 years (1), would bear out the relationship between high infant mortality rates, which result from those killer diseases, and lowered life expenctancy. The average U.S. citizen at the turn of the century had a life expectancy of 47 years and a death rate among children between 1 and 14 of 100 per 1000 live births.

Three topics will be considered in this paper:

(a)   The international scope of excessive, prevent-
       able infant and maternal morbidity and mortality;
(b)   The causes of infant and maternal morbidity and
       mortality in developing and developed nations; and
(c)   Successful interventions, previously applied, which
       offer solutions to problems we face.

SCOPE OF INFANT MORBIDITY AND MORTALITY

     Dr. Jacques Vallin (2), a research fellow with the
National Institute of Demographic Studies in Paris,
published an estimate of world trends in infant mortality
since 1950. Where possible, he used officially registered
mortality data. Otherwise, data was produced from surveys
and other observations as reliable as possible. In some
cases, he used UN estimates of life expectancy and the
Princeton mortality models to reach an estimate. Accord-
ding to Dr. Vallin's report, if infant mortality were to
be estimated for mankind as a whole, it would probably
stand at between 80 and 90 deaths per thousand. However,
a look at mortality by continents and regions gives a more
meaningful impression of the situation. In Africa, for
which the least reliable data are available, infant
mortality has been estimated at about 200 deaths per 1000
live births. Other rates range from 150 per 1000 in Me-
lanesia, to 95 per 1000 in tropical South America, and 65
per 1000 in China. As an example of current progress in
China, a recent study in Shanghai county showed infant
deaths to be 10 per thousand. Southern Europe has a rate
of 40 per 1000, the British Isles 18 per 1000, and the
Scandinavian countries and Japan at a rate close to 12 per
thousand. As a general guide, it has been estimated that
neonatal mortality rates in Africa and Asia are about 50
percent of the infant mortality rates (2).

Causes of Excessive Mortality in Developing Nations

     Infections and parasitic diseases play a major role,
with poor nutrition complicating many other contributing
factors. It has been estimated that up to 80 to 90 percent of infant mortality in developing nations (3) is
attributable to infections and parasitic diseases, though
that figure varies from country to country from one year
to the next. By contrast, countries with low infant
mortality, attribute most deaths to "perinatal mortality"
which accounts for between 50 and 60 percent of infant
deaths. This fact seems connected with the concentration
of deaths in the first few days after birth. In these
nations, the second group of causes is "congenital anomal-

ies" which become more apparent where mortality is very
low. This is followed by pneunmonia which accounts for a
lower proportion of deaths when mortality is low.

Neonatal tetanus is a major preventable cause of high
infant death rates in the developing nations. Studies in
Bangladesh and Indonesia have shown that up to 50 percent
of neonatal deaths can be attributed to tetanus - a figure
which translates into 5 percent of all births. In Haiti,
where a succession of prevention programs immunized all
women with tetanus toxoid, tetanus of the newborn disap-
peared as a public health problem between 1940 and 1970.
According to a study by W & G Berggren, frequency of death
from tetanus of the newborn diminished from 25 percent of
live births to none. Education, as well as vaccination,
may be the prescription of choice in this case. Following
age-old traditions, many in developing nations cut the
umbilical cord with bamboo or other easily accessible
instruments from nature, and thus introduce tetanus
spores. Simple instruction of mothers and midwives
about hygiene and handling of the umbilical cord with
aseptic instruments and bandaging could be effective in
lowering the rates of death from tetanus.

Malaria is another major cause of high unneccessary
morbidity and mortality among infants and pregnant women
in the developing nations. The child's under-developed
immune system, often complicated by his nutritional
status, makes him an easy target for the age-old scourge
of the tropics. It has been estimated that mortality in
the 6-months to 5-year age group reaches 10 percent from
malaria.

Pertussis, a relatively minor childhood disease in
the developed countries, has a case fatality rate of 65 to
70 percent in children less than 12 months of age in the
developing countries. Complications arise because pertussis is difficult to diagnose in small infants in whom the
characteristic cough is frequently absent. Whooping cough
can be the first step in a downward tract leading to
severe illness and death. Coughing followed by vomiting,
loss of appetite, and parents' unwillingness to feed a
child until vomiting has stopped, can increase the danger
from this disease.

Repeated attacks of diarrhea in developing countries
lead to malnutrition and growth retardation because of
associated food restrictions by the family, loss of
appetite and malabsorption. A 1975 study estimated 500
million episodes of diarrhea per year in children below

five years of age in Africa, Asia and Latin America.
These episodes led to an estimated 5 million deaths. The
peak incidence of these attacks is between 6 months and 2
years of age.

Measles, targeted for elimination in the United
States by October 1983, is another prominent killer of the
young in developing nations, where children over 9 months
are at the greatest risk. The case-fatality rate for
measles in these countries is estimated at between 3 and 7
percent. When complicated by diarrhea, pneumonia, blindness and loss of weight, measles is a dread visitor to
families of the developing world.

Low birth weight, no matter where a child is born -
be it in a developed or developing nation - will be an
important determing factor in his or her fate. It has
been estimated that infants who weigh less than 2500
grams, or 5-1/2 pounds, account for 54.3 percent of stillbirths and 52.6 percent of neonatal deaths (4). Low birth
weight children have an infant mortality rate 20 times
greater than other babies. Low birth weight increases a
child's chances of growth and developmental problems as
well as increasing his chances of death.

In the developing nations, highly prevalent infectious diseases of the mother occupy a prominent place as
cause of low-birth weight and infant death. A 1975 study
of infections in pregnant women in a developing country
(5) showed a high incidence of malaria, respiratory infection, diarrhea and dysentery, urinary tract infections and
similar conditions. Other illnesses in pregnant women,
including conjunctivitis, otitis media, stomatitis, and
skin infections, affected developing fetuses. Vaginal
infections of many kinds were also responsible for low
birth weight babies. A recent National Institute of
Allergy and Infectious Diseases study group reported that
if primary and secondary syphilis is untreated during
pregnancy, half of the infants will be stillborn, premature, or will suffer neonatal death while the other half
will develop congenital syphilis. The significance of
this risk is confirmed by a recent study in an African
country in which higher RPR titers were nine times
greater for mothers of stillborn infants than for mothers
of live-born infants.

In developed nations, other maternal factors such as
lack of prenatal care, poor nutrition, smoking, alcohol
and drug abuse, age (especially youth of the mother),
social and economic background and marital status are

associated with low infant birth weight. Infants born to
women experiencing complications of pregnancy such as
toxemia and infections of the uterus have a four to five
times higher mortality rate than others in both developing
and developed countries (6).

     Undernutrition is a complicating factor with any of
the infectious diseases of mothers and children in
developing nations. As fewer mothers breast feed their
children, the possibility of unnecessary morbidity and
mortality increases. There is much evidence to support
breast feeding of the young in developing nations. Among
these:

(a)   Breast-feeding appears to be a way to improve
      nutritional status;
(b)   It transfers antibodies from the mother to the child;
(c)   It may be an important means of preventing diarrheal
      diseases; and
(d)   It provides better health for both child and mother
      by frequently serving as a way to increase intervals
      between birth of children.

According to data from the World Health Organization, in
developing nations, bottle fed babies are five times more
likely to die than are their breast fed cousins and
playmates.

Causes of Infant Mortality in Developed Nations.

     In the developed nations, a different picture of
childhood illness and death appears (7). Infants die primarily of birth injuries, congenital anomalies, influenza
or pneumonia and enteritis or diarrheal disease. Children
1 to 4 years old in the developed nations die from
accidents, congenital anomalies, malignant neoplasms and
influenza or pneumonia, while children of the same age in
developing nations are still dying of infectious diseases.

     Though infant and perinatal mortality rates have
continued to decline in the developed countries during the
past decades, there are still great differentials according to socioeconomic status in those nations. This is a
challenge to all of us in public health. Health and
longevity should be a matter of choice for all of our
people instead of a matter of chance for those who live in
poverty. The urban and rural poor of many developed
nations are living history as they fall prey to diseases
which killed their grandparents and great-grandparents,
but not their more affluent neighbors.

SCOPE OF MATERNAL MORBIDITY AND MORTALITY

The burden of excess maternal mortality, as with infant mortality, falls most heavily on developing nations. It is estimated that Africa has 10 maternal deaths per 10,000 live births; Asia has 52 per 10,000; Latin America 12 per 10,000 and North America 1 per 10,000 live births. These estimates are based on known data for these regions and undoubtedly underestimate mortality in Africa.

Maternal mobidity and mortality in developing countries, as in developed countries, is based on a number of factors, many of which are common to all nations. Maternal age, specially if it is less than 15 years or more than 40 years, is a factor in premature morbidity and mortality. The first pregnancy is the period of highest risk to any mother. A study in Bangladesh (8) indicated maternal mortality of 9 per 1000 first live births. The risk of death for the mother drops with the second, third and fourth child, and then increases steadily from the fifth and succeeding children.

Anemia, traced to undernutrition, malnutrition or other causes, is a risk factor in maternal mortality. Malaria and other infectious diseases also take their toll on pregnant women, particularly in developing nations. Inadequate antenatal care, including lack of tetanus toxoid, exacts its price.

Eclampsia is responsible for 25 percent of maternal deaths, with hemorrhage, obstructed labor and a retained placenta accounting for another 40 percent.

In both developed and developing nations, sexually transmitted infections have been shown to cause maternal morbidity, if not mortality, and illness or death of the child. The organisms B streptococci, chlamydia, ureaplasma (a newly identified agent), Herpes virus hominis and cytomegalovirus infections can all be responsible for a defective intrauterine growth, pre-term delivery and neonatal mortality. Chlamydia has frequently been found with other potential pathogens, which suggests strong relationship between chlamydia infection and a puerperal maternal infections - endometritis, amnionitis and salpingitis (9).

SUCCESSFUL INTERVENTIONS

Infant and maternal mortality is without question a

universal problem. In all nations, infections and infectious diseases still play a part in the unacceptable
outcomes of too many dead and damaged children and too
many mothers unable to care for themselves in order to
protect their own lives and those of their children. What
recourse do we have to solve these problems?

One recourse is to return to mothers their confidence
in playing the role of provider of primary health care.
By giving them information, successful formulas for care,
and access to medical assistance as necessary, it is possible to greatly supplement scarce medical professionals.
Formal projects in Indonesia, India and Mexico have shown
that mothers are able to tell when children need special
attention; many times they are able to provide needed
care, and with sufficient information, can prevent
children's illnesses.

The parasitic and infectious diseases have responded
to techniques used during the first public health revolution in the Western World. Improved sanitation, clean
water supplies, improved food supplies for mothers and
children, immunizations, are all known, long-successful
methods for dealing with these problems.

We are embarking, through the United Nations Development Program, World Bank, World Health Organization, and
other international agencies, on a program designed to
provide clean water for many of the people of developing
countries during this decade. By assuring that supplies
of fresh water are available within reasonable distance of
village and urban dwellers, we can greatly improve the lot
of mothers and children in developing nations. In some
cases we can also expect the bonus of doing away with
illness from guinea worm disease, directly attributable to
impure drinking water. Access to clean water will also
reduce the work load of women in developig countries who
invest great amounts of energy and time in carrying water.
In some villages in Africa, women walk 2 to 3 hours every
day to water sources and carry about 50 pounds of water on
their heads. The process burns off as much as 600 calories per day, about one-third of their average food
intake.

If we meet the targets set by 1990 for the clean
water decade, hundreds of millions of urban and rural
dwellers in Asia, Africa, and Latin America will have
access to clean water and improved sanitation.

Early diagnosis and treatment of respiratory or

intestinal infections, and supportive care such as oral
rehydration and feeding during illness, should be possible
through an accessible system almost anywhere. Low-cost
methods for diagnosis of vaginal infections should be
available through local health facilities or personnel.
Improved personal hygiene can be taught to expectant
mothers and could help reduce incidence of amniotic fluid
infections.

In developing countries, the provision of antimalarials within easy access of mothers and other family
decision makers would cut down on the incidence of
malaria, which strikes adults and children without
discrimination.

Epidemiologic tools should be employed to identify
women at highest risk of delivering pre-term babies and a
follow-up system should be employed to provide necessary,
easily accessible assistance. Nations from around the
world are working together in the Expanded Program of
Immunization. As we solve the problems of the cold chain
for protecting vaccine potency, and improve the stability
of vaccines, we will be able to bring immunization against
tetanus, measles, poliomyelitis, pertussis and other
death-dealing diseases to children and others previously
unprotected. With the U.S. about to eliminate measles and
other nations approaching historically low number of
cases, it may be time to seriously consider global
elimination of that disease. This would have potentially
dramatic results in developig nations, where measles
causes high mortality.

Today there are simple, effective rehydration methods
which can be taught to mothers to combat the effects of
diarrhea. Our greatest contribution can be made by teaching the use of available materials within easy reach of
the mother who can then make fluids for rehydration. We
can go a step further by teaching the mother to continue
feeding her child even though it continues to lose some
nutrients through diarrhea. If we can make her understand
that what is absorbed will make the difference between the
strength to battle for life and the inevitable complications of diarrheal depletion, she will become an even more
effective provider of primary health care.

It is also possible to combat low birth weight
throughout the world. Mothers in developing countries can
be taught the need for good nutrition during pregnancy,
they can be shown that an extra portion of rice allocated
to the meal for themselves is a necessary nutrient for

successful deliveries and safer infancies for their children.

Mothers can be taught the consequences of excessive smoking and abuse of other substances during pregnancy. The price for their life-style choices will be paid by the infant who are born at a low birth weight. Antenatal counseling of mothers at every age can give them an active, meaningful role in the birth and parenting process.

Family planning information should be made available to teenagers to prevent pregnancies in those whose youth is a liability to themselves and to their children of whom many are unwanted and mistreated. About 70 percent of expectant mothers under 15 receive no care during the first months of pregnancy, the period most important to fetal development; 25 percent of their babies are premature, a rate three times that for older mothers.

Mothers the world over can also be taught the importance of spacing their children to give them the best start in life. UNICEF has estimated that the infant mortality rate in developing countries is 200 deaths before the age of one year per 1000 live births if there is less than a year between successive children born to the same mother. That number drops to 80 deaths per 1000 live births when children are spaced 3 to 4 years apart.

In addition to education, which allows mothers and families to be basic health care providers, and to use what is locally available when possible, mothers and babies in developing nations need access to some health care facility within a reasonable distance. Though it may be a simple clinic, providing immunization and emergency help or other medical services when needed, if it is easily accessible it may be more valuable than the most sophisticated medical facility in the world, located in a nation's capital. Such a clinic can be a source of teaching for those in a community who can provide some primary health care or who can function in some public health role. It can also be a source of reassurance for families emerging into a new sense of responsibility and maturity as they assume some control over their own destinies.

CONCLUSION

Primary prevention and cure of infection in the mother and the newborn is a critical step in controlling the destiny of our nations and our people. As we set

priorities for our own nations we must keep an eye always
to the future: for what we do now will be the mark by
which history and our chidren will judge our ability to
provide a rational, healthy world for generations to come.

REFERENCES

1. United Nations (1977): World population prospects as
    assessed in 1973. Department of Economic and Social
    Affairs, Population Studies No. 60, United
    Nations, New York.
2. Villin J (1976): World rends in infant mortality
    since 1950. World Health Stat Rep, 29:646-674.
3. (1982): Health: the facts. UNICEF News, Issue
    108/2:8-9.
4. WHO (1976): New trends and approaches in the delivery
    of maternal and child care in health services.
    Sixth report of the WHO Expert Committee on Maternal
    and Child Health. WHO Tech Rep Ser, No. 600.
5. CIBA Foundation Symposium (1980): Perinatal
    infections. 77 New Series, Excerpta Medica, New
    York.
6. (1975): Malnutrition and infection during pregnancy.
    Determinants of growth and development of the child
    (Conclusion). Am J Dis Child, 129:249-580.
7. U. S. Department of Health, Education, and Welfare
    (1979): Healthy people. The Surgeon General's
    report on health promotion and disease prevention.
    U. S. Government Printing Office, Washington.
8. Chen LC et al (1974): A perspective study of birth
    intervals - Dynamics in rural Bangladesh.
    Population Studies, No. 28, 277-297.
9. Thompson S, Lopez B, Wong KH et al (1982): A prospec-
    tive study of chlamydia and mycoplasma infections
    during pregnancy: relations to pregnancy outcome
    and maternal morbidity. In: Chlamydial Infec-
    tions, P. A. Mardh, editor, Fifth International
    Symposium on Human Chlamydial Infections, Lunde,
    Sweden. Elsevier Biomedical Press, Amsterdam, 155.

PREVENTION AND MANAGEMENT OF MATERNAL INFECTIOUS
DISEASES DURING PREGNANCY

R. R. Trussell

Professor of Obstetrics and Gynecology
St. George's Hospital
London, United Kingdom

INTRODUCTION

Infection is an excellent example of an area where
maternity care and child health care are impossible to
separate because of a great deal of overlap. In many
ways, action that will improve one will also improve the
other. All health personnel must be prepared to consider
both mother and child. In discussing the prevention and
man- agement of maternal infectious diseases during
pregnancy, it is necessary to emphasize a number of
general points before dealing with specifics.

GENERAL PRINCIPLES

Many actions that may be taken to reduce infection
will be far removed from the administration of drugs. It
is probably true in most parts of the world that a greater
impact has been made on the health of a given community by
a general improvement in living standards than by any specific medical remedy. This has certainly been true of the
United Kingdom. A good clean water supply and the
adequate disposal of excreta are more important than the
contents of a bottle of medicine on the shelf of a dis-
pensary. Similarly, the ability of a woman or her baby to
withstand an infection may depend as much on her
nutritional status as on the particular infective agent
involved, or the remedy prescribed.

A woman's reproductive performance will depend on her

previous well-being, going back as far as her own intrauterine existence. Maternal deprivation, so often
associated with infections and infestations, will be at
least partly responsible for the problems of the next
generation.

Much can be achieved by antenatal care, but certain
adverse factors can be dealt with before pregnancy; the
40 weeks of pregnancy itself is not long enough. It may
well be said that this is a counsel of perfection - the
concept of a pre-parental clinic is a very sophisticated
one. However, when we have dealt with a particular high-
risk pregnancy to the best of our ability, we have a
responsibility not to allow that patient to leave our
supervision until her deficit, be it nutritional, hemato-
logical, infective, etc., has been corrected. The time to
consider about the next pregnancy is when the last one has
been reviewed.

We need to know the particular taboos and customs
that surround the pregnant woman. She may be isolated,
deprived of her usual diet, or excluded from sun and air
for part of her pregnancy. She may be encouraged to sit
over steam baths to prepare her pelvis for delivery. In
Northern Nigeria for example, there is a practice of providing excessively hot baths in an overheated room during
the puerperium, which may lead to burns and scalds, which
is turn may be complicated by infection, gangrene and
fulminating septicaemia. Caustic substances may be placed
in the vagina after delivery to restore it to a presumed
"virgin" condition. The umbilical cord may have been cut
by a traditional spear or panga as it may be in East
Africa in the case of twin pregnancy. Customs may be
useful and encouraged, neutral and ignored, or harmful and
exorcised. But we need to know.

It is as true of the hygiene of pregnancy as it is of
so many other aspects of medicine; we often know what
needs to be done, but this knowledge has not been transmitted to where it is most needed. There are a number of
maxims tht must be uppermost in our minds if we are to be
successful in putting into practice the principles of
hygiene with which we are all familiar.

(a) It must be our aim to ensure that every pregnant
mother in our country be seen at least once in her pregnancy. This principle is inescapable and should be given
at least as much emphasis as the development of more
ambitious programs on antenatal care for the selected few.

(b)   It must be accepted that on a global basis at present, only one-third of the world's population has skilled assistance of any sort in pregnancy and delivery. In line with the previous recommendation therefore, we must ensure that every birth attendant, from hospital specialist through the trained midwife to the traditional birth attendant (TBA), must be made to appreciate members of the same health team and be given clear encouragement and training appropriate to their level of capability. The facilities of the TBA maybe limited but they must be defined and recognized. The need for supervision and encouragement applies equally to the newly qualified doctor working in an isolated rural area as well as to the village health worker.

(c)   Each level of worker must know his or her limitations. All must be made aware of the high-risk concept and know when a patient should be transferred to a more central part of the service with better facilities and greater skills.

(d)   After training of an individual to a certain standard, the tools necessary to ensure these standards must be made available, such as sterile razor blades, tapes, antiseptic powders for management of the umbilical cord, or appropriate drops to instill into the eyes of the newborn.

SPECIFIC PRINCIPLES AND MEASURES

Important details of some infections and infestations that may plague the pregnant woman are discussed. The relative importance of these will vary from one region to another. It will be necessary to identify the agents in any one area which demand particular attention. In parts of the world where resources are limited, we must concentrate on the essentials.

The initial evaluation of the pregnant patients should be early, unhurried and accurately recorded. It should include in particular the outcome of previous pregnancies, renal infections, chest infections particularly tuberculosis, rubella, venereal disease, and cardiac problems.

Examination will be detailed and should include a total review of the patient, including skin, teeth, chest and cardiovascular system. Cervical studies, including a smear and swab should be carried out where possible and

relevant. A vaginal swab is of little use in looking for
gonorrhea, thus stool must also be examined for infestations, and the urine for infection. Serology will include
a VDRL test for syphilis, and tests for rubella and
toxoplasmosis. This is the time when advice on hygiene of
pregnancy should be given.

In general, the pregnant patient is as well equipped
as anyone else in the community to deal with infection
and infestation. The process of adaptation to pregnancy,
however, leaves her vulnerable in a few respects. It is
well to remember that the urinary system is affected by
the smooth muscle effects of progesterone and by pressure
from the developing uterus on her ureter where they cross
the pelvic brim. The net result is a degree of hydro-
neprosis and hydroureter leading to urinary stasis. The
joint effects of these two factors are often maximal at
about 24 weeks of pregnancy and it is at this time that
urinary infections, usually pyelitis is most common.

The pulmonary system is not impaired in normal pregnancy but there is nevertheless an increased "awareness of
the need to breath" - an increased respiratory effort, and
a chest infection will be more serious than in the non-
pregnant.

The immune system undergoes changes in pregnancy. A
good example of this is represented by malaria. In endemic areas where there is high incidence of acquired
immunity, this is reduced by the 20th week of pregnancy,
resulting in the appearance of parasites in the blood
stream, and the possibility of hemolytic anemia, premature labor and impaired birth weight of the fetus.

Malaria

In malaria, prescribing will have to take into
account the relevant species of plasmodium in an area.
Local knowledge of this and the degree of local resistance
will be invaluable. Residents of a holoendemic area
already taking antimalarial drugs should continue to take
them during pregnancy. Residents who become pregnant and
who do not normally take antimalarials should be given an
initial therapeutic dose to clear any preexisting parasit-
emia (e.g. chloroquine 600 mg) and this should be followed
by regular prophylaxis (300 mg weekly), which should
continue for six weeks after the confinement. The resulting drop in immunity will not be dangerous, but the first
reinfestation may be clinically apparent.

Chloroquine resistant parasites are becoming a major hazard, especially in Indochina, Malaysia, India and East Africa, and are also known in the Amazon basin.   Chloroquine resistant strais of P. falciparum are also commonly resistant to phyrimethamine thus maloprim is the preparation of choice. Folinic acid may be added in the first trimester and it is wiser to continue prophylaxis up to and after delivery, since fetal and neonatal hazard of the drug is probably less than the risk of an attack of malaria. P. vivax is occasionally resistant to chloroquine, in which case high doses of proguanil is the drug of choice. Visitors to a holoendemic area should take prophylactic medication for the duration of their stay and for six weeks after their return, as delayed attacks of P. vivax malaria can occur.

No antimarlairal drug is entirely safe in pregnancy. Pyrimethamine and proguanil are folate antagonists, and should be avoided if possible during the first trimester. If folate deficiency or malnutrition are likely to be present, calcium folinate (15 mg daily), can prevent pyrimethamine-induced hemolytic changes without affecting its antimalarial activity. Pyrimethamine is present in breast milk but is not known to be harmful to the breast fed infant. Chloroquine has been suspected of causing neonatal deafness in the first trimester, but the evidence is poor, and it is certainly safer than quinine. Primaquine, along with sulfanomides and dapsone, produce hemolysis in patients with glucose-6-phosphate dehyrogenase deficiency and may do so in neonates even without this deficiency. These drugs should not be used in the last week of pregnancy. There may also be a small risk in the breast fed neonate.

Toxoplasmosis

This infestation has a world-wide distribution but has a greater prevalence in the tropics. The organism is acquired by the ingestion of raw meat or other food contaminated by cat feces. The disease is not often recognized clinically but previous infection can be detected by screening for specific antibodies. If infections occur for the first time in pregnancy, cysts or oocytes may cross the placenta and infect the fetus, causing abortion, stillbirth or neonatal toxoplasmosis. The fetus is not affected by infection acquired before pregnancy, as it is protected by transplacental maternal antibody. It is unnecessary to treat pregnant woman who acquired the disease before pregnancy, and women giving birth to an

affected child in one pregnancy will not have problems in
subsequent pregnancies. Treatment is by pyrimethamine (1
mg/kg body weight up to a maximum of 75 mg every 24
hours), together with sulfadiazine (1 mg every 6 hours for
14 days). The problems associated with the administration
of pyrimethamine and sulfadiazine in pregnancy have been
discussed.

Schistosomiasis

The gastrointestinal tract and liver are the organs
mainly affected by S. mansoni; while the bladder,
pelvic organs and bowel take the brunt of attack by S.
haemotobium. Pregnancy has no effect on these parasites
and the adverse effect on the pregnancy is mainly the
longstanding tissue scarring and tissue destruction of the
genital tract which may interfere with vaginal delivery.

Intestinal Infestations

Attention is given to hookworm and amebiasis. Infection with Ankylostoma duodenale or N. americanus is
found throughout the tropical and subtropical regions.
Manifestations are directly proportional to the number of
worms and the related tissue destruction and blood loss.
Every 1000 eggs per g of feces is associated with a loss
of 2 ml of blood a day and a heavily infested individual
may lose 100 ml of blood in 24 hours. A previous asymptomatic infestation may become significant in pregnancy.
Befenium is the drug of choice in pregnancy. A single
dose (5 g) is effective in duodenale, but must be repeated on 3 successive mornings to eradicate N. americanus.
A 100 percent eradication is never achieved, but eliminating the bulk of the parasite burden in pregnancy is worthwhile. Mebendazole, which is used particularly when
hookworm is part of a mixed infection, e.g. with whipworm,
is probably best avoided in the first trimester of
pregnancy, although teratogenicity has been described only
in rats.

Amebiasis does not usually affect pregnancy but may
run a severe course. Latent infections may be exacerbated
and new infections may rarely prove fatal. The same
reaction has been seen when patients who have unsuspected
amebiasis are given corticosteroids. Metronidazole (800
mg three times daily), is given for 5 days. Diloxamide
(500 mg three times daily, 10 to 14 days), will increase
the rate of elimination of parasites from the bowel.

Trichomonas vaginalis

This flagellate protozoa is found in the vagina of 10 to 25 percent of all women. It is a cause of severe local discharge and irritation, but perhaps of interest is the frequency with which it coexists with other organisms, whose presence may be more significant. Thus, candida, gonorrhea and chlamydia are all seen in association with it. Donne first described it in 1886 and believed it could only exist in the presence of a vaginitis caused by another infection. A related urethritis is often found in the male partner of an infected patient. Metronidazole is effective and can be given either as a 2 g single dose or 200 mg three times a day for 7 to 10 days. The affected partner should also be treated. Side effects are uncommon and include nausea, rashes and alcohol intolerance. Local preparations such as acetarsol should be used in the first three months of pregnancy, although there is no direct evidence of teratogenicity.

Candida albicans

This yeast-like fungus is widespread in nature and is found in one-third of women of child-bearing age. It flourishes in pregnancy because of the high estrogen levels and increased glycogen content of the vaginal cells. The most severely infected patients are those in whom pregnancy and diabetes coincide. Obesity and the administration of broad spectrum antibiotics may be contributory. It is surprising that amniotic infection is not more common. The neonate should be examined if a known infection of the mother exists. Current treatment is with nystatin vaginal pessary (each containing 100,000 units, twice daily for 10 to 15 days). The male partner should wear a sheath or is given nystatin cream. Recurrence is common and in these circumstances a stool specimen should be examined and oral treatment with nystatin given where appropriate. More recently, canesten has been found to be effective in a shorter 3-day course.

Chlamydia

Chlamydia is another intracellular obligate parasite mainly inhabiting the cervix. It has already been mentioned that it may be associated with trichomonas and gonorrhea. The major risk to the fetus is an eye infection and less commonly, pneumonia. Infection of mother and child responds to sulfonamides and erythromycin. The use of silver nitrate for the prophylaxis of gonococcal ophthalmia will not protect the eye of the newborn from infection with chlamydia.

Bacterial Infections

Several principles must be enumerated in discussing
the problem of bacterial infection in pregnancy, labor and
puerperium. It is not necessary to wear masks during
normal vaginal delivery and a simple regime of hand washing and sterilization of equipment should be worked out
and adhered to for each level of maternity care. Cathe-
terization should be avoided unless absolutely necessary.
On the other hand, abnormal deliveries shuld be afforded
the care and precautions appropriate to any surgical
procedure.

There is little doubt that the development of uro-
genital infection in labor and the puerperium are directly
related to the duration of labor, and in particular to the
length of time the membranes have been ruptured. Intact
membranes are no guarantee against infection and certain
authorities believe that invasion of the fetal membranes
by organisms from the vagina, even before labor, constitute a major hazard to the fetus, particularly where
malnutrition is present. "Let not the sun go down upon
your labor twice" is an old wives maxim. The majority of
labor should be over within 24 hours and most are considerably less than this. Vaginal examination should be
restricted to every 4 hours and be carried out with full
aseptic precautions. If the uterus is known to be infected, both the penicillins and cephalospirins reach the
fetus and are known to be safe. Amoxycillin has better
tissue penetration than ampicillin. Materials should be
sent for bacterial examination, the delivery expedited and
the pediatrician informed. In our setting, it simply
means reminding ourselves to treat the baby.

In case of premature rupture of membranes before 36
weeks gestation, antibiotics should be given only if there
is evidence of infection. There is no place for prophylaxis here. Vaginal examination should be avoided. After
36 weeks, the sooner the patient is delivered the better.
Over the last 10 years, interest has developed in the
presence in the vagina of a group of ß-hemolytic streptococcus, capable of developing a fulminating septicemia in
the infant within a few hours of delivery, fatal in 50
percent of the cases. There is no consensus of agreement
on how to deal with this problem which probably occurs in
about 1 to 2 per 1000 deliveries. It has been suggested
that prophylaxis should be concentrated on the small number of high-risk mothers, for example, those with a past
history of unexplained stillbirth and previous newborn
with severe septicemia.

In elective caesarean section, infection rate is low but this rate increases dramatically when the membranes have been ruptured for any length of time. It has been suggested that in these cases where the membranes have been ruptured for more than 6 hours, antibiotics be given. Amoxycillin and metronidazole would be appropriate. Prophylactic antibiotics are unnecessary and unwise for the elective operation, but recently a pre-operative vaginal pessary of povidone-iodine, has been used with advantage.

Septicemic shock most often follows abortion, but can accompany spontaneous abortion, caesarean section or present in the puerperium. Apart from the gram negative organisms which release endotoxins, the chlostridia and Streptococcus pyogenes can produce an overwhelming infection. Blood coagulation problems and renal failure may follow. After taking maternal blood sample for bacteriology, a high tissue concentration of broad spectrum antibiotics is necessary. A combination of gentamycin, amoxycillin and metronidazole is effective.

In urinary tract infection, nitrofurantoin will deal with the asymptomatic bacteruria and amoxycillin with the majority of cases of pyelonephritis. Gentamycin would be suitable if there was a history of penicillin anaphylaxis. There is high recurrence rate in pregnancy and thorough renal evaluation is necessary for cases which do not respond.

Tuberculosis treatment should be as in the non-pregnant, with isoniazid and ethambucil as the first line of defense. Rifampicin is probably safe. Protection for the baby in the past has been by separation from the mother. However, the baby is now protected with isoniazid and vaccinated with BCG. Isoniazid is continued until tuberculin test is positive. Breast feeding is contraindicated where there is recent active infection. Gonorrhea in pregnancy usually is limited to the lower genital tract including the cervix, urethra, periurethral and bartholins glands and sometimes the rectum. It is said that in the first three months of pregnancy before the chorion fuses with the decidua, salpingitis can still occur but it is so rare as to be dismissed. The infection may antedate the pregnancy; it may have been acquired at the time of insemination or subsequently. Failure of, or inadequate treatment, will allow the patient to infect sexual partners, suffer gonococcal arthritis or other desseminated disease and infect the infant at the time of delivery, causing ophthalmia, and developing an ascending infection of the genital tract after delivery. Therefore even

asymptomatic disease should be treated. Diagnosis consists of examination of material from the cervix, urethra
and rectum. A high vaginal swab is useless. A suspicion
may be aroused by the discovery of gram negative intracellular diplococci in a smear. Definitive diagnosis
involves culture in an appropriate medium (Thayer-Martin).
It is best to inoculate the material directly onto a
plate, but failing this, Stewart's transport medium may be
employed.

The drug of choice is penicillin. Effective treatment requires a high blood level (0.35 units of penicillin
per ml) maintained over 24 hours. While noting different
degrees of sensitivity, some authorities would state that
there is no such thing as a penicillin-resistant
gonorrhea, and that all patients will respond if enough
penicilln is given. Prior to treatment, the patient must
be questioned for history of allergy and should be kept in
the clinic 30 minutes after injection. Epinephrine, an
antihistamine and a steriod should be available in case of
an anaphylactoid response. To achieve adequate dosage,
procaine penicillin G in aqueous suspension should be
given by the intramuscular route, divided between the two
buttocks. The dose (2.4 to 4.8 million units), will vary
according to the local organism. If probenecid (1 g) is
given shortly before the injection, the drug acts by
interfering with the renal tubular excretion of penicillin
and helps to maintain the blood levels. The long-acting
penicillins have no place in the treatment of gonorrhea.
If for reasons of allergy pencillin cannot be used, erythromycin (1.5 g orally followed by 0.5 g four times daily
up to a total of 9.5 g) may be used. The estolate forms
of erythromycin are contraindicated. More effective than
erythromycin are cefazolin and spectinomycin but they
have not been clearly established to be safe for the
fetus. The infant whose mother has gonorrhea requires
treatment with aqueous pencillin G, 50,000 units for term
sized infants, and half of this for infants that are
small.

Syphylis

The health worker must be aware that pregnancy is not
only a critical time to detect syphilis because of the
need to protect the mother and her sexual partner from the
many complications of pregnancy, but especially important
in preventing the extensive pathological changes that characterize congenital syphilis. In this connection the
health worker will be concerned mainly with the primary,
secondary and latent syphilis. The incubation time in

pregnancy is often short, and in the presence of other local lesions such as herpes genitalis, it may be as brief as six days. The Hunterian chancre is classically a single painless nodule and is often missed. A non-tender solitary lymph node is often present. The chancre heals in about 5 weeks and may be followed by secondary characteristics which may be very slight and confined to the genitalia; there may be condylomata which may ulcerate. A highly variable skin rash may be seen but is by no means universal. A stillborn or congenitally abnormal baby may be the first indication of syphilis. It is important that a suitable serological screening test at the first antenatal visit be performed on as large a percentage of the population as possible. The VDRL slide test is one such test. This will almost certainly be positive 4 to 6 weeks after contracting the disease. Confirmation of a positive result is accomplished by a Fluorescent Treponema Antibody Absorption test.

Of the many congenital infections, syphilis is the easiest to prevent and the most amenable to therapy. Patients exposed to an infected partner should be treated for early syphilis. The treatment described for gonorrhea will be effective for incubating syphilis. Serology should be carried out after 3 months.

Treponema pallidum divides every 30 to 33 hours in early syphilis and while lower blood levels of penicillin are treponemicidal, the blood levels have to be maintained to cover sufficient division times to be effective. Thus treatment may consist of 2.4 million units of benzathine penicillin G half in each buttock; or 600,000 units of aqueous procaine penicillin G per day for 8 days. For patients allergic to penicillin, oral erythromycin 2 g per day for 15 days is recommended. If clinical signs persist, cerebrospinal fluid examination should be done.

For syphilis of indeterminate length or more than a year's duration, benzathine penicillin G (2.4 million units divided between each buttock) is given weekly for 3 successive weeks, or aqueous procaine penicillin G (600,000 units), intramuscular each day for 14 days. If the cerebrospial fluid is positive, more intensive therapy is done and the spinal fluid is tested every 6 months for three years. Those allergic to penicillin are given erythromycin at a dose of 500 mg 4 times a day for 30 days. Women in pregnancy are susceptible to reinfection. Serology should be carried out monthly for the remainder of the pregnancy and a rise in titre of 4 dilutions warrants further treatment.

Congenital Syphilis

Every infant with suspected or proven syphilis should have their cerebrospinal fluid examined. Following treatment, infants should be followed up at monthly intervals until serology is negative. Symptomatic infants or those with positive spinal fluid should be treated with aqueous penicillin G (500 units/kg intramuscular or intravenous in 2 divided doses each day for 10 days). For asymptomatic seropositives with negative spinal fluid, a single dose penicillin G is given (50,000 units/kg intramuscularly). Infants born of mothers treated by erythromycin should be treated as if they had congenital syphilis.

CONCLUSION

Preventive management of infectious diseases in pregnancy needs strict observation and adherence to general principles. The specific pinciplesof therapy vary according to the nature of the infectious agent.

REFERENCES

(Available by correspondence from R. R. Trussel)

SYNERGISM BETWEEN MALNUTRITION AND INFECTION IN INFANTS

Y.W. Cho and R.M. Suskind

Departments of Medicine, Pharmacology and
Pediatrics, University of South Alabama
Mobile, Alabama, U.S.A.

INTRODUCTION

In developing countries, malnutrition and infections
are the most important causes of infant mortality and
morbidity. Although there are separate incidence and
prevalence rates for the two groups of diseases, it should
be recognized that there is a synergism between both (1).
Nearly all infections have detectable adverse effects of
the nutritional status of infants, and malnutrition increases the severity of infection. Public health programs
should be concerned with this synergism to break the
vicious interaction between infection and malnutrition.
The emphasis of this review is the mechanism of synergism
which will in turn dictate the nature of the public health
programs designed to reduce infant and neonatal mortality
and morbidity.

ADVERSE EFFECTS OF INFECTIONS ON NUTRITIONAL STATUS

It is generally known that nearly all infections,
even when they are not associated with overt disease, can
influence the nutritional status of infants. The adverse
effects can occur during three phases of the infections:
incubation period, acute illness, and convalescent period.
During each phase, there are metabolic endocrine,
biochemical and immunologic responses, some of which
relate to the adverse effects of the infection on the
nutritional status of the infant (2).

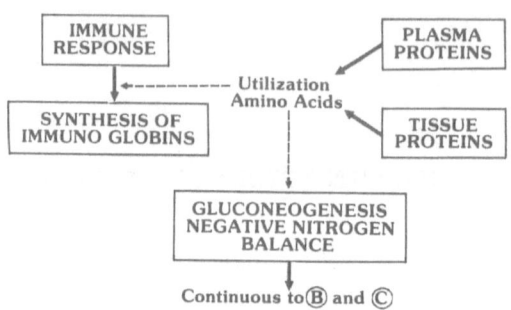

Figure 1:   Immunologic Response During
            Incubation Period.

A.   Immunologic Response During Incubation Period

     Following the exposure to an infectious agent, a
complex sequence of nutritionally important phenomena is
initiated. As part of the immunologic response to the
invading infectious agent, there is an increase in utilization of amino acids for the synthesis of proteins,
specially immunoglobins. Although the primary source of
amino acids is plasma protein, there is generalized mobil-
ilization from peripheral tissues including skeletal
muscles. The negative nitrogen balance occurring from
infections start during the incubation period and continues through the acute phase when amino acids are also
utilized for gluconeogenesis (Fig. 1).

B.   Nutritional Consequences of Acute Infection

     After the incubation period, the acute illness starts
with fever and signs and symptoms of organ involvement:
coughing if respiratory or diarrhea if gastrointestinal.
The physiologic and biochemical responses during the acute
phase of the infection influence the nutritional status in
the following manner   (Fig. 2):

     First: Fever and Sweating. The rise in body
temperature is followed by an increase in metabolism which
contributes to energy loss. Sweating associated with
fever undoubtedly leads to further loss of fluid, electrolytes and amino acids. The end result is loss of body
weight.

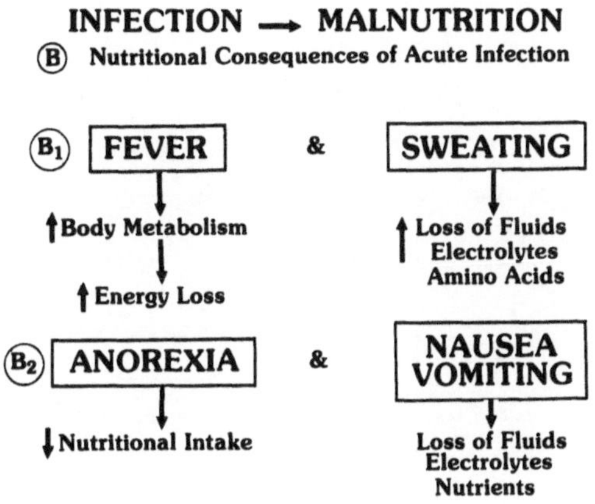

INFECTION → MALNUTRITION

Ⓑ Nutritional Consequences of Acute Infection

(B₁) FEVER   &   SWEATING

↑ Body Metabolism   ↑ Loss of Fluids
                                 Electrolytes
                                 Amino Acids

↑ Energy Loss

(B₂) ANOREXIA   &   NAUSEA
                               VOMITING

↓ Nutritional Intake   Loss of Fluids
                               Electrolytes
                               Nutrients

Figure 2:   Nutritional Consequences of
            Acute Infection.

Second: <u>Anorexia, Nausea and Vomiting.</u> There is a
reduction in food intake following infections, regardless
of etiology. It is not known if the anorexia is caused
directly by the infectious process, or by the febrile response and the resulting stress syndrome. The reduction in
food intake can occur even with an infection as mild as
immunization with a vaccine (3). Even though the infant
is institutionalized with ad libitum feeding, it is impossible to maintain a normal dietary intake during the
anorexia of acute infection. The vomiting from serious
infections signifies an acute loss of fluids and electrolytes which further threatens the nutritional status of
the sick infant.

Third: <u>Dietary Change.</u> There is an almost
universal tendency to change the character of the diet
during an acute infection. For older infants, almost all
solid foods are commonly withdrawn and the replacements
are lower in calories and protein content. If the substitutes are sweetened beverages or diluted cereals, this may
contribute to the development of clinically evident
malnutrition (Fig. 3).

Fourth: <u>Reduced Nutrient Absorption.</u> Diarrhea of
infectious diseases leads to an increase in caloric loss
in excess of 500 to 600 calories per day (4). In addition
to decreased absorption of protein, fat, and carbohydra-
tes, there is also malabsorption of vitamin A, vitamin
B-12 and folic acid. The difficulties in absorption of
vitamins may result not only from direct effects of
bacterial toxins but from the presence of intestinal

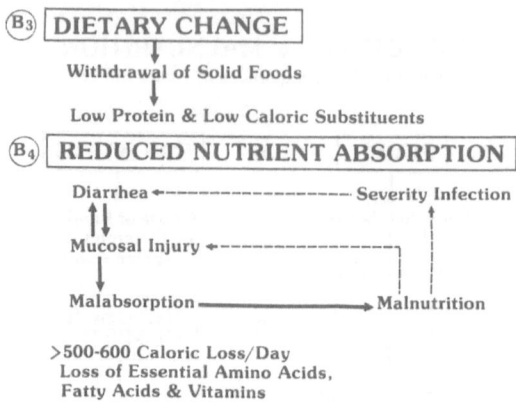

Figure 3:   Dietary Change and Reduced
            Nutrient Absorption.

parasites. Systemic infections of bacterial or viral
origin cause malabsorption of nutrients which may outlast
the duration of fever and diarrhea (Fig. 3).

        Fifth: Stress Response. Infection triggers the
hypothalamic-pituitary stimulation to secrete growth
hormone, thyrotropin and corticotropin (Fig. 4). The end
result is catabolism, wasting of muscle and weight loss.
During the negative nitrogen balance characteristic of the
acute phase of the illness, there is also an increased excretion of potassium, magnesium, zinc, phosphate, sulfate
and some vitamins (A and C).

C. Disease Consequences During Convalescent Period

        When infections episodes are superimposed on infants

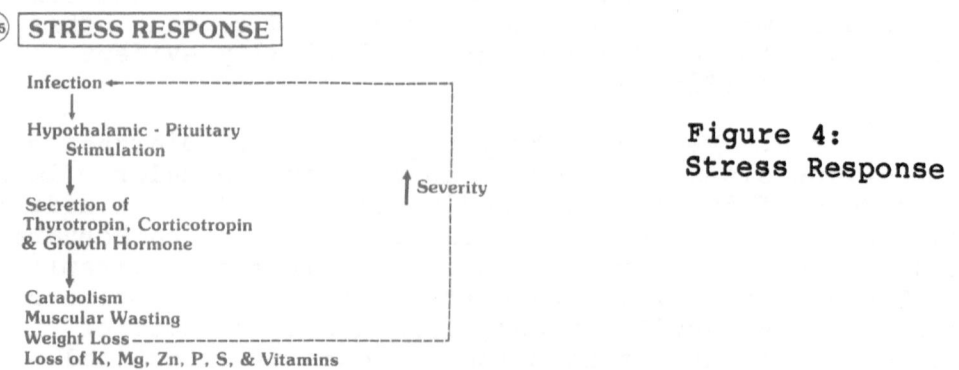

Figure 4:
Stress Response

(C) **DISEASE CONSEQUENCES DURING CONVALESCENCE**

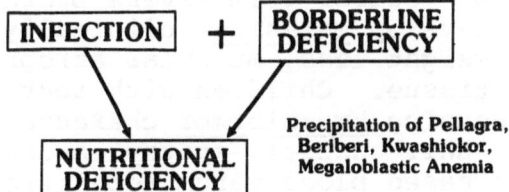

(D) **IMPAIRED GROWTH & DEVELOPMENT**

Explained by Synergism between Infection & Malnutrition
Correct Negative Nitrogen Balance

Figure 5:   Disease Consequences
            During Convalescence

When infectious episodes are superimposed on infants who are on a diet borderline in one or more essential nutrients, then nutritional deficiency occurs (Fig. 5). For instance, kwashiorkor prevalence increases after a month following epidemics of infectious diseases, particularly of gastroenteritis (5). Pellagra and beriberi are precipitated by infectious episodes. Megaloblastic anemia from fish tapeworm becomes more severe when there is superimposed infection (6). These examples illustrate the debilitating action of infection on infants who are already predisposed to diseases of nutritional deficiency.

D.   Impairment of Physical Growth and Development

During convalescence, the diet should be sufficient to correct the negative nitrogen balance sustained during the acute phase of infection. The period of accelerated growth rate during recuperation may be disrupted when there are additional episodes of acute infection. The end result is impairment in physical growth and development. Studies show a correlation of frequency of infection with growth impairment (7). However, it is not possible to determine how much of the correlation is due to the effect of infection on nutritional status and how much to the diarrhea of malnutrition. The most acceptable explanation for impairment of growth and development is synergism between infection and malnutrition.

MALNUTRITION AND THE IMMUNE RESPONSE

Protein-calorie malnutrition occurs either in its primary form (reduced intake) or secondary to other

diseases (congenital or acquired involving gastrointestinal, hepatorenal or cardiopulmonary systems). Infants
and children who suffer from severe protein-calorie
malnutrition develop <u>marasmus</u>, clinically with growth
retardation, weight loss, muscular atrophy, and loss of
subcutaneous tissue. Children with acute protein loss or
deprivation develop <u>kwashiorkor</u> characterized by edema,
skin lesions, hair changes, apathy, anorexia, and enlarged
liver and decreased blood serum total proteins. The less
severe forms of protein-calorie malnutrition have a feature common to marasmus and kwashiorkor; the malnourished
child is susceptible to infection which is a major factor
in the high mortality and morbidity rates.

Clinical observations suggest that the malnourished
infant's immune system may respond to infection differently from that of the well-nourished individual. An
infectious organism that it is relatively harmless to the
well-nourished infant, may give rise to a severe or even
fatal infection in an individual with protein-calorie
malnutrition. For example, a localized infection in the
extremities would spread and cause gangrene in the
individual with malnutrition. Furthermore, septicemia is
a more frequent complication in children with protein-
calorie malnutrition. In the malnourished infant, several
host defenses have been adversely affected including cell-
mediated immune response, namely: humoral immune response, phagocytic function of polymorpho-nuclear leukocytes and macrophages, and complement system. The remainder of this review is devoted to a discussion of how much
of the four components of the immune response is influenced by malnutrition which in turn can explain the
increased susceptibility to infection of the infant or
child with protein-calorie malnutrition.

A. Cell-Mediated Immune Response

In 1925, Jackson noted at autopsy that children with
kwashiorkor had atrophied thymus glands, lymph nodes,and
tonsils, and that the spleen was smaller (8). The phenomenon of lymphoid atrophy in cases of protein-calorie
malnutrition has been repeatedly seen by other investigators. More recently, technics have been developed to
evaluate the response of lymphocytes in malnourished
children. An in vivo test is by intradermal skin testing
using dinitrofluorobenzene. A positive test is characterized by the appearance of inflammation of the site of skin
injection, indicating that the sensitized lymphocyte is
able to recognize the foreign antigen and respond with the
release of lymphokines. In a group of children suffering

Ⓐ CELL-MEDICATED IMMUNE RESPONSE

Autopsy Findings (Jackson 1925)
    Kwashiorkor & Protein - Calorie Malnutrition
    Atrophy of Thymus, Lymph Nodes, Tonsils & Spleen
    Generalized Lymphoid Atrophy

IMMUNE RESPONSE IN PROTEIN - CALORIE MALNUTRITION
Dinitrofluorobenzene
↓
Lymphocytic Response
Lymphokines Release
↓
Dermal Inflammation
Postive Skin Test

DAY TESTED	No. PATIENTS	POSITIVE	NEGATIVE
1	30	4 (13%)	26
15	5	3 (60%)	2
56	8	6 (75%)	2

Figure 6: Cell-mediated Immune Response.

from protein-calorie malnutrition, the results were as
follows: positive skin test in 13 percent when tested on
day 1, 60 percent on day 15, and 75 percent on day 56.
These results indicate that the malnourished children were
unable to develop normal inflammatory response, whereas
nutritionally recovered children were able to respond (9).
In vitro test of lymphocytes from malnourished children
react poorly to antigens such as phytohemagglutinin-A (9).
The results show recovery to normal cell-mediated immune
response in the course of recovery from malnutrition (Fig.
6).

B. Humoral Immune System

     The bursa cell also known as B-lymphocyte is respon-
sible for immunoglobulin production. We undertook a study
to examine the antibody response in malnourished children
to typhoid antigen (10). Ten malnourished children
(kwashiorkor or marasmus) and ten recovered patients were
evaluated for antibody response to intradermal typhoid
antigen, 8 and 20 to 29 days after immunization. The
anti-H antibody was measured by radio- immunoassay.
Children with protein-calorie malnutrition who were
immunized on admission showed essentially no increase in
antibody titer in the first week, during which they received 100 Cal and 1 g protein per kg. The nutritionally
recovered children who were receiving 175 Cal and 4 g
protein per kg showed a significant increase in antibody
activity over the preimmunization level within a week
after immunization (10). This response to an antigenic
stimulus, such as typhoid antigen, is a sensitive and
reliable evaluation of the humoral immune system (Fig. 7).

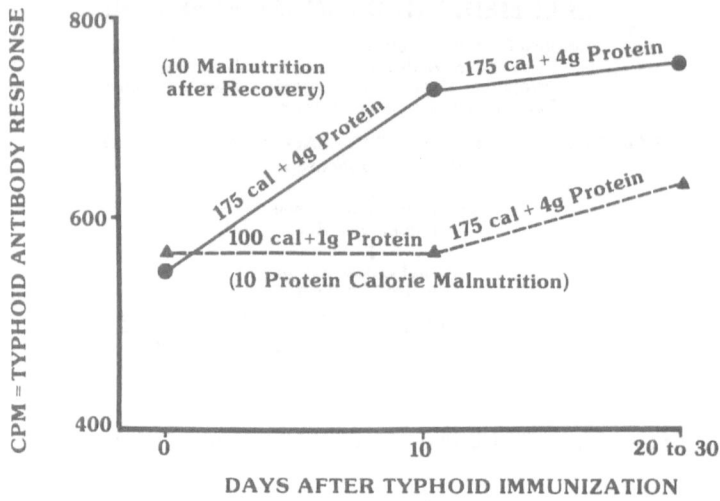

Figure 7:   Humoral Immune System.

C.   Phagocytosis by Polymorphonuclear Leukocytes and Macrophages.

Polymorphonuclear leukocytes and macrophages are phagocytic cells which are important in controlling bacterial infections. Studies indicate that malnourished infants and children do not show any interference of phagocytic function-chemotaxis and engulfment. The postphagocytic events were unchanged in malnourished individuals. Bacterial phagocytes is therefore adequate in patients with protein-calorie malnutrition (Fig. 8).

D.   Complement System

Defects in the complement system have been associated with increased susceptibility to bacterial infection. Studies show that nutritional status of the child influences the activation of the complement system and the formation of complement fragments which are involved in host defenses including viral neutralization, opsonization of fungi, endotoxin inactivation, lysis of virus-infected cells and bacteriolysis (11). In other words, malnutrition causes decreased complement values which accounts in part for the increase in susceptibility to, and severity of infection. In summary, protein-calorie malnutrition influences three of the four system relating to the host defense mechanisms; cell-mediated immune response, humoral immune system and complement system, but not on phagocytosis by polymorphonuclears and macrophages (Fig. 8).

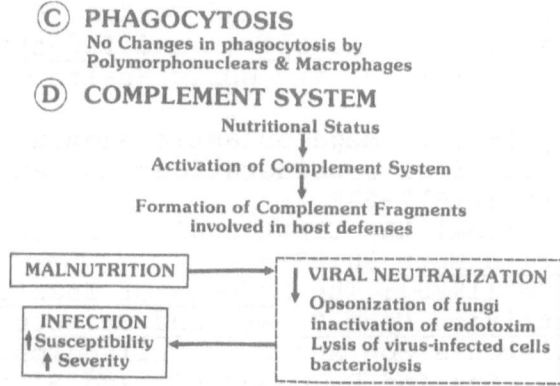

Figure 8: Phagocytosis and Complement System.

CONCLUSION

As pediatric pharmacologists, we can only comment on the therapeutic implications of the synergism between infection and malnutrition. Therapy includes the use of antibiotics and the treatment of malnutrition. It should be recalled that the net loss of nitrogen during an acute infection can vary from 0.6 to 1.2 g/kg/day, depending on the nature and severity of the illness. This loss can be overcome more effectively during the recuperation period, since oral feeding is impractical during the acute phase of severe infection. The efficacy of antibiotics is questionable unless malnutrition is corrected.

REFERENCES

1. Scrimshaw NS (1981): Significance of interactions of nutrition and infection in children. In: Textbook of Pediatric Nutrition, Edited by R.M. Suskind, pp. 229-240, Raven Press, New York.
2. Beisel WR (1976): In: Nutrient Requirements in Adolescence, Edited by J.I. McKigney and H.N. Munro, pp. 257-275, MIT Press, Cambridge, MA.
3. Gandra YR and Scrimshaw NS (1961): Infection and nutritional status. II. Effect of mild virus infection induced by 17-D yellow fever vaccine on nitrogen metabolism in children. Am J Clin Nutr 9:159-163.
4. Rosenberg IH, Solomons NW and Schneider RE (1977): Malabsorption associated with diarrhea and intestinal infections. Am J Clin Nutr 30:1248-1253.

5.   Scrimshaw NS, Taylor CE, and Gordon JE (1968):
      Interactions of Nutrition and Infection, WHO
      Monogr Serial No. 57, World Health Organization,
      Geneva.
6.   Luhby AL (1959): Megaloblastic anemia in infancy.
      III. Clinical considerations and analysis. J
      Pediatr 54:617-632.
7.   Mata LJ, Kromal RA, Urrutia JJ, and Garcia B (1977):
      Am J Clin Nutr 30:1215-1217.
8.   Jackson CM (1925): The Effects of Inanition and
      Malnutrition Upon Growth and Structure, p. 285,
      Blackiston's Son and Co., Philadelphia.
9.   Edelman R, Suskind R, Olson RE, and Sirisinha S
      (1973): Effect of infection on food intake and
      the nutritional state: perspectives as viewed
      from the village. Lancet 1:506-508.
10.   Suskind R, Sirishinha S, Edelman R, Vithayasai V,
      Damrongsak D, Charupatana C, and Olson RE (1977):
      In: Malnutrition and the Immune Response,
      Edited by R.M. Suskind, pp. 185-190, Raven Press,
      New York.
11.   Sirisinha S, Suskind R, Edelman R, Kulapongs P, and
      Olson RE (1977): In: Malnutrition and the
      Immune Response, Edited by R.M. Suskind, pp.
      309-320, Raven Press, New York.
12.   Suskind RM (1981): Textbook of Nutrition, pp.
      241-262, Raven Press, New York.

EPIDEMIC OF NECROTIZING ENTEROCOLITIS:

ITS POSSIBLE VIRAL ORIGIN

C. Sureau

Department of Obstetrics and Reproductive
Physiopathology, Université René Descartes
Clinique Universitaire Baudelocque
Paris, France

INTRODUCTION

During the period 1978 to 1980, an epidemic of necrotizing enterocolitis was observed at the Maternity Unit of the Baudelocque University Clinic. A total number of 46 cases occurred during three different periods, among 3988 deliveries.

A study from a clinical, therapeutic and prophylactic point of view of these cases is presented. The circumstances which imply that these cases are probably the result of infection by the corona virus is also described.

CLINICAL FEATURES

Between August 1978 and May 1979, thirty cases occurred in two successive waves among 1800 deliveries: August to November, 5 cases; February to May, 25 cases. A clear relationship exists between the occurrences of the cases and the activities in the ward.

The time of occurrence was between day 4 and day 14 in twenty-six cases, but mostly during the 2nd week of life. However, three children became sick before the 3rd day and one premature baby after a month. Nine babies were premature, four were small for dates at term and seventeen had been born after 37 weeks and weighed more than 2500 g.

Among these thirty cases, the diagnosis was certain in 17, on the basis of radiographical and/or histological evidence. In thirteen cases however, because of the lack of characteristic findings, the diagnosis was presumptive. In every case, specimens were taken for bacteriological examination.

The treatment was chiefly medical, consisting of aspiration, parenteral nutrition, and antibiotics. Among the seventeen certain cases, 8 children were cured by medical treatment; 4 children were operated upon (resection and/or colostomy) in the acute stage of the disease, with one death after operation for bowel perforation; 3 children had secondary closure of the colostomy carried out without further problem; and 5 children were operated upon later for scar stenosis. One died because of staphylococcal septicemia which occurred in the intensive care unit.

Among the thirteen probable cases, 12 were cured and 1 died on day 5. The postmortem examination failed to demonstrate the cause of death or the presence of an enterocolitis.

Among these 30 children, only one received complete direct breast feeding. Human milk from a bottle was given to 14 and formula or mixed feeding to 15.

Bacteriological studies were positive in nineteen children with the following various organisms in the fecal, gastric, blood and peritoneal specimens: E. Coli 2, Enterobacter 2, Klebsiella 1, Ristella 1. In seven cases, one or several Clostridia were found in the stools (butyricum, perfringens, tertium, difficile). Virological studies were negative at that time. A retrospective epidemiological study was conducted and compared with two control groups. All the information concerning the three groups had been stored previously using the process of data acquisition for computerization.

RESULTS

Twenty-nine were premature babies with 40 percent being less than 2500 g as against 6 and 11 percent respectively in the controls. All the other parameters such as age of the mother, socio-economic status, parity, third trimester hemorrhage, number of antenatal consultations, length and location of antepartum hospitalization, and composition of the medical personnel are not significantly

different. As expected, the only significant differences
were the complications occurring at the delivery and the
neonatal state (only one umbilical catherization in the
enterocolitis group). Treatment against infection during
pregnancy has been more frequently observed in the study
group compared to controls. Summarizing these observations, it may be said that an epidemic occurred abruptly
in a department where no such case had been observed
previously. Term and premature babies were involved
simultaneously.

Administrative and medical measures were taken in
order to stop the epidemic. These included reinforcement
of hygienic measures; closure, cleaning and sterilization
of the neonatal unit and delivery rooms; complete separation between mother and newborn; use of disposable
bottles; and encouragement of breast feeding (from 45 to
80 percent). These measures seemed to be effective since
no further case occurred after May 12th until the month of
September. The origin of the epidemic remained a mystery.

In September 1979, 5 new cases occurred. One of them
was relatively severe and needed surgery due to perforation. After the reopening of the unit in November that
same year, eleven new cases occured; all cases were mild
and recovered.

For psychological reasons, it was necessary to close
the department completely for two months, during which,
both complete disinfection and architectural changes were
made. One measure in particular may have been effective.
All the postnatal rooms were converted to single rooms,
with the baby staying day and night in the same room with
the mother, in order to avoid contact with other infants.
Despite these measures, the epidemic persisted.

As stated above, the virological studies made in May
had been unsuccessful. In September, studies completed in
two other laboratories (Dr. Chany, Hôpital St. Vincent de
Paul, Paris, and Dr. Laporte, National Institute for
Agronomic Research, Grignon) were able to document the
presence of the corona virus in the 4 cases studied. Such
a virus was also observed in 5 of the 11 cases occurring
after the reopening of the unit, and in 6 of the 7 mothers
studied.

DISCUSSION

The seven reasons in favor of implicating the corona
virus are as follows:

(a) Observation of the corona virus by electron micro-
     scope in the feces and digestive tract specimens from
     sick newborn infants. Such an observation is quite
     unusual and is different from the frequent observa-
     tion of the rotavirus in the feces of newborns with
     mild diarrhea.
(b) Culture of the corona virus from the feces of sick
     newborn.
(d) Similarities with enteritis due to the corona virus
     in animals.
(e) Simultaneous occurrence of digestive tract epidemics
     among adults or infants in the Paris area.
(f) Observation of the corona virus in the feces of
     mothers of sick newborns.
(g) Observation of a large number of carriers among the
     nursing and medical staff. There was an overall
     occur- rence of 10 percent of which 3 percent were
     doctors and 7 percent were nurses. Interestingly
     enough, the person in charge of the laundry had also
     been contaminated.

     Although it is clear that no definite proof that the
corona virus is responsible for this specific epidemic, it
does seem a reasonable assumption. This does not mean
that no other organism can be associated with the viral
infection. On the contrary, such an association appears
to be quite probable particularly in the production of
intestinal gas giving rise to the characteristic
radiological signs.

CONCLUSION

     Necrotizing enterocolitis is no longer restricted to
babies' intensive care units. It may occur in maternity
departments. It affects normal term infants as well as
those premature and small for dates.

     Preventive measures are effective to some extent,
particularly isolation of the newborn to the room of their
mothers and also breast feeding. Immunologic protection
of the bowel may encourage normal bacterial colonization.

     It is recommended that when such epidemics do occur,
a rapid exchange of information be organized. Also, a
central register could be established at the IAMANEH
office.

REFERENCES

1. Amiel TC, Lebrun F, Diallo P, Sureau C (1980):
    L'entérocolite ulcéronécrosante du nouveau-né.
    Une épidémie en maternité. _Méd Hyg_ (Genève)
    38:1706-1710.
2. Sureau C (1982): Round table discussion. To be
    published Proceedings of XI Journées de la
    Société Franciase de Médecine Péwrinatale
    Marseille 12-14 Novembre 1981, G. Barrier, Editor,
    Arnette Publishing, Paris.
3. Lebur F, Amiel TC, Sureau C (In Press): L'entéroco-
    lite ulcéronécrosante. Etude de 46 cas survenus
    en maternité.
4. Maria B, Nguyen R, Breart G, Boujard J (1980): Etude
    des facteurs de risques pré et pernataux de
    l'entérocolite ulcéro nécrosante du nouveau-né.
    Méd Hyg (Genèva) 38:1712-1714.
5. Moscovici O, Chany C, Lebon P, Rousset S, Laporte J
    (1980): Association d'infection à corona virus
    avec l'entérocolite hémorragique du nouveau-né.
    C.R. Acad Sci (Paris), 290 Série D:869-872.
6. Sureau C, Amiel TC,m Moscovici O, Lebon P, Laporte J,
    Chany C (1980): Une épidémie d'entérocolites
    ulcéronécrosantes en maternité. Arguments en
    faveur de son origine virale. _Bull Acad Nat Med_
    164:286-293.

VERTICAL TRANSMISSION OF HEPATITIS B VIRUS

AND ITS PREVENTION BY HBIG

T. Kawana and K. Shiraki

Department of Obstetrics and Gynecology
University of Tokyo, Faculty of Medicine
Tokyo, Japan

INTRODUCTION

Research on hepatitis B has been enhanced by the discovery of Australia Antigen by Blumberg in 1964, resulting in the discovery of HB virus (HBV) as well as in the elucidation of its immunological, virological and clinical features. Many Japanese investigators have taken part in this research. Based on data reported by some of the leading Japanese researchers and by our group, the recent progress in the study of vertical transmission of HBV is presented in this paper.

CHARACTERISTICS OF HB VIRUS INFECTION

There are two types of infection of HB virus: transient or acute, and persistent or chronic. The former is an asymptomatic infection and is called acute Hapatitis B; the latter signifies a carrier state called chronic hepatitis characterized by cirrhosis and hepatoma. Usually, the former responds to HB antigen while the latter does not. From the etiological point of view, the former is caused by horizontal transmission of HB virus and the latter mainly by vertical transmission or by horizontal transmission among children under 4 years. The prevalence rate of HBV chronic infection is high (Table 1). Three-fourth of HB carriers are living in the Asia-Oceana region. These data explain why Japanese researchers have investigated HBV.

Table 1. Distribution of HB Virus Carriers From a
          Global Point of View (WHO).

Continent	Percentage
Africa	13.8
Europe	2.9
North America	0.6
Middle South America	1.2
Asia-Oceania	75.7
USSR	5.8
Total	100.0

Table 2. HBs Antigen Prevalence in General Population
          and Pregnant Women of Various Countries.

	Japan	Taiwan	Caucasian
General population	2-3%	15-20%	0.2-0.4%
Pregnant women	2%	16%	0.2-0.4%

Table 3. Comparison of Factors Related to Vertical
          Transmission of HB Virus Among Various Countries.

	Japan	Hong-Kong	Taiwan	Caucasian
HBs carrier in pregnant women	2-3%	6.6%	16%	0.2-0.4%
Prevalence of HBe Ag among HBs Ag carrier mothers	20-30%	49%	43%	25%
Rate of vertical transmission	30%	52%	46%	20%
Carrier infants born to HBe Ag positive carrier mothers	80-90%	84%	75-80%	80%

From the epidemiological study, it has been shown
that HB virus carriers resulted from infection of their
mothers in 30 percent, from their fathers in 20 percent,
and from their siblings or other individuals in the
remaining 50 percent.

The prevalence of HBs Antigen positive carriers, in the general population and pregnant women is shown in Table 2. In pregnant women, almost the same prevalence rate is detectable, as in the general population. In Japan, 2 to 3 percent of pregnant women are HBV carriers, whereas in Taiwan the rate is 16 percent, and in Caucasian countries, it is 0.2 to 0.4 percent, lower than in Japan.

The HBV particles contain three antigen systems which have corresponding antibodies, namely HBs, HBc, and HBe. The clinical significance of these three antigen-antibody systems when detected in the serum may be summarized as follows: HBs in the serum signifies current infection of HBV, while the presence of anti HBs signifies past infection. Low titer of HBc antibody indicates past infection while a high titer means present infection. The third antigen system, HBe, was discovered by Magnius et al in 1972, and is closely related to infectivity of HB virus. For instance, HBs antigen positive serum with HBe (one to a hundred million diluted blood) was infectious when injected to chimpanzees (Fig. 1).

In the vertical transmission of HB virus, these antigen-antibody systems play a role. In a follow-up study of 75 infants born to carrier mothers, 21 became positive for HBs antigen of whom 18 were continuously positive while 3 were only transient. Nine infants developed HBs-antibody. Thus, thirty of the 75 infants, or 40 percent, were infected by HB virus (Fig. 2).

Several risk factors have been proposed in relation to vertical transmission. The first factor shown to be closely related to vertical transmission of HBV is the presence of HBe antigen in carrier mothers resulting in infants having the highest risk. Among infants born to HBe antigent positive carrier mothers, 82 percent developed HBs antigenemia and 14 percent developed HBs antibody, so that a total of 96 percent of infants were infected. On the other hand, among infants born to carrier with HBe antibody, only 6 percent developed HBs antigenemia and 11 percent antibody, thus only 17 percent were infected as seen in Figure 3. Moreover, the important point is that 86 percent of infants born to carrier mothers with HBe antigen became carriers of HB virus, whereas none of infants born to mothers with HBe antibody became carriers.

It is interesting to note that in some countries, the same relationship of HBe antigen with transmissibility of HBV exists. Also, that almost 80 to 90 percent of infants

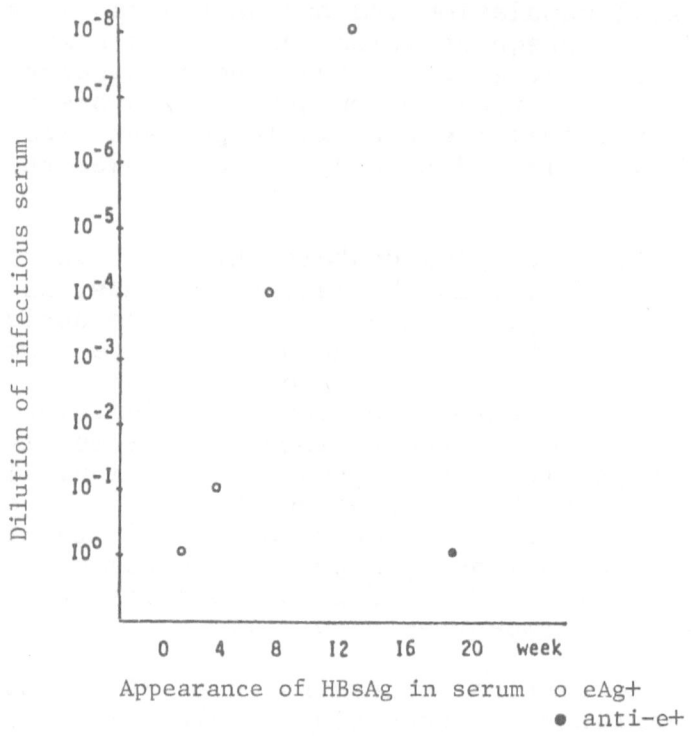

Figure 1.   Infectivity of HBs positive blood to
chimpanzees in relation to HBe antigen-
antibody.

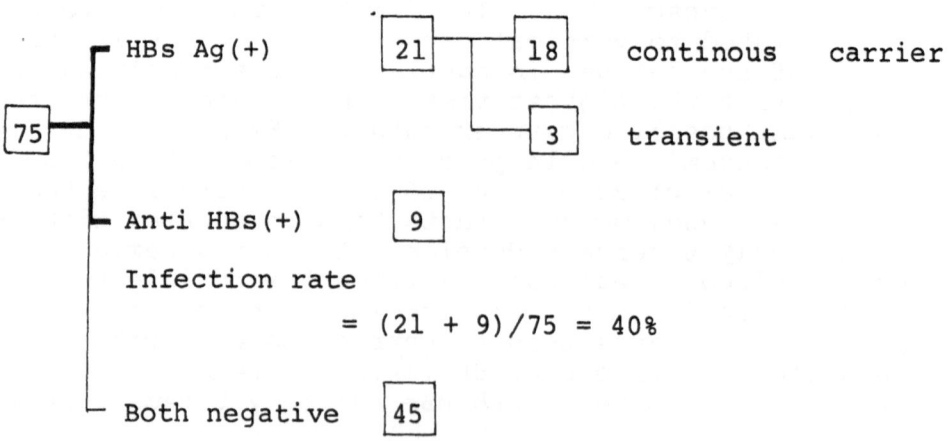

Figure 2.   Follow-up study of 75 infants born to HBV
carrier mothers.

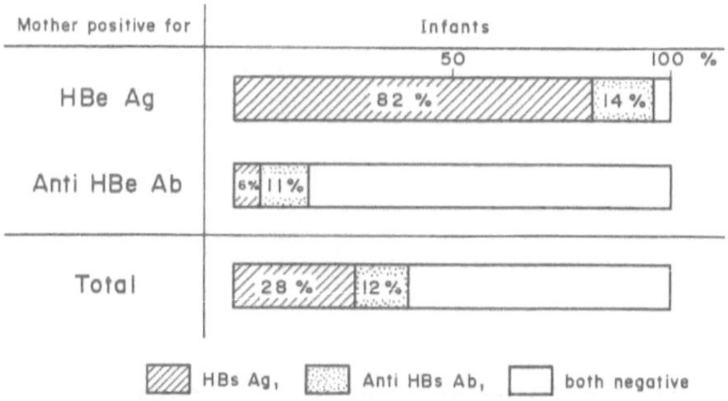

Figure 3.   Outcome of infants born to HBV carrier mother
            positive for HBe antigen or HBe antibody.

born to HBe antigen positive mothers became carriers in
these countries (Table 3).

     As far as age distribution of HBe antigen-antibody
system is concerned, the antigen is dominant in the younger generation (Fig. 4).   This event seems to reflect the
relationship between age of carrier mother at delivery and
incidence of carrier children.   It has been shown that the
older the mother at delivery, the less is the incidence of
carrier children (Fig. 5).

VERTICAL TRANSMISSION

     Some important problems are involved in vertical
transmission of HBV.   First, individuals who are infected
in the perinatal period are prone to develop carrier
state.   Second, some infants develop acute or chronic hepatitis.   Third, about 10 percent of HB carriers have been
shown subsequently to develop chronic hepatitis when they
have grown up;   some of them may develop liver cirrhosis
and still later, in some cases, hepatoma.   Thirty-eight
percent of infants born to HBe antigen positive mothers
developed chronic hepatitis B, while 6 percent of infants
born to HBe antibody positive mothers developed acute
hepatitis B.

     An explanation on the outcome of vertical transmis-
sion has been proposed.   When blood contains a high titer
of HB virus, it may induce immunological tolerance due to
the high dose of antigen.   Therefore, the infected infants
cannot eliminate the HB virus, resulting in chronic persistent infection.   On the other hand, when the mother is
HBe antibody positive, the transmitted dose of HB virus is

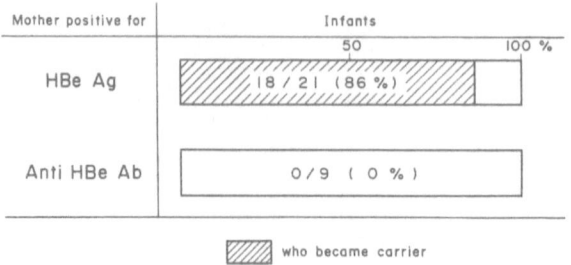

Figure 4. Distribution of cases who became carriers among infected infants.

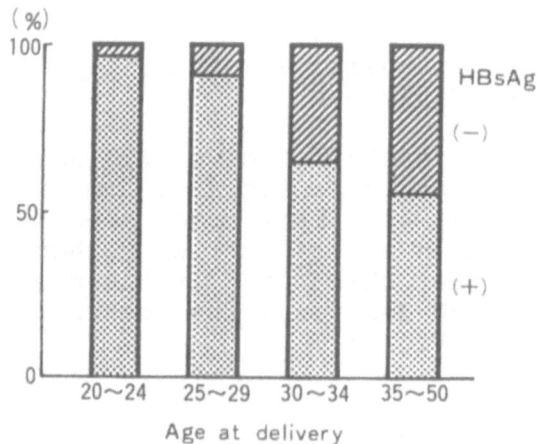

Figure 5. Relationship between age of carrier mothers at delivery and incidence of HBs carrier children.

so low that it may induce immunological response in infected infants resulting not only in elimination of HB virus but also in the development of acute hepatitis B caused by antigen-antibody reaction.

　　Generally speaking, there are three possible routes of the vertical transmission of infectious agents: transplacental, infection in the birth canal, and trans-colostral. As for HB virus, the main route seems to be infection in the birth canal; transplacental infection seems to occur in less than 10 percent, and transcolostral infection seems to be negligible. The following observations support birth canal infection: First, most of the infants became positive for HBs antigen one to three months after birth, suggesting that infection of HB virus occurred during birth, since this period is almost the

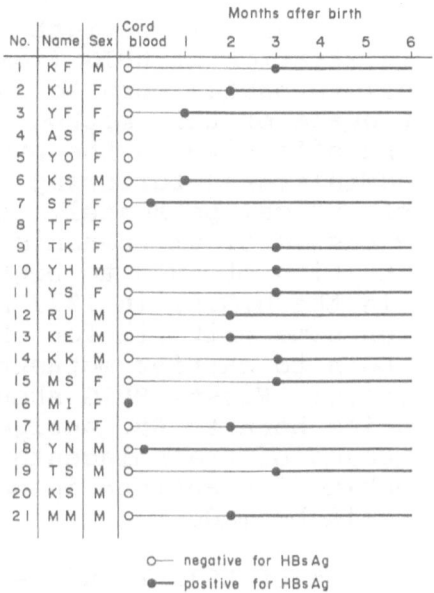

Figure 6.   Time of appearance of HBs antigen in infants after birth.

same as the incubation time in HB virus infection. Second, in more than 90 percent of cases, HBs antigen is not detectable in the cord blood, suggesting that trans- placental infection may occur less frequently. Only three cases became positive at or very soon after delivery, suggestive of transplacen- tal transmission (Fig. 6).

The influence of the type of infant feeding on HBs antigen and antibody was studied. Among 40 infants who were breast fed, eight (20 percent) developed HBs anti- genemia, whereas among 15 non-breastfed infants, four (27 percent) developed HBs antigenemia. From these data, breast feeding is unrelated to development of carrier state.

PREVENTION OF VERTICAL TRANSMISSION

In order to prevent vertical transmission of HB virus, two methods have been proposed. One method is the administration of Interferon to HBe antigen positive carrier mother with the intention of reducing active HB virus. However, this method is not available at present, because adequate amounts of interferon is difficult to

obtain; besides, the effect of interferon on the developing fetus has not been fully investigated. The other
method is the administration of HBIG (immunoglobulin with
high anti HBs titer) to babies born to carrier mother at
delivery. The rationale of this method is that the HBIG
has been shown to be effective in the prevention of acute
Hepatitis B when administered following accidental exposure of HB virus of medical personnel. As for the
prevention of HB virus vertical transmission, a successful
attempt of administration of HBIG to high risk babies have
already been made in the U.S.A. in 1977 by Kohler's group.
Our group has set up some criteria for the administration
of HBIG to babies born to carrier mothers to prevent them
from becoming carriers: First, HBIG should be administered to high risk babies born to HBe antigen positive
mothers; Second, cases of transplacental infection should
be excluded by checking HBs antigen in cord blood; Third,
close follow-up should be made.

The administration of HBIG requires a time sequence:
the first time is within 24 hours after birth followed by
a second dose, 5 days after birth. Thereafter, in order
to prevent horizontal transmission from their mother when
antibody HBs titer falls to 1:4 or less, repeatedly HBIG
is given until the baby is a year old.

The preventive effects of HBIG on vertical transmission of HBV in high risk infants are demonstrated in the
finding that out of 22 treated infants, 20 were free of
HBs antigen. As far as these cases are concerned, HBIG
were thought to be very effective, since 82 percent of
non- treated babies born to carrier mother with HBe antigen developed HBs antigenemia. Other Japanese researchers
also reported the effectiveness of HBIG, showing that in
the treated group, carrier status was found at significantly lower incidence. However, during our long term
follow-up, a serious problem occured: some of the seemingly successful cases later developed HBs antigenemia
after cessation of HBIG. Of nine cases that were followed
for more than 13 months, four cases became carriers (these
were un- successful), two developed HBs antibody (these
were successful), and three were both negative. Two
possible explanation for the unsuccessful cases are
propounded: First, HBIG might have only delayed the
proliferation or the immunological expression of HBV. The
same situation had been demonstrated in the personnel who
had been exposed to HB virus by accident and given HBIG.
Second, horizontal transmission from their mother might
have occurred.

Additional problems involved in HBIG administration for prevention of vertical transmission of HB virus require further investigation. First, how long should it be administered? Second, how can horizontal transmission from carrier mother be prevented? In this regard, one possible solution may be active immunization by HB vaccine after cessation of passive immunization by HBIG. HB vaccine prepared from components of HB virus is now under development and will probably be available in the near future. Third, the most serious problem which seems to be the most difficult to solve is that HBIG cannot be used for cases with transplacental transmission of HB virus, on whom a different mode of treatment should be developed.

The identification of the characteristics of HBV infection and its probable prevention is a step towards the eradication of HB virus. Obstetricians and pediatricians and others who are taking part in maternal and child health care could all contribute towards this goal, which has become of global concern.

CONCLUSION

In Japan, Hepatitis B Virus (HBV) carriers are found in 2 to 3 percent of pregnant women. The vertical transmission of HBV from these mothers to their infants was studied. Among 75 babies born to HBV carrier mothers, 21 babies developed HBs antigenemia one to three months after birth, and 9 babies developed HBs antibody. Therefore, vertical transmission occured in 40 percent (30/75). Since HBe antigen was shown to be closely related to hyperactivity of HBV, relationship between HBe antigen-antibody system and vertical transmission was studied. In 21 out of 22 babies born to HBs carrier mothers (positive for HBe antigen), vertical transmission occurred. It is worthwhile to mention that of these 21 babies, 18 became HBV carrier infants. On the other hand, among 53 babies born to HBV carrier mothers positive for HBe antibody, vertical transmission occurred in 9 (17 percent) infants, none of whom became a carrier. As regards to time and route of infection, about more than 90 percent of affected infants appeared to be infected in the birth canal during birth and the remaining less than 10 percent through transplacental route.

Prevention of vertical transmission in high risk babies treated with hepatitisb B immunoglobulin (HBIG) has been attempted. HBIG was administered to babies born to carrier mothers positive for HBe antigen within 24 hours

of birth, in case HBs antigen was not detected in their
cord blood. The HBIG preparation was administered several
times until was one year old. Among 22 treated cases, 20
did not develop HBs antigenemia by one year old.

However, after cesstion of HBIG administration, 4 out
of 9 babies who were followed for more than one year
developed antigenemia. This phenomenon seems to be caused
either by the horizontal transmission of HBV from their
mother or by the appearance of transplacental transmitted
HBV which has been prevented from reactivation during the
administration of HBIG.

MONITORING INCOMPLETE ABORTION CARE

AT DACCA MEDICAL COLLEGE

S. F. Begum, A. R. Khan, S. Jahan, and
F. A. Jahan

Population Planning Commission and
Fertility Research Program
Dacca Medical College Hospital
Dacca, Bangladesh

INTRODUCTION

Induced and spontaneous abortions are known as global problems of social, health and demographic significance. The issue is increasingly drawing closer attention of health professionals because of the recent awareness about the nature and magnitude of abortion-related problems (1). Consequences of induced abortion now constitute a major cause of death among women of reproductive age in developing countries (2). It is estimated that 4 to 70 percent of all maternal deaths in developing countries are due to complications of induced abortion. In Bangladesh an estimated 7800 women die annually due to such complications (3).

Abortion is defined as termination of gestation before the fetus is viable (usually 28 weeks), and interruption of the normal course of pregnancy subsequent to this is considered a premature birth (4). Termination of gestation or deliberate attempt to do so by human interference is known as induced abortion, and when the same phenomenon occurs unintentionally we call it spontaneous abortion.

While spontaneous abortion basically represents a health problem, the incidence of which is not likely to

vary much between societies, induced abortion represents a
social problem of greater magnitude, and is likely to vary
widely between societies.   Bangladesh is not immune to
tnis problem (5, 6).

Incomplete abortion, either induced outside the hospital or occuring spontaneously, poses increasingly as a
medical care problem for urban hospitals in Bangladesh
(7).   A sizeable fraction of the admissions in the obstetric wards of these hospitals are for treatment of
incomplete abortion.   Inspite of a restricted legal provision, many desperate women in Bangladesh undergo induced
abortion usually performed by unqualified personnel with
unsafe procedure and in clandestine and unsanitary circumstances frequently leading to serious complications (6, 8,
9).   Women even with serious complications do not seek
hospital admission until they are subjected to considerable suffering that cannot be relieved outside the
hospital.   Thus the patients we do see in hospitals only
represent a fraction of what happens in the society.

METHOD AND MATERIALS

During the period May 1977 to April 1978 a total of
1003 cases of complicated abortion were admitted in the
Dacca Medical College Hospital and were treated for
threatened, inevitable, incomplete or missed abortion.
This report presents the socio-demographic profile, pattern of complications, contraceptive practice history and
other clinical and non-clinical experiences of these 1003
women with induced or spontaneous abortions, in a comparative frame.   In this report, induced abortions are
categorized as those cases which were either definitely or
probably induced outside the hospital according to the
patient's own statement.   Of the 1003 patients, 243 (24.2
percent) reported as having deliberately induced the
abortion process and 760 (75.8 percent) were reported as
having spontaneous abortions.   However, there were reasons
beyond the structured questionaire to suggest that an
unknown fraction of the reported spontaneous abortion
cases were in fact induced.

Follow-up data were recorded for 97.0 percent of the
patients.   Data were recorded on standard hospital abortion study forms, which was monitored by the Bangladesh
Fertility Research Programme (BFRP) staff and subsequently
computer analyzed at the International Fertility Research
Program (IFRP), Research Triangle Park, North Carolina,
USA.

RESULTS

Table 1. Socio-demographic Characteristics for Induced
          and Spontaneous Abortion Patients Treated at
          Dacca Medical College in Dacca, Bangladesh.

| | Type of Abortion | | |
	Induced (N=243)	Spontaneous (N=760)	Total (N=1003
Residence			
Urban	56.8	68.8	65.9
Rural	30.0	23.6	25.1
Slum	13.2	7.6	9.0
Age			
<19	2.1	11.5	9.3
20 - 29	36.2	61.5	55.3
30 - 39	50.6	23.7	30.2
40 - 44	11.1	3.3	5.2
Mean	30.5	25.4	26.6
Marital Status			
Single	0.0	0.1	0.1
Married	97.5	99.3	98.9
Formerly married	2.5	0.6	1.0
Patient's Education			
None	84.4	72.8	75.6
1 - 6	8.2	10.9	10.3
7 - 9	3.7	7.2	6.4
10 - 12	3.3	8.0	6.9
13+	0.4	1.1	0.8
Mean	1.1	2.1	1.9

Socio-demographic Characteristic

Table 1 presents the socio-demographic profile of the
induced and spontaneous abortion patients. Nearly two-
thirds of the patients lived in urban areas. A somewhat
higher proportion of spontaneous abortion patients as compared to induced abortion patients (68.8 percent compared
to 56.8 percent) lived in urban areas. A greater percentage of women living in the slum area had induced
abortions (13.2 percent) than those who had spontaneous
abortion (7.6 percent). Nearly all the women (98.9
percent) in this study were married.

Most of the patients (55.3 percent) were in the age
group from 20 to 29 years. The induced abortion group is,

Table 2. Selected Reproductive Characteristics For
          Induced and Spontaneous Abortion Patients
          Treated at Dacca Medical College.

	Type of Abortion		
	Induced (N=243)	Spontaneous (N-760)	Total (N=1003)
Parity			
0	4.1	28.4	22.5
1	2.5	15.7	12.5
2 - 3	11.5	31.8	26.9
4 - 6	53.5	19.5	27.7
7+	28.4	4.6	10.4
Mean	5.4	2.2	3.0
No. of Additional Children Wanted			
0	91.8	23.1	39.1
1	3.5	12.1	10.1
2 - 3	3.0	34.8	27.4
4+	1.7	30.0	23.4
Mean	0.2	2.9	2.3
No. of Previous Induced Abortions			
0	93.5	99.9	98.3
1	4.9	0.1	1.3
2	1.6	0.0	0.4
Mean	0.1	0.0	0.1
No. of Previous Spontaneous Abortions			
0	68.0	70.1	69.6
1	23.0	17.4	18.7
2	5.3	7.5	7.0
3+	3.7	5.0	4.7
Mean	0.5	0.5	0.5
No. of Stillbirths			
0	84.4	89.9	88.5
1	13.6	7.5	9.0
2+	2.0	2.6	2.5
Mean	0.2	0.1	0.2

on the average, about five years older than the
spontaneous abortion group, with the mean ages of 30.5
years and 25.4 years respectively.

Overall, three-fourths of the women (75.6 percent) did not have any education. The mean educational attainment was 1.1 years for the induced abortion group and 2.1 years for the spontaneous abortion group. Compared to this low educational attainment of only 1.1 years for the seekers of indigenous abortion service, the acceptors of modern pregnancy termination services as reported from the Mohammadpur Model Clinic, had an average of 8.5 years of formal schooling (10, 11).

Reproductive Characteristics

The induced abortion patients had on the average 5.4 live births as compared to only 2.2 live births for the spontaneous abortion patients. Presuming 15 years of age as the beginning of reproductive period for both groups of patients, the induced abortion patients had an average 5.4 live births in the 15.5 years, as compared to 2.2 live births in 10.4 years for the spontaneous abortion patients. Thus the women in the induced abortion group were subject to a large family burden, which apparently made them feeling desperate not to have the next birth. The underlying patient motive is also reflected in the desire for additional children, showing that the induced abortion patients wanted an average of only 0.2 additional children, as compared to 2.9 for the spontaneous abortion patients. As would be expected, the mean parity in both groups increases with advancing age. However, the mean parity is higher for induced abortion patients than spontaneous abortion patients in each age group.

Overall, 6.5 percent of induced abortion patients and only 0.1 percent of spontaneous abortion patients reported having induced abortion previously. Majority of patients (69.6 percent), and nearly equal proportion in both groups, reported having no previous spontaneous abortions. The mean number of previous spontaneous abortions was 0.5 for both groups. One or more stillbirth was reported by 15.6 percent of induced abortion patients and 10.1 percent of spontaneous abortion patients. The mean number of stillbirths was not much different in both groups (0.2 for the induced abortion group compared to 0.1 for the spontaneous abortion group).

Abortion Status at Admission

A large majority of the patients (79.4 percent) were categorized as having incomplete abortion at the time of admission, and the remaining patients were categorized as having inevitable abortion in 9.8 percent, threatened

Table 3.   Admission Complications By Type of Abortion For
           Induced and Spontaneous Abortion Patients
           Treated at Dacca Medical College.

Major Complications at Admission	Type of Abortion		
	Induced (N=243)	Spontaneous (N=760)	Total (N=1003)
Sepsis/pelvic infection	35.8	2.2	10.4
Fever	23.0	0.4	5.9
Uterine perforation (Suspected)	1.6	0.0	0.4
Cervical laceration	2.1	0.0	0.5
Excessive blood loss	6.6	13.4	11.8
Serious hypotension	2.5	0.7	1.1
No major complication	28.4	83.3	69.9

abortion in 7.8 percent, complete abortion in 2.3 percent
and missed abortion in 0.7 percent of cases. Pregnancy
duration was estimated as 12 weeks or less in 61.4 percent
of the patients. The mean duration of pregnancy was longer for the spontaneous abortion patients (13.9 weeks) than
the induced abortion patients (11.5 weeks). A plausible
reason for this difference may be that in case of induced
abortion the gestational age is subject to a limitation by
the non-availability of a suitable technology for termination of pregnancy after 12 weeks of gestation. But the
gestational age in case of spontaneous abortion is not
subject to similar limitation.

Complications Upon Admissions

     A relatively greater proportion of spontaneous
abortion patients (83.3 percent) than induced abortion
patients (28.4 percent) did not have any major complication at the time of admission (Table 3). A large
proportion of women with induced abortion were admitted
with sepsis or pelvic infection (35.8 percent) and with
above normal temperatures (23.0 percent). The most frequent complication among spontaneous abortion patients was
excessive bleeding (13.4 percent). The significantly
greater incidence of complications (specially sepsis) in

Table 4. Method of Initiation of Abortion Process as Per
         Statement of Induced Abortion Patients Treated
         at Dacca Medical College.

Method of Initiation	Induced Abortion	
	Number	Percent
Chemical installation	1	0.4
Insertion of solid objects	46	18.9
Oral abortification	189	77.8
Dilation and/or evacuation	3	1.2
Other	3	1.2
Total	242*	100.0

One case excluded due to missing data

the induced abortion group is an obvious consequence of
the unsanitary procedure they had. In most of these cases
the patient was admitted with an already gross septic
condition.

Abortion Procedure Prior to Hospital Admission

     Table 4 shows the indigenous methods of induction of
abortion. The most frequently used method to induce abortion as per statement of the patients, was the intake of
oral abortifacients (77.8 percent). In 18.9 percent cases, solid objects were introduced through the cervix to
termi- nate the pregnancy. There was however reason to
believe that in an unknown proportion of cases this information could have been misrepresented. Women would be
more hesitant to admit a physical intervention than any
oral medication, because physical intervention is more
likely to be perceived as legally inappropriate. The
abortion procedure was initiated by a non-medical person
in about 54.7 percent of the cases. In many instances
the non-medical person was the mother-in-law of the
patient.

Abortion Treatment During Admission

     The treatment of the largest proportion of cases
consisted of curettage with antibiotic therapy. Sharp or
suction currettage was used in 82.3 percent of cases and

antibiotic was given in 99.1 percent of cases of induced
abortion cases. Considering the fact that induced abortion patients were all in either gross septic condition or
were potentially infected, the use of antibiotics was
almost universal. The procedure was repeated for 2.5
percent of the induced abortion and for 13.1 percent of
the spontaneous abortion patients, mainly due to retained
products of conception. A second procedure was also required mainly for patients with longer period of gestation
and for the spontaneous abortion patients who had longer
menstrual delay. Slightly over half of the patients (50.6
percent) were given only analgesia. General anesthesia
was used in a relatively higher proportion of induced
abortion cases (35.3 percent) than spontaneous abortion
cases (14.9 percent). Blood transfusion of 250 ml or more
were given to 22.2 percent of the induced abortion
patients and to 22.9 percent of the spontaneous abortion
patients. The mean time spent in the operating room was
38.1 minutes for the induced abortion and 41.0 minutes for
the spontaneous abortion patients.

A significantly lower percentage of spontaneous
abortion (22.1 percent) than induced abortion patients
(99.2 percent) were given antibiotics therapeutically,
while a significantly higher percentage of spontaneous
abortion (22.4 percent) than induced abortion (3.7 percent) patients were given oxytocics for therapeutic
purpose.

Mortality Risk

The overall mortality rate for these cases was 18 per
1000 admissions, and was primarily due to complications
present at the time of admission. The mortality rate was
49 per 1000 admissions for the induced abortion patients
and 6 per 1000 admissions for the spontaneous abortion
patients.

Six deaths which occurred among patients with
spontaneous abortions were not septic at the time of admission. In each of these cases the patient had excessive
blood loss with severe hypotension, and the cause of
death was listed as hypovolemic shock. Except in the case
of one patient who died during the procedure, all other 5
patients died before any procedure could be administered.
One of the six patients who died had an ectopic pregnancy
of eight week's gestation. The patient had internal
bleeding in the tube without any external bleeding. Another patient, 14 weeks pregnant with severe anemia, had

been bleeding for two days. A third patient, 18 weeks pregnant, also had two days of bleeding prior to admission. Two of the deaths occurred among patients 20 weeks pregnant, one of whom had one day of bleeding, and the other had eight days of bleeding prior to hospitalization. The sixth patient was 22 weeks pregnant with 15 days of bleeding prior to coming to the hospital.

Twelve patients died from among the induced abortion patients (4.9 percent). These patients had septic abortions at the time of admission and all died of septic shock. In one of these 12 cases, abortion was initiated by a nurse/midwife and in another, by a physician, and in all the other 10 cases by a non-medical person. Insertion of solid objects was the method of initiation in all but one case. The physician used injection of synlacinon by intravenous drip. Except in the patient whose abortion was initiated by the physician and who died after the procedure was given in the hospital, all the patients died before any procedure could be administered. For these 12 maternal deaths, the duration of pregnancy ranged from 8 to 20 weeks, and the time duration from onset of bleeding to admission ranged from 3 to 45 days.

There was no real difference in the duration of pregnancy and in the time from onset of bleeding to admission, between patients who died and those who were discharged recovered. Patients who died had pregnancy duration from 8 to 26 weeks and time from onset of bleeding to admission ranged from zero to 45 days. Patients who lived had pregnancy duration from 4 to 27 weeks, and time from onset of bleeding to admission ranged from 1 to 90 days. Among patients who lived, there were some women for whom the total number of days from onset of bleeding to admission was reported to be longer than the pregnancy duration. This may have been due to problems with estimating gestational age, poor patient recall or coding error.

One should remember that not all cases of induced abortion are hospitalized. It is likely that relatively more complicated and serious cases would seek admission. The above death rate therefore represents the mortality risk of only the hospitalized induced abortion cases.

The total duration of hospital stay for most women (78.9 percent) was two to three nights. However, duration of hospital stay was significantly shorter for the spontaneous abortion patients.

Table 5. Contraceptive Practice Prior to Abortion (within
          a month) and After Discharge at Follow-up Time.

Types of Contraceptive Method	Before		After	
	Induced (N=243)	Spontaneous (N=760)	Induced (N=227)	Spontaneous (N=747)
None	39.5	82.8	4.0	61.4
Oral	34.2	6.7	77.1	34.5
Condom	26.3	10.3	–	–
Sterilization	–	0.1	18.9	3.7
IUD	–	–	–	0.1
Injection	–	0.1	–	–
Others	–	–	–	0.1
Total	100.0	100.0	100.0	100.0

Number of missing observation = 29

Follow-up Complications

     At follow-up, two patients had only fever requiring
antibiotics. These patients were not re-admitted to the
hospital. Fourteen patients were readmitted from 1 to 6
nights because of complications such as bleeding, retained
products of conception and/or fever in spite of treatment
with antibiotics. Except for one patient with retained
products of conception for whom no treatment was recorded,
all were treated by using sharp or suction curettage.
Patients with shorter gestations were mainly the ones with
retained products at follow-up. An early pregnancy is
more easily missed than a late one.

Pre- and Post- Abortion Contraceptive Practice

     Contraceptive practice status in the month before
admission and at follow-up after discharge from hospital
for both induced and spontaneous abortion patients were
studied and summarized in Table 5. Among the induced
abortion patients 60.5 percent practiced contraception in
the past, as against only 17.2 percent among the spontaneous abortion patients. This past contraceptive practice
rate in the induced abortion group is comparable to the
past contraceptive practice rate found among the acceptors

of pregnancy termination and MR in Mohammadpur Model
Clinic, which were about 60 percent and 68 percent respectively (10, 11). The past contraceptive practice among
nduced abortion patients is considerably higher than the
known rate of contraceptive practice among urban women,
which was estimated at 19.5 percent by Bangladesh Fertility Survey (12). Thus many of the women in the induced
abortion group had already demonstrated their intention to
avoid the last pregnancy and consequently took steps to
terminate the same. Occurrence of pregnancy despite high
rate of contraceptive practice also reflects poor
effectiveness.

The post-abortion contraceptive practice was significantly higher than the pre-abortion rates, particularly
among the induced abortion group. Ninety-six percent of
induced abortion patients, as compared to only 38.6 percent of spontaneous abortion patients, were found to have
accepted contraceptives at follow-up. This indicates that
after having experienced an unwanted pregnancy, women are
likely to be more careful in their reproductive behavior.
Relatively low practice rate among spontaneous abortion
group, both pre and post abortion, is a testimony of lack
of motivation to prevent pregnancy. The frequency of use
of different methods may perhaps reflect the popularity of
individual methods. It is also noticed that after the
traumatic experience of suffering from the consequences of
induced abortion, women tend to choose more effective and
preferably female method, which may indicate that they
wanted to assume the responsibility of contraceptive protection in their own hands rather than leaving the same to
their husbands. Before abortion, about a third (34.2 percent) of the induced abortion patients used oral pill and
little over a fourth (26.3 percent) used condom. After
abortion, 77.1 percent of these women favored the use of
oral pill and none was for condom. The acceptance of oral
pills has also increased sharply among the spontaneous
abortion patients, from 6.7 percent before admission to
34.5 percent after. About one-fifth (18.9%) of the women
in the induced abortion group accepted sterilization.

DISCUSSION

In this study, the patients with induced abortions
were older and had more children than the spotaneous
abortion patients. A higher percentage of spontaneous
abortion patients wanted additional children. This is
expected since they had fewer children. Also most of them
refused contraception following the procedure, whereas

most of the induced abortion patients accepted it. While
sepsis and infection was the most frequent complication
among the induced abortion patients, excessive blood loss
was most common among spontaneous abortion patients. This
determined largely the pattern of treatment and trend and
cause of mortality. Sharp or suction curettage was used
in mose cases in both groups. Antibiotic use was almost
universal among induced abortion patients.

A third of the women who had induced abortion reported that they were using oral contraceptives during the
month of conception. The fact that they resorted to
induced abortion indicates that their pregnancies were
unwanted.   A question arises as to why such a high percentage of women who wished to avoid pregnancy and who
were reportedly using an effective contraceptive method
became pregnant. They may have been taking pills incor-
rectly, may have run out of supplies, or may have stopped
taking pills due to experienced or feared side effects.
The provider should attempt to determine the reason for
this high rate of unwanted pregnancy among this group, and
take steps to improve patient education or other aspects
of contraceptive services to ameliorate the problem.

There were 18 deaths in this study, which is a very
high number. However, these deaths were due to severe
complications at admissions. It appears that the procedures used in the hospital to treat the patients are quite
safe and effective without the use of general anesthesia.

CONCLUSION

A method of monitoring care for induced and spontaneous abortions is exemplified in this study. As a result,
one is able to evaluate the magnitude of health care
problems arising from incomplete abortion admissions in
hospitals, thus appropriate health and medical care policies for the management and prevention of threatened,
incurable and incompete abortions, are formulated.

REFERENCES

1. Potts M et al (1977): In: Abortion, Cambridge
       University Press, p. 2
2. Liskin LS (1980): Complications of abortion in
       developing countries. Population Reports Series
       F, No. 7.
3. Measham AR et al (1981): Complications from induced

abortion in Bangladesh related to types of
practitioners and methods, and impact on mortality.
<u>Lancet</u>, 8213:1199-202

4. Krupp MA et al (1976): <u>Current medical diagnosis and
    treatment</u>. Lange Medical Publications,
    California, p. 461.

5. Hassan S (1976): Should abortion be legalized?
    Desperate women seek quack's help. <u>The Bangladesh
    Times</u> December 13-14.

6. Anonymous (1977): Abortion (in Bengali). <u>Weekly
    Bichitra</u>, Dacca, July 22.

7. Begum SF et al (1978): A study of 1003 induced and
    spontaneous abortion patients treated at Dacca
    Medical College, Dacca, Bangladesh. <u>BFRP
    Technical Report</u>, No. 8.

8. Burhanuddin AFM (1974): Abortion as a measure of
    population planning and its relevance for
    Bangladesh. <u>Int J Gyn Obstet</u>, 12:93-100.

9. Director of FP Evaluation Division (1975):
    Memorandum. Center for Disease Control, August 6,
    p. 37-42.

10. Khan AR et al (1977): Pregnancy termination by vacumn
    aspiration and D & C for 344 patients at Model
    Clinic, Mohammadpur, Dacca. <u>BFRP Technical
    Report</u>, No. 3.

11. Kahn AR et al (1977): Menstrual regulation services
    in Bangladesh: Model clinic experience. <u>BFRP
    Technical Report</u>, No. 6.

12. Anonymous (1978): <u>World fertility survey, Bangladesh
    fertility survey</u>. Population Control and Family
    Planning Division, December.

STUDY ON THE ONSET OF THE FIRST OVULATION

DURING THE PUERPERIUM

R. Okai, T. Fukuiya, Y. Kanakura, M. Morisada,
S. Kawakami, T. Takahashi, and R. Iizuka

Department of Obstetrics and Gynecology
School of Medicine, Keio University
Tokyo, Japan

INTRODUCTION

There is no sufficient data on the physiology of women in postpartum as compared to that of pregnant women because of less opportunities of periodic check-ups of mothers in the postpartum period. Therefore, although various studies have been made on the reappearance of ovulation in postpartum (1-7), these are rather fragmentary and no report is available dealing with the correlation between the general physical condition and the process of resumption of ovulation. This paper is an attempt to study the pattern and process of reappearance of postpartum ovulation.

MATERIALS AND METHODS

Endocrinological studies in postpartum women include diencephalon, pituitary and ovary. In this study, we used the following observations:

(a) The basal body temperature (BBT) in 146 cases after delivery until the first ovulation in postpartum;
(b) The correlation between the general physical condition (body weight, anemia, galactorrhea) and the changes of prolactin levels in the course of regaining ovulations; and
(c) The LH-RH tests, and changes of prolactin levels in the course of resuming ovulations in postpartum.

Table 1.   First Menstruation and Reappearance of Ovulation
           in Non-lactators Postpartum.

Postpartum Days	0-28	29-56	57-84	85-112	113-140	Total
First Menstruation						
No. of Cases	0	36	12	12	9	66
Percent	0	54.5	18.2	18.2	9.1	100
Reappearance of Ovulation						
No. of Cases	0	14	34	12	6	66
Percent	0	21.2	51.5	18.2	9.1	100

Table 2.   First Menstruation and Reappearance of Ovulation
           in Lactators, Postpartum.

Lactating Period Days	0-28	29-56	57-84	85-112	113+	Total/ Average
Number of Cases	30	14	16	12	8	80
First Menstruation						
Average Days	59.8	61.0	98.5	100.2	178.7	81.0
Reappearance of Ovulation						
Average Days	61.9	82.5	113.0	143.3	171.0	96.5

RESULTS

Nursing Condition and Reappearance of Ovulation and
Menstruation in Postpartum

        The average period from delivery until the reappear-
ance of ovulation for mothers who did not breast feed was
76 days, ranging from 56 days (8 weeks) to 84 days (12
weeks), representing 21.2 percent and 73 percent of the
women respectively (Table 1). The shortest period was 36
and the longest was 186 days. The average period til the
reappearance of menstruation was 67.2 days.

        The average period from the delivery to the re-
appearance of ovulation and menstruation in postpartum for
mothers who breast fed was 96.5 and 81.0 days respectively
(Table 2). The average period till the reappearance of
ovulation and menstruation grouped according to period of
breast feeding indicates that the longer the period of
breast feeding, the longer it took for the reappearance of

Table 3.   Relation Between Age and Average Days For
Reappearance of Ovulation in Postpartum.

	Non-Lactators		All Cases	
	Less than 34	Over 34	Less than 34	Over 34
Number of Cases	44	22	108	38
Average Days	72.6	75.0	93.7	88.9
(M ± S.E.)	±8.2	±10.6	±7.1	±8.5

ovulation or menstruation. The first menstrual cycle in
postpartum was found ovulatory in 38.5 percent of the
total.

Mother's Age and First Ovulation in Postpartum

Investigations on the relationship between maternal
age and the number of days elapsed til the first ovulation
in postpartum was made by dividing the mothers into two
groups: one group whose age was less than 34, and the
other over 34 (Table 3). It was revealed that regardless
of breast feeding or not, the younger group of mothers had
reappearance of ovulation at shorter intervals than the
older group (34 and above). In other words, the younger
group showed shorter recovery period of the ovulatory
function.

Method of Delivery and Initial Ovulation in Postpartum

The first ovulation in postpartum appeared approximately two weeks earlier in the group with cesarean
section than in the group who had transvaginal deliveries
(Table 4). This difference is attributable to the high
rate of bottle feeding among mothers delivered by cesarean
section.

Maternal Obesity and First Ovulation In Postpartum

The effect of change of body weight on postpartum
ovulation is significant. There are women who increase
their body weight at a fairly high rate at each pregnancy.
Those women who are obese had a delay in the onset of initial ovulation in postpartum. Thus, we consider increased
body weight at postpartum one of the important factors, in
addition to the effects of nursing, as conditions affecting the onset of ovulation. Thin women were less affected
(Table 5).

Table 4.   Postpartum Reappearance of Ovulation in
           Vaginal and Cesarean Section Delivery.

	Non-Lactators		All Cases	
	Days of Onset of Ovulation (M + S.E.)	No. of Cases	Days of Onset of Ovulation (M + S.E.)	No. of Cases
Cesarean section	65.7 $\pm$ 15.9	10	68 $\pm$ 9.6	18
Trans-vaginal	79.9 $\pm$ 7.1	56	90.5 $\pm$ 5.4	128

Table 5.   Postpartum Reappearance of Ovulation in Relation
to Maternal Body Weight.

	Obese (days)	Normal (days)	Thin (days)
Lactators	224	154	175
Non-lactators	126	84	91

Table 6.   Anemia and Postpartum Reappearance of Ovulation.

	Non-Lactators		All Cases	
Hemoglobin Value 4th day Postpartum	Less 9.0 g/dl	Over 9.0 g/dl	Less 9.0 g/dl	Over 9.0 g/dl
Number of Cases	12	54	32	114
Days of Onset of first Ovulation (M $\pm$ S.E.)	105.8 $\pm$21.4	69.9 $\pm$5.5	114.8 $\pm$13.9	86.0 $\pm$5.7

Anemia and Postpartum Reappearance of Ovulation

        Markedly anemic women showed a delay in the onset
of initial ovulation in postpartum (Table 6).   This may be
a phenomenon caused by one of the factors under general
physical condition that influence ovulation.   Most of the
anemic women showed poor lactation.

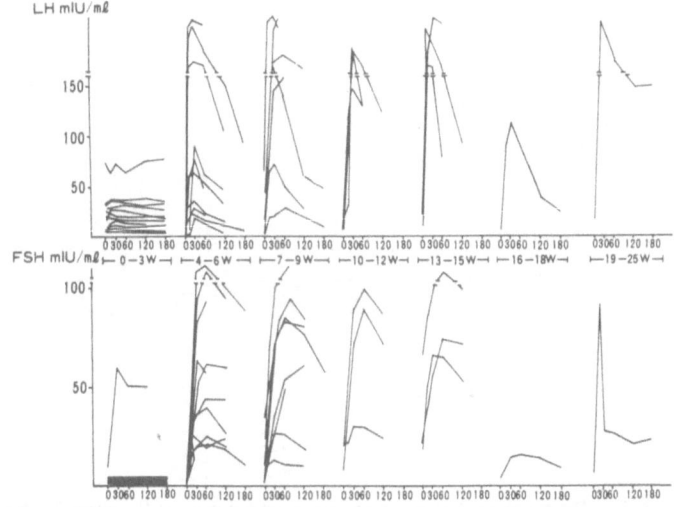

Figure 1.   LH-RH test in postpartum.

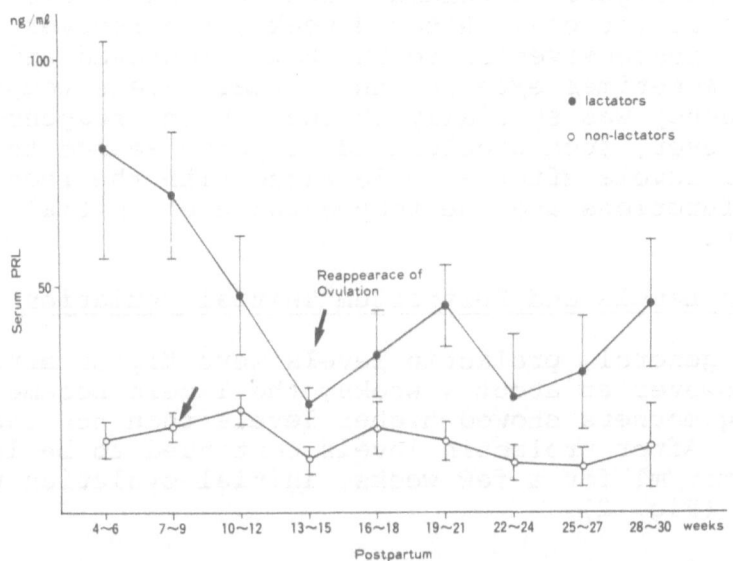

Figure 2.   Serum levels of prolactin (PRL) in postpartum.

LH-RH Test for Postpartum Women

Figure 1 summarizes the results of LH-RH test administered to postpartum women. No response was observed until the 3rd week to both LH and FSH at which time LH

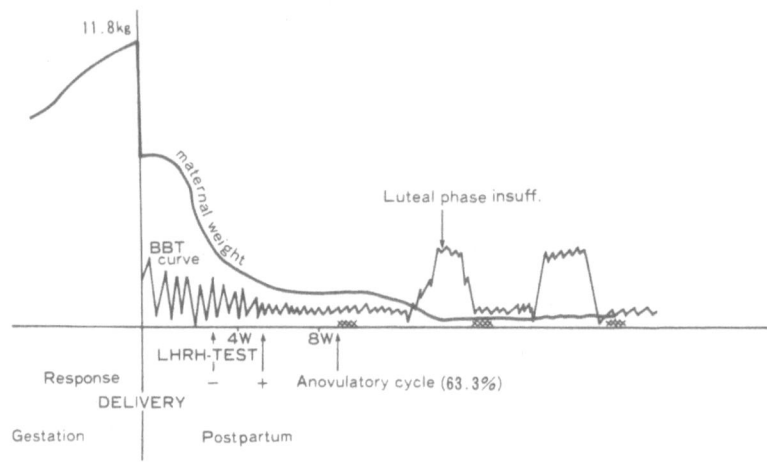

Figure 3.   Postpartum reappearance of ovulation and
            maternal weight reduction.

levels were higher in general than the FSH levels in all
cases except for one. After 4 weeks, the recovery of
pituitary responsiveness to LH-RH was improved and the
response sometimes exceeded the normal levels temporarily.
This tendency was specially obvious in the response to
FSH. However, such accelerated response seemed to return
to normal levels after a while along with the recovery of
ovarian functions and the reappearance of initial
ovulation.

Prolactin Levels and Postpartum Initial Ovulation

        In general, prolactin levels were higher after deli-
very; however at about 4 weeks, the levels became lower.
Lactating mothers showed higher levels than non-lactating
mothers. After prolactin levels continued to be lower
than 30 miv/ml for a few weeks, initial ovulation was
observed (Fig. 2).

BBT Curve in Postpartum

        To confirm that the reappearance of ovulation serves
as one of the indicators of ovarian function recovery, we
made studies into the correlation between the reappearance
of ovulation and maternal body weight alterations on 110
women by keeping the patterns of the basal body temperature (BBT). Correlation of the reappearance stage of
ovulation on BBT and body weight alterations (which are
compared with those of pregestational period) are shown in

Figure 3. By analyzing this figure, we learn the general trend that re-appearance of ovulation after delivery coincides with the time when body weight returns to their respective pre-gestational level. Moreover, it was observed that the reappearance of ovulation was sooner among those who recovered normal body weight. Those who were obese or emaciated in postpartum showed delay in recovery of ovarian function. Another characteristic found was that the first menstruation in postpartum is anovulatory.

CONCLUSION

        The pattern and process of postpartum ovulation as assessed primarily by means of basal body termprature and LH-RH test in 66 non-lactators and 80 lactating women is characterized by the following:

        (a) The average onset of ovulation is delayed when lactation continues over 4 weeks.
        (b) In general, the first menstruation in post-partum is anovulatory.
        (c) The onset of the first ovulation is delayed in obese and anemic mothers.
        (d) LH level regains its normal range during the 3rd week.
        (e) Pituitary response to LH-RH is not recognized until the 4th week postpartum.
        (f) Ovulation is delayed when prolactin levels are high.

REFERENCES

1. Kawakami S, Iizuka R et al (1977): Alteration of maternal body weight in pregnancy and postpartum. Keio J Med, 26:53-62.
2. Kawakami S, Iizuka R et al (1971): Study of the secondary sterility with the alteration in female body weight. Jpn J Fert and Steril, 16:4.
3. Kawakami S (1969): Study on the reproductive function of obese female with special reference to estrogen metabolism. Jpn J Fert and Steril, 14:4.
4. Fukunaga T, Iizuka R et al (1980): Study on hyper-prolactinemic anovulatory syndromeandtreatment with Bromocriptine. Acta Obstet Gyn Jpn, 33:No. 2.
5. Kawakami S, Fukuiya T, Iizuka R (1980): Study on the reproductive function of obese female. Proc First Congress of Obesity.

6. Kawakami S, Fukuiya T, Iizuka R (1981): Women in
      postpartum and anemia. <u>Obstet Gyn Practice</u>,
      30:No.30.
7. Ko T (1974): Study on the onset of first ovulation
      during the puerperium. <u>Jpn J Fert Steril</u>, 19:4.

SMOKING AND REPRODUCTION

R. T. Ravenholt

Director, World Health Surveys
Centers for Disease Control
Rockville, Maryland, U. S. A.

INTRODUCTION

Wise elders intuitively knew that smoking was a harmful practice (1, 2), and their apprehension and general disapproval helped constrain this practice by pregnant women until the twentieth century. But during this century, the combination of intense commercial promotion of cigarette smoking and inadequate measurement of its harmful effects, resulted in women adopting the habit of smoking so generally and enthusiastically that by mid-century it was viewed as ordinary behavior - even if the woman was pregnant (2, 3).

Yet, when subjected to actual measurement of pregnancy outcome, severe deleterious effects associated with smoking upon fetal development and survival are readily discernible - specially the greater losses of fetuses (3), with consequent reduction in the proportion of live born male offspring (4, 5), the marked reduction in average birth weight of infants (2-5), and the many more subtle impairments of the health and development of children (3). But despite the now overwhelming evidence of ill effects associated with smoking during pregnancy (3), this practice has continued and even increased during recent decades (2), and there is urgent need for all who attend this First International Congress on Maternal and Neonatal Health to promulgate a number of simple principles and facts on smoking and health to women throughout the world.

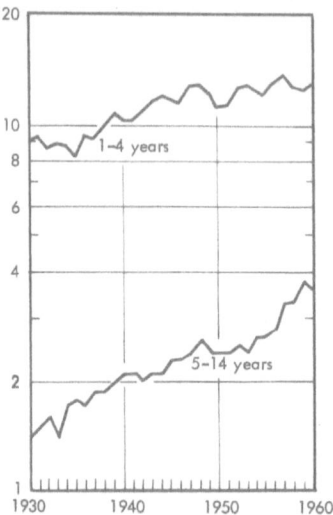

Figure 1.   Congenital malformation mortality, United
            States, ages 1 to 4 and 5 to 14, from 1930
            to 1960.

PRINCIPLES OF CIRCULATING MUTAGENS FROM SMOKING

        When optimal gametes combine to form an optimal
zygote and the resultant organism develops in an optimal
intrauterine environment, the result is a healthy newborn
infant. But there are many deleterious agents in the
general and uterine environments which may assail germ
cells and the developing organism and deviate cells from
their primeval purpose (6). These environmental agents
known to deviate heritable cellular characteristics from
optimal normal are <u>mutagens</u> - ionizing radiation,
certain chemicals, and viruses - with capacity for
increasing heritable differences among cell populations of
tissues (7).

        Many carcinogenic agents were identified in tobacco
smoke by earlier animal assay methods of measurement (8,
9, 11), and recent application of newly-developed short
term tests of mutagenicity has demonstrated that a high
proportion of these carcinogenic compounds are mutagens
(9). But the most notable mutagen identified in tobacco
smoke remains the radioisotope, Polonium 210, a volatile
alpha particle emitter and a most powerful contact mutagen
(10), which has been consistently identified in tobacco
smoke in the respiratory mucosa and urine of smokers (2,
11). Transport of such mutagenic agents from the respira-

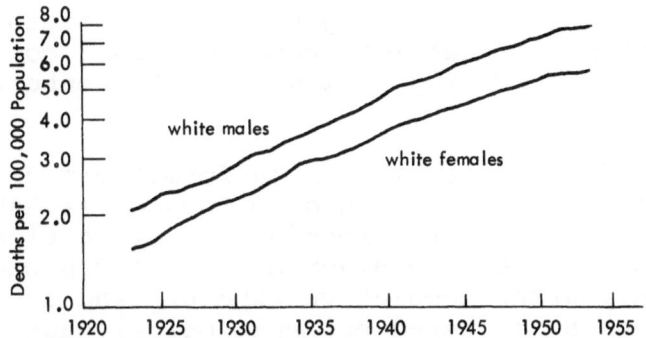

Figure 2a.   Leukemia mortality trends, all ages, United
             States, 1921 to 1955.

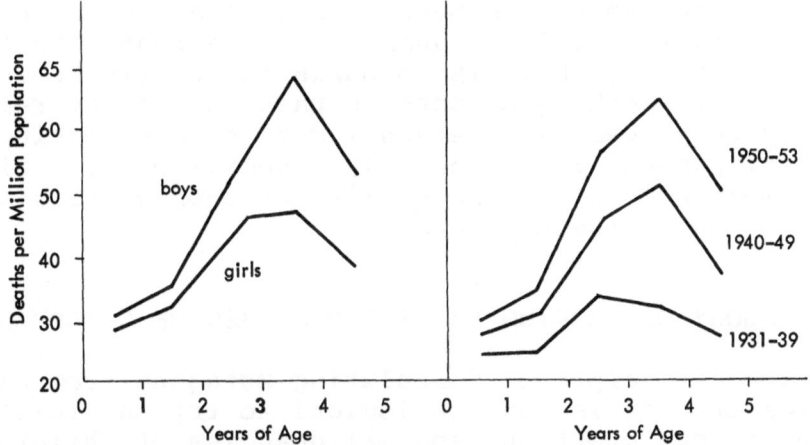

Figure 2b.   Childhood leukemia mortality by age, sex,and
             time.   Children under 5 years, England and
             Wales, 1931 to 1953.

tory tract to the urine necessarily occurs via the blood
stream, and germ cells as well as somatic cells are
inescapably exposed to the blood-borne mutagens.

     Likewise the embryo and fetus are exposed to damage
by mutagens and other harmful substances entering the
circulation of pregnant women who smoke (4, 5).   Thus,
inhalation of smoke exposes the entire body of the smoker
- every tissue and cell, including uterine contents - to
genetic damage analogous to that suffered by radiologists
and others chronically exposed to X-rays and other kinds
of ionizing radiation (12).

     Is it, then, any wonder that childhood diseases of

genetic aberration i.e., congenital malformations, leukemia, and other malignancies, have increased concurrently
with the rise in smoking during the 20th century (Figures
1 and 2)?

How much of this rise in malformations and malignancies can justly be ascribed to tobacco is unknown.
Circulatory mutagens from smoking are symmetrical systemic
poisons; and because the diverse ill effects become discernible only after cumulative exposure and long latent
intervals, on a cluttered epidemiological base, the probable contribution of smoking thereto has thus far largely
eluded measurement. But because it is known that tobacco
smoke contains mutagens, that these are absorbed through
the pulmonary circulation and circulated throughout the
body, and that there has been a large increase in congenital malformations and malignancies concurrent with the
smoking pandemic, there is no basis for public health
complacency. Smoking by persons past the age of reproduction may be viewed as a personal matter, but smoking by
potential parents is inescapably a social matter, with
large implications for the quality of reproduction and the
health of future generations.

EPIDEMIOLOGY OF SMOKING-RELATED DISEASES OF CHILDREN

The "Principle of Circulating Mutagens from Smoking"
dictates that it is just as logical to try and relate
congenital malformations and malignancies of children to
the smoking experience of mothers and other progenitors,
as it is to relate these conditions to exposures to
diagnostic and therapeutic X-rays, nuclear explosions,
drugs, and other environmental hazards.

The fact that a large and progressive increase in
congenital malformations and childhood leukemia occurred
concurrently with the great increase in smoking by women
during this century (Fig. 1, 2) makes it imperative that
the possible role of smoking in the causation of these
diseases be thoroughly studied. Ideally, such studies
should measure the prenatal exposure of the child to
maternal smoking, the preconceptual smoking experience of
both parents, the smoking experience of grandparents and
other progenitors, and the non-smoking mutagenic
experience of all concerned.

However, many of these data are unobtainable and so

fully comprehensive studies are not feasible. But because
smoking is ordinarily the dominant source of mutagenesis
for smokers, as measured by longevity and mortality patterns (11, 13) and the Polonium 210 content of tobacco
smoke - which may expose smokers to as much as 200 rems
per average lifetime (16) - studies focusing mainly upon
fetal and parental smoking experience relative to disease
occurrence may yield valuable findings.

Therefore, an attempt was made by the author and
coworkers (5,6) some years ago to measure by careful
quantitation of parental smoking experience the effects of
smoking upon reproduction generally (Fig. 3) and the possible contribution of smoking to congenital malformations
and childhood leukemia in Seattle. Data were obtained by
public health nurse-telephone interviews from mothers of
2,023 infants born in Seattle during 1964; from mothers of
164 children hospitalized with diverse congenital malformations in Fircrest School (Seattle), during 1965; and
from mothers of 57 children with leukemia, identified
through the Children's Orthopedic Hospital in Seattle
during 1965. Cooperation of the mothers with the
interviewers was almost complete: 98.4 percent of the
mothers of normal newborns contacted by telephone co-
operated, and only two of 223 mothers of children with
congenital malformations or leukemia declined to be
interviewed.

Although the findings of this study (Tables 1, 2),
do not demonstrate a striking relationship of congenital
malformations and childhood leukemia to the smoking experience of their parents, the data patterns do suggest a
clustering of children with leukemia to women who smoked
most heavily (4,000+ cigarettes) during the index pregnancies. Such studies need repetition and enlargement to
yield firm understanding of the role of smoking in the
causation of congenital malformations and childhood leukemia; but lack of a strikingly obvious relationship, such
as exists between phocomelia and thalidomide, provides
little reassurance that smoking is an unimportant cause of
such diseases. Rather, the relationship may be so com-
plexified by the generality and diffuseness of smoking
effects on multiple generations, that a more comprehensive, meticulous, multigenerational approach, which
quantitatively considers all mutagenic experience and
hereditary disease patterns, may be needed to fully
elucidate the role of smoking in the production of these
diseases.

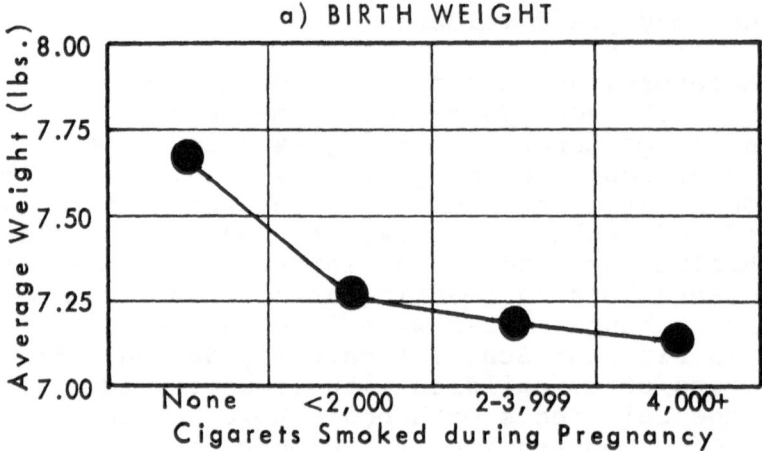

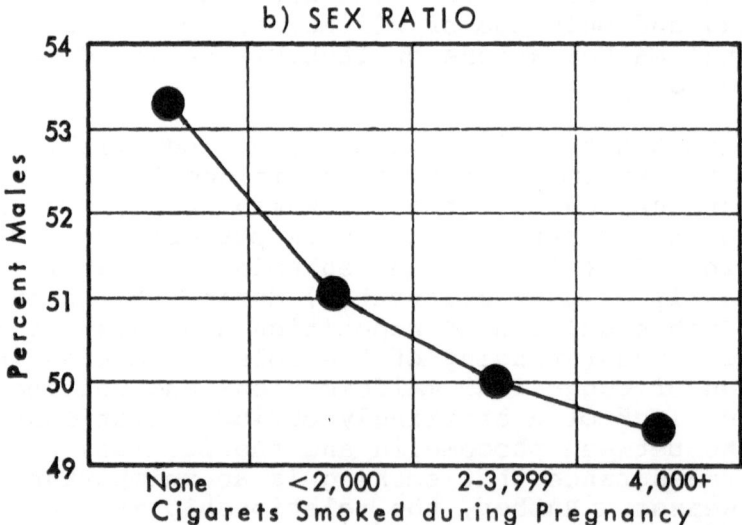

Figure 3.   Weight and sex of offspring by smoking of
            mothers during pregnancy.

Table 1. Cigarette Smoking Experience of Mothers of Children With Mongolism, Other Mental Retardation, or Leukemia (Seattle, Washington).

CIGARETS SMOKED BY MOTHER BEFORE CONCEPTION	NUMBER CIGARETS SMOKED BY MOTHER DURING PREGNANCY				SMOKING DURING PREGNANCY COMBINED	ALL CONDITIONS COMBINED	
	None	2,000	2-3,999	4,000+	COMBINED	No.	%
None	20M 47X 8Y 3Z 2P,T 30L				20M 47X 8Y 3Z 2P,T 30L	111	50.2%
32,000	4M 4X Y Z 2L	4M 11X 2Y 2Z P 5L	3X 3Y 2L	4X 4L	8M 22X 6Y 3Z P 13L	53	24.0%
32-63,999	M 2X z	M X z	2X 2Y 2Z L	2M 7X z 7L	4M 12X 2Y 4Z 8L	30	13.6%
64,000+	M X R	2Y	2M X L	3M 8X Y E 5L	6M 10X 3Y R,E 6L	27	12.2%
Smoking Before Conception Combined	26M 54X 9Y 4Z 2P,R,T 32L	5M 12X 4Y 3Z P 5L	2M 6X 5Y 2Z 4L	5M 19X Y Z E 16L	38M 91X 19Y 10Z 3P,E,R,T 57L	221	100%
Total Number	129	30	19	43	221		
Percent	58.4%	13.6%	8.6%	19.4%	100%		

M = Mongolism; X = Congenital mental retardation, cause unknown; Y = Congenital mental retardation, birth injury mentioned; Z = Probable post natal cause; P = Phenylketonuria; E = Ectodermosis; R = Rubella; T = Tuberous schlerosis; L = Leukemia (3 of the 57 children dying of leukemia were mongoloid).

EPIDEMIOLOGY OF SMOKING BY PREGNANT WOMEN

When supporting development of a standardized Maternity Record for use by many hospitals cooperating with the Maternity Care Monitoring Project of the International Fertility Research Program (IFRP) (17), Dr. Roger Bernard and the author insisted that one question be devoted to "Tobacco Smoking During Pregnancy". This was done, and the data collected by the IFRP from 108 hospitals in 34 countries from 1977 to 1980, are presented in Table 3.

Apparently, large proportions of women delivering in European countries and the United States smoked during their index pregnancies, with highest maternal smoking rates in Scotland with 36.7 percent, Ireland with 35.8 percent, and Sweden with 34.0 percent; while in developing countries, the highest rates were in Latin America: Chile with 25.1 percent, Venezuela with 24.0 percent, Brazil with 20.1 percent, and Colombia with 18.8

Table 2. Condition of Offspring by Smoking Experience of
          Mother During Pregnancy.

CONDITION OF OFFSPRING		NUMBER CIGARETS SMOKED BY MOTHER DURING PREGNANCY				SMOKING DURING PREGNANCY COMBINED
		None	2,000	2-3,999	4,000+	
Normal	No.	1,248	241	196	338	2,023
	%	61.7%	11.9%	9.7%	16.7%	
Mongoloid	No.	26	5	2	5	38
	%	68.4%	13.2%	5.3%	13.2%	
Other Mental Retardation (Institutionalized)	No.	71	20	13	22	126
	%	56.3%	15.9%	10.3%	17.5%	
Childhood Leukemia	No.	32	5	4	16	57
	%	56.1%	8.8%	7.0%	28.1%	

percent. Elsewhere in the developing world, especially
Africa and Asia, few women smoked during pregnancy.

     But commercial tobacco forces are determined to
exploit potential buyers everywhere, and unless stout
barriers are quickly built, all the developing countries
are destined to suffer the same spectrum of "Western
diseases" which now so greatly afflict Europeans and
Americans. As shown in Table 3, many Philippine women
(5.5 percent) smoked during their index pregnancies.
Strong preventive action is needed in the Philippines to
protect future generations from the cigarette plague now
pandemic in the world.

     A recent birth survey in Nevada, U.S.A. (18), found
that 28 percent of the mothers had smoked during their
index pregnancies an average of 4100 cigarettes per
pregnancy, or 15 per day. The average birth weight of
their offspring (6.9 pounds) was 0.9 pounds less than the
average (7.8 pounds) birth weight of the infants of Nevada
women who did not smoke. It was further calculated that
the average birth weight of offspring of mothers who
smoked during pregnancy was approximately 1 gram less per
10 cigarettes smoked.

CONCLUSION

     Smoking is now the foremost environmental hazard to
the health and longevity of smoking Americans and their
progeny. For persons smoking a package or more of cigarettes per day from adolescence on, smoking is a greater

Table 3.   Smoking During Pregnancy.
By Region and Country*.

Regions and Countries	Number Participating Hospitals	Number MCM 903 Records Analyzed	Number Responding to Smoking Question	Women Smoking During Index Pregnancy Number	Percent
Less Developed Countries					
Africa					
Egypt	6	10,278	10,273	120	1.2
Sudan	3	1,180	1,155	8	0.7
Tunisia	1	148	143	1	0.7
Zaire	1	1,033	1,032	0	0.0
Asia					
Bangladesh	12	9,261	9,249	311	3.4
India	12	16,848	16,847	62	0.4
Indonesia	12	33,566	33,563	252	0.8
Iran	1	19,932	19,932	188	0.9
Jordan	1	458	452	12	2.7
Pakistan	2	1,257	1,254	1	0.1
Philippines	1	199	199	11	5.5
Sri Lanka	3	4,092	4,090	5	0.1
Taiwan	1	2,916	2,916	18	0.6
Thailand	2	6,275	5,808	32	0.6
Latin America					
Brazil	9	11,520	11,424	2,301	20.1
Chile	4	16,858	16,833	4,223	25.1
Colombia	-	580	580	109	18.8
Costa Rica	1	1,600	1,600	139	8.7
El Salvador	1	4,299	4,293	92	2.1
Honduras	2	17,482	17,472	891	5.1
Mexico	7	7,562	7,560	663	8.8
Panama	1	6,934	6,934	445	6.4
Venezuela	1	11,874	11,771	2,824	24.0
LDC Subtotal	84	186,152	185,380	12,708	6.9
More Developed Countries					
Austria	1	4,477	4,465	782	17.5
Belgium	2	1,157	1,054	261	24.8
Canada	1	972	971	250	25.7
Hungary	2	11,400	11,398	1,512	13.3
Ireland	1	999	998	357	35.8
Italy	6	3,749	3,745	977	26.1
Japan	2	794	785	63	8.0
Scotland	1	799	777	285	36.7
Sweden	1	1,991	1,967	668	34.0
United States	2	1,246	1,124	218	19.4
West Germany	3	2,071	2,041	645	31.6
Yugoslavia	2	2,832	2,832	552	19.5
MDC Subtotal	24	32,487	32,157	6,570	20.4
Grand Total	108	218,639	217,537	19,278	8.9

*These data were collected by the Maternity Care Monitoring program of the International Fertility Research Program, Research Triangle Park, North Carolina, with support from the Office of Population, U.S. Agency for International Development; from 108 participating hospitals in 34 countries during 1977-1980.

threat to health and life than all other environmental
hazards to life combined - and actually doubles the
chances of the smoker dying during middle age.

Smoking by pregnant women is a double hazard to
social health, because it exposes both the mother and
fetus to noxious products of burning tobacco. Hence,
among the tens of millions of Americans diminishing their
health by smoking this year, highest priority for social
action should be directed toward the million currently
pregnant smokers. Because heavy smoking during pregnancy
increases fetal losses by roughly one-third, and approximately one-fourth of pregnant American women smoke, it
is estimated that this practice will cause the loss of
more than 50,000 fetuses by miscarriage in the U.S. this
year and adversely affect the health of additional
hundreds of thousands of live born offspring. Surely,
such subtrac- tion from the quality of reproduction is
intolerable and there is urgent need that every cigarette
package promi- nently display the warning: "Not For Use
By Pregnant Women".

REFERENCES

1.   Editorial (1889): Lancet, 1:709.
2.   Surgeon General (1980): The Health Consequences of
        Smoking for Women, A report of the Surgeon
        General. Office of Smoking and Health, U.S. De-
        partment of Health and Human Services, Washington.
3.   Population Information Program (1979): Tobacco -
        hazards to health and human reproduction.
        Population Reports, Series L, 1:40, Johns Hopkins
        University, Baltimore.
4.   Ravenholt RT, Levinski MJ (1965): Smoking during
        pregnancy. Lancet, 1:961.
5.   Ravenholt RT, Levinski MJ, Nellist DJ, Takenaga M
        (1966): Effects of smoking on reproduction. Am J
        Obstet Gyn 96:267-281.
6.   Ravenholt RT, Clark OE, Levinski MJ, Nellist DN
        (1965): The role of tobacco in cellular deviation.
        Presented to the American Public Health Associa-
        tion, Chicago, October. (Unpublished)
7.   Ravenolt RT (1966): Malignant cellular evolution. An
        analysis of the causation and prevention of cancer.
        Lancet, 1:523-526.
8.   Larson PS, Hoag HB, Silvette H (1961): Tobacco:
        Experiental and Clinical Studies. Williams and
        Wilkins Co., Baltimore.

9. Ames BN (1979): Identifying environmental chemicals causing mutations and Cancer. <u>Science</u>, 204:587-593.
10. Redford EP, Hunt VR (1964): Polonium 210: A volatile radioelement in cigarettes. <u>Science</u>, 143:247-249.
11. Surgeon General (1979): <u>Smoking and Health</u>. A report of the Surgeon General, U.S. Department of Health, Education and Welfare, Washington.
12. Washington (1961): <u>Longterm effects of ionizing radiation from external sources</u>, Washington.
13. Pearl R (1938): Tobacco smoking and longevity. <u>Science</u>, 87:216-217.
14. Ravenholt RT, Applegate J (1965): Measurement of smoking experience. <u>New Eng J Med</u>.
15. Ravenholt RT (1980): The real villains: Cigarettes (A Letter). <u>The Washington Star</u>, June 27.
16. Little JB, Radrod EP Jr (1967): Polonium 210 in bronchial epithelium of cigarette smokers. <u>Science</u>, 155:606-607.
17. Bernard RP, de Watteville H, Kessel E, Ravenholt RT, Kendall EM (1979): International Maternity Care Monitoring: Results of a pretest. <u>Int J Gyn Obstet</u>, 17:24-39.
18. Ravenholt RT, Ravenholt OH, Payne D, Arrington H (1981): Multi-state birth studies. Presented to the Annual Meeting, American Public Health Association, Los Angeles, November 4.

ENVIRONMENTAL CHEMICALS AND DRUGS INFLUENCING THE FETUS

D. M. Aviado

Department of Pharmacology, University of
Medicine and Dentistry of New Jersey and
Atmospheric Health Sciences, Inc.
Short Hills, New Jersey, U.S.A.

INTRODUCTION

In recent years, it has become apparent that maternal medication and environmental chemicals can influence the development of human embryo and cause birth defects (1). Until forty years ago, the prevalent opinion was that congenital malformations were caused by genetic and chromosomal factors inherited from the parents. The possible etiologic role of environmental factors was demonstrated by four events: Gregg's classical demonstration in 1941 that rubella infection in the mother caused congenital cataract in the newborn (2); the Minamata mercury poisoning in the 1950's (3); the thalidomide disaster in the 1960's (4); and the discovery of transplacental carcinogenesis in the 1970's associated with the maternal use of diethylstilbestrol (5).

Presently, obstetricians and pediatricians generally agree that the maternal environment does not confer absolute protection to the human embryo against all adverse influences. Toxicologists have compiled a growing list of several hundred chemical substances that are suspected of influencing the fetus prior to and after conception. The chemical substances that potentially influence maternal health, and in turn affect the newborn, include medications, cosmetics, alcohol and nonalcoholic beverages, food and water contaminants, and air pollutants in the work environment, dwellings, public buildings, and the outdoors. It has been estimated by Wilson (6) that appoximately one-third of all birth defects can be attributed to either genetic and chromosomal factors (25 percent) or to environmental chemical factors (10 percent). The causation of two-thirds of congenital malformation (65 percent) is still unknown and some experts have the opinion that a majority can be attributed to chemicals in the environment. In other words, the suspected role of environmental chemicals in the causation of birth defects ranges from 10 to 75 percent.

The seven-fold difference (10 to 75 percent) in estimation of the role of environmental chemicals in the causation of birth defects is also applicable to other parameters that measure perinatal mortality, neonatal morbidity, and subsequent growth and development. It is difficult to obtain a consensus because the estimations are derived from a variety of studies that include:

(a) epidemiologic studies designed to separate maternal constitutional factors (inherited genetic factors, malnutrition and socio-economic status) from environmental chemicals; unfortunately, such studies are suggestive but do not establish a cause-and-effect relationship;
(b) case reports that are limited in number and may be a spontaneous occurrence with coincidental exposure to a chemical substance; and
(c) animal studies designed to test the reproductive and fetal effects of maternal exposure to large doses of drugs or chemicals.

In spite of the disagreement among clinicians, epidemiologists and toxicologists, it is possible to separate the fetotoxic drugs and environmental chemicals to: First, those that are certain or noncontroversial or established in their causal relationship; from Second, those that are uncertain, controversial or suspicious. The criteria for recognizing a fetotoxic drug or environmental chemical are as follows:

(a) an abrupt increase in the incidence of perinatal mortality or birth defects;
(b) coincidence of this increase with a known environmental change or introduction of a new drug;
(c) known maternal exposure either early or late in pregnancy;
(d) exclusion of other risk factors that influence perinatal mortality or cause birth defects; and
(e) confirmation of fetotoxicity or teratogenicity by animal experimentation.

Unfortunately, the majority of drugs and chemicals that are suspected of causing adverse effects on the fetus do not fulfill the above criteria and are regarded as uncertain, controversial or suspicious fetotoxins and teratogens. The general plan of this article is to review maternal medications administered prior to and during pregnancy that can positively be verified from interviewing the mothers. The chemicals in the food, water and air are discussed separately because maternal exposure is difficult to recognize by either the interviewer or even the patients.

MATERNAL MEDICATION

It would have been anticipated that the thalidomide disaster in the 1950's would have significantly reduced the use of drugs during pregnancy. However, in subsequent decades the level of therapeutic drug usage during the course of pregnancy has not been appreciably reduced (7). In a survey conducted in the late 1970's, the consumption of 93 percent American pregnant women was five or more drugs. The order of frequency of usage is as follows: almost all women took iron and vitamin preparations and analgesics; more than half used topical ointments, suppositories, douches and oral antacids; a significant portion of pregnant women received antiemetics, barbiturates and antihistaminics. Approximately a tenth of the group were taking medication because of medical reasons prior to pregnancy. The fetotoxic effects of medications discussed below are grouped according to their usage, namely before, during the early stage, and during the late stage of pregnancy.

Drugs to Inhibit Preterm Labor

Although recent improvements in neonatal intensive care have resulted in reductions in neonatal morbidity and death, the impact of preterm delivery on perinatal mortality rate is still staggering. Preterm infants (born prior to 37th week of amenorrhea) account for a majority of neonatal deaths, including stillbirths (8). In addition, a large percentage of preterm infants suffer significant neonatal morbidity and long-term sequelae such as motor and intellectual handicaps. When adequate prenatal care fails to prevent preterm labor, then pharmacologic suppression of labor is commonly undertaken since there have been reported decreases in neonatal morbidity and death, with the addition of one or two weeks of existence in utero (Fig. 1).

MATERNAL MEDICATION

(A) Drugs to Inhibit Preterm Labor

- Sympathomimetic Uterine   Tachycardia
      Relaxants ------------------→ Lactacidosis

- Prostaglandin Inhibitors   Premature Closure of
      Indomethacin ------------------→ Ductus Arteriosus
      Aspirin   Pulmonary Hypertension

- Diazoxide ----------------------→ Hypoglycemia
                                     Alopecia
                                     Hypertrichosis

- Ethanol --------------------→ Fetal Intoxication

Figure 1.   Drugs that inhibit preterm labor.

Sympathomimetic uterine relaxants. Epinephrine,
the primary constituent of the adrenal medulla, is a
potent drug that inhibits uterine hyperactivity. However,
its use in the treatment of preterm labor is limited by
its cardiovascular side effects. In recent years, several
synthetic drugs have become available that are predominantly smooth muscle relaxants, with minimal cardiac
stimulant or pressor effects. The drugs identified as
selective beta-two adrenergic receptor activators include
isoxsuprine, mitodrine, salbutamol, terbutaline and
fenoterol (9). It should be recalled that these beta-two-
mimetic drugs were developed for the oral therapy of
peripheral arterial disease and of bronchial asthma.
Their additional usefulness in the inhibition of uterine
hyperactivity is understandable because beta-two adrenergic receptors are located on the surface of smooth muscle
cells, such as the uterus, the arteries and the bronchial
airways. The selectivity of these drugs for the beta-two
adrenergic smooth muscle receptors is not absolute because
intravenous infusion can still activate beta-one adrenergic cardiac receptors. Thus, tachycardia and low blood
pressure may occur, although less intense than the adverse
effects seen with epinephrine. The fetal heart may also
be accelerated by the maternal injection of sympathomimetic uterine relaxants. In addition, these drugs cause
metabolic changes in the liver and skeletal muscle, mani-
fested by lactacidosis in the fetus. These effects on the
fetus are mild and transient in nature and are unlikely to
adversely affect the fetus. Most of these uterine relaxants have been shown to be effective in the inhibition of
preterm labor, when compared to the use of placebo-saline
injection.

Prostaglandin inhibiting drugs. Since prostaglandins occupy a pivotal role in human reproduction, the inhibition of prostaglandin synthesis has been suggested as a means of modifying the process of parturition. The two widely-known synthetase inhibitors are aspirin and indomethacin and both are effective suppressants of uterine hypermotility. Inhibition of prostaglandin synthesis may influence the normal mechanism of transition from fetal to neonatal life. By its vascular action, the prostaglandin inhibitor may cause premature closure of the ductus arteriosus. In animal experiments, the maternal injection of indomethacin caused intrauterine contraction of the ductus (10). Furthermore, neonatal animals treated with indomethacin demonstrate a higher level of pulmonary hypertension in response to hypoxia (11). Two case reports of transient primary pulmonary hypertension in human neonates whose mothers received indomethacin prior to delivery have been reported (12). On the other hand, congenital anomalies, premature closure of the ductus arteriosus and pulmonary hypertension were not reported in those infants exposed to prostaglandin inhibitors during pregnancy (13). However, the number of cases studied was so small that the potentially serious side effects militate against the widespread routine use of these agents to prevent or treat preterm labor.

Diazoxide. In the management of hypertension or toxemia of pregnancy, diazoxide is administered intravenously to reduce blood pressure and dramatic inhibition of uterine contraction. The most common adverse reaction is hypoglycemia, occurring both in the mother and in the neonate. Alopecia and hypertrichosis lanuginosa have been reported in some infants exposed to diazoxide in utero for several weeks. In sheep and goats, high doses of diazoxide produce cataracts, skeletal muscle fibrosis and necrosis of the pancreas (14), but these effects have not been observed in human neonates whose mothers received diazoxide during pregnancy. The significance of these findings remains uncertain.

Ethanol by infusion causes labor inhibition by several mechanisms, namely: suppression of endogenous oxytocin secretion, preventing prostaglandin synthesis, releasing catecholamines, and direct relaxation of uterine smooth muscle. Alcohol freely traverses the placenta so that the neonate may become intoxicated. Although neonatal respiratory depression or apnea has not been a problem, small premature infants may show lethargy, apnea, poor muscle tone and abnormal reflexes.

Oxytocics for Medical Induction of Labor

The posterior pituitary extract containing oxytocin, can be infused for the induction of labor. Continuous monitoring of the mother and fetus is necessary to avoid overstimulation of the uterus that can threaten the life of the fetus. Fetal bradycardia and neonatal jaundice have been reported. The ergot-derived oxytocics are not used for medical induction of labor and their indications are limited to treatment of postpartum hemorrhage.

Obstetrical Analgesics

There is no exception to the general rule that inhalational, intravenous, and local anesthetics, pre-anesthetic medications and anesthetic adjuvants including curareform drugs, readily cross the placenta. The most common fetal reaction is respiratory depression and even apnea. When recognized, respiratory resuscitation in-cluding oxygen inhalation is initiated and continued until the neonate is able to respire spontaneously and adequately.

Medications Prescribed During Early Pregnancy

The confusion on the interpretation of studies on as-pirin illustrates the difficulties in composing a list of proven or likely teratogens. Aspirin is a positive tera-togen in several animal species. Although retrospective studies in humans suggest that maternal use of aspirin may produce congenital malformations, a prospective study of mothers consuming aspirin throughout pregnancy did not increase the incidence of malformation. The effect of aspirin on perinatal mortality is controversial; both a positive increase and a lack of effect have been reported. Wilson (6) has referred to aspirin as a "Possible Terato-gen", defined as a drug of widespread use, but only rarely implicated in human teratogenesis. The positive animal results of teratogenicity is in conflict with the contro-versial results in humans, thus the term "Possible Teratogen". The other widely used drugs belonging to this category are antibiotics, antituberculous drugs, quinine and some antimalarials, imipramine and insulin.

"Probable or Suspected Teratogens" are drugs that are occasionally associated with malformations in the neonates of women treated during early pregnancy. The occurrences of birth defects constitute only a small portion of the total number of women known to have been treated so that the occurrence has been interpreted in one of three ways: (a) Spontaneous malformation with coincidental use of drugs; (b) maternal disease-related that prompted the use

Ⓔ **MEDICATION PRIOR TO PREGNANCY**
Disease Related Fetal Effects
Maternal Medication & Envirnomental Chemicals
Paternal Medication & Environmental Chemicals

	HUMAN OBSERVATIONS	ANIMAL EXPERIMENTS
Estrogens	●	●
Thalidomide	●	●
Anethetic Gases	●	●
Alcohol	●	●
Caffeine	●	●
Lead	●	●
Morphine	—	●
Methadone	—	●

Figure 2.   Medications administered prior to pregnancy.

of drugs;   or (c) a real but weak teratogenic potential of
the drug. The list of "Probable or Suspected Teratogens"
includes anticonvulsants, dextroamphetamine and related
anorexic drugs, oral hypoglycemics and alkylating-antineo-
plastic drugs. Like medications belonging to the two
other categories, this group of "Probable or Suspected
Teratogens" are positive teratogens in animal studies.

     "Likely or Positively Implicated Teratogens" include
thalidomide, steroid hormones, and folic acid antagonists.
There is a consensus in interpretation of human and animal
studies (6, 15, 16), indicating that these drugs are positive teratogens. The congenital defect may be apparent
not only at birth, but also as changes in behavior in
childhood and as cancer at puberty.

Medications Prescribed Prior to Pregnancy

     Most of the drugs prescribed during early pregnancy
are likely to be used prior to its onset (Fig. 2). A
consideration of the drug-related fetotoxicity is complex
because of the problem of distinction between disease-
related effects and drug-induced toxicity. For example,
if a diabetic patient treated with either oral hypoglycemics or insulin prior to and during pregnancy has a
neonate with birth defects, several interpretations may be
considered: (a) that diabetes or its complications cause
poor supply of blood and nutrients to the reproductive
system; or (b) insulin or oral hypoglycemics cause chromosomal or genetic defects. In addition to congenital
malformations, the adverse effects of medication include
miscarriages or spontaneous abortion and even persistent
infertility. There is also the possibility that paternal

drug use may influence the viability of the developing embryo. Environmental chemicals also exert similar effects on the reproductive system of males and females, as discussed in the next section.

ENVIRONMENTAL CHEMICALS

Prior to a review of maternal exposure to environmental chemicals, a discussion of paternal exposure is in order. The clinical and animal experimental data are scant. However, the available information suggests that use of or paternal exposure to thalidomide, anesthetic bases, alcohol, caffeine and lead is associated with increased spontaneous abortions and higher incidence of congenital anomalies (17). The animal experiments also indicate persistent effects on spermatogenesis leading to sterility. There are observations in animals indicating that opiates cause paternal sterility and adverse effects on the offsprings but there are no human observations verifying that the association also occurs in humans.

In the above discussion of fetal effects arising from paternal exposure, half of the examples relate to environmental chemicals. The list of potential fetotoxins and teratogens in the maternal environment is more extensive and includes food additives, water contaminants, occupational inhalants, and air pollutants.

Food Additives

Heavy metals may be introduced inadvertently into foods through the equipment in which food is processed, prepared or served. Although many countries have regulations for the control of metals in cookware and serving dishes, the problem still exists. Glazes on earthenware, decals on the inside of cocktail glasses, and lead in homemade stills have been found to be sources of lead poisoning (18).

A more frequent and serious source of heavy metals in food is the result of environmental pollution. The concentration of lead, zinc, cadmium and nickel in roadside soil and vegetation is significantly higher near heavily traveled roads. The contamination is believed to be related to the composition of gasoline, motor oils, and tires, and to the roadside deposition of vehicular waste products. It is difficult to determine the human toxicity to these metals that persist in edible plants. Outbreaks of mercury poisoning in Minamata (Japan) have been traced

ENVIRONMENTAL CHEMICALS

Ⓐ **Food Additives**
- Metals: Lead, Mercury, Zinc, Cadmium, Nickel
- Sweeteners, Colorings, Flavorings, Preservatives
- Food Packaging & Containers

Ⓑ **Water & Soil Pollutants**
- Metals
- Pesticides
- Herbicides
- Fertilizers
- Chlorinated Hydrocarbons

Figure 3. Food additives, water and soil pollutants suspected of causing fetal malformations.

to the high mercury content of fish from water heavily polluted with industrial waste. Mercury can also enter the food chain at other points, such as birds eating seeds treated with mercury as fungicides, hogs fed mill sweepings of mercury-treated grain, and ingestion of mercury treated grains for planting.

The list of potential teratogens includes a wide variety of food additive compounds used as artificial sweeteners, colorings, flavorings, and preservatives. Chemicals that leech or migrate from packaging materials are also suspected teratogens (18). The packaging of foodstuffs in plastic materials presents very complex problems that are being investigated at the present time. Although the plastic itself may be relatively insoluble, partially reacted polymers, plasticizers and manufacturing contaminants can migrate into the food (Fig. 3).

Water and Soil Pollutants

The toxic metals contained in the food are also likely to pollute the soil, naturally occurring bodies of water, and ulimately drinking water. In addition, there are agricultural products such as pesticides, herbicides, and fertilizers that reach food and water (Fig. 3). In the process of water purification by chlorination, chlorinated hydrocarbons are formed. There are animal experiments showing that these chemicals contained in water cause infertility and birth defects in offsprings. However, there are no human observations that would assist in proving or disproving a causal relationship between ingestion of water pollutants and fetotoxicity or teratogenicity (19).

ENVIRONMENTAL CHEMICALS

Ⓒ **Occupational Inhalants**
- Metals
- Pesticides
- Halogenated Organic Chemicals
- General Anesthetics - Operating Rooms

Ⓓ **Air Pollutants**
- Vehicular Emissions
- Fuel Combustion

Figure 4. Occupational inhalants and air pollutants
            suspected of causing fetal malformations.

Occupational Inhalants

The industrial use of heavy metals and the manufacture of pesticides are suspected of causing adverse
health effects to mothers and their offsprings. Halogenated organic chemicals are also suspected of causing
maternal and fetal toxicity. Health professionals exposed to general anesthetics in the operating room have a
higher incidence of spontaneous abortions and occurrence
of congenital anomalies in their offsprings, compared to
other professionals (20). Work standards for pregnant
women are presently being revised to respond to the increasing number of positive animal teratogens that are
being identified in the work environment (Fig. 4).

Air Pollutants

Vehicular emissions contain lead, carbon monoxide,
sulfur oxides, nitrogen oxides, and hydrocarbons. The
long-term exposure of mothers to products of fuel combustion are not known, although animal experiments
suggest fetotoxicity, teratogenicity and transplacental
carcinogenesis. As with other forms of environmental
chemical contamination, it is difficult to separate environmental toxicity from nonenvironmental, spontaneous or
genetically induced adverse effects on the fetus.

CONCLUSION

At the present time, the list of suspected or possible teratogens and fetotoxins far exceed the number of
likely or probable human teratogens and fetotoxins. The
proven ones are supported by results of epidemiologic
studies and human case reports with confirmation from

animal studies. The most overwhelming problem is the
resolution of the status of medications and environmental
chemicals that are fetotoxic and teratogenic in animal
experiments. There are no human observations to prove or
disprove their adverse effects on the fetus. Should these
drugs and chemicals be banned completely to prevent maternal exposure? Or, should such a drastic action await
proof from human studies?

Regulatory agencies in the United States have taken
a conservative attitude of prohibiting the maternal use of
drugs that are proven human teratogens, such as thalidomide. Possible or suspected animal teratogens are not
banned from use because their therapeutic benefits far
exceed the health risk. However, the suspected teratogens
are properly labeled to warn the physician of the reported
fetal effects in animals that have not been observed in
humans. For environmental chemicals, the Environmental
Protection Agency and the Occupational Safety and Health
Admnistration have recommended animal testing for reproduction and teratogenicity. The experimental results are
considered together with other toxicologic information to
determine the acceptable ambient and work environment
standards. In a Congress devoted to maternal and neonatal
health, toxicologists seek the cooperation of health professionals. On the Maternal Care Minitoring Questionaire,
it may be possible to include questions relating to maternal exposure to medications and environmental chemicals.
The questions can readily be formulated from the results
of animal studies reviewed above.

REFERENCES

1. Cho YW, Aviado DM: Clinical Pharmacology for
        Pediatricians. IV. Maternal Medication
        Influencing the Fetus. J Clin Pharmacol,
        (Submitted)
2. Gregg NM (1941): Congenital cataract following german
        measles in the mother. Trans Ophthalmol Soc
        Amst, 3:35.
3. Tsubaki T, Irukayama K, Editors (1976): Minamata
        Disease, North-Holland, New York.
4. Slone D, Shapiro S, Mitchell AA (1980): Strategies
        for studying the effects of the antenatal chemical
        environment on the fetus. In: Drugs and Chemical
        Risk to the Fetus and Newborn, Edited by RH
        Schwarz, SJ Yaffe. Alan R. Liss Inc., New York,
        pp. 1-7.

5. Herbst AL, Scully RE (1970): Adenocarcinoma of the vagina in adolescence; A report of seven cases including six clear cell carcinoma. Cancer, 25:745.

6. Wilson JG (1977): Environmental Chemcals. In: Handbook of Teratology. Edited by JG Wilson, FC Fraser. New York Academic Press.

7. Schwarz RH (1980): The obstetrician's view. In: Drug and Chemical Risks to the Fetus and Newborn. Edited by RH Schwarz and SJ Yaffe. Alan R. Liss Inc., New York, pp. 153.

8. Caritis SN, Edelstone EI, Mueller-Huebach E (1979): Pharmacologic inhibition of preterm delivery. Am J Obstet Gynecol, 133:557.

9. Aviado DM (1970): Sympathomimetic Drugs. Charles Thomas, Springfield.

10. Sharpe GL, Thalme B, Larsson KS (1974): Studies on closure of the ductus arteriosus. IX. Ductal closure in utero by a prostaglandin synthetase inhibitor. Prostaglandins, 8:363.

11. Tyle T, Wallis R, Leffler C, Cassin S (1975): The effects of indomethacin on the pulmonary vascular response to hypoxia in the premature and mature newborn goat. Proc Soc Exp Biol Med, 150:695.

12. Manchester D, Margolis HS, Sheldon RE (1976): Possible association between maternal indomethacin therapy and primary pulmonary hypertension of the newborn. Am J Obstet Gynecol, 126:467.

13. Zuckerman H, Reiss U, Rubinstein I (1974): Inhibition human premature labor by indomethacin. Obstet Gynecol, 44:787.

14. Boulos BM, Davis LE, Almond CH, Jackson RL (1971): Placental transfer of diazoxide and its hazardous effect on the newborn. J Clin Pharmacol, 11:206.

15. Pomerance JJ, Yaffe SE (1973): Maternal medication and its effect on the fetus. Curr Probl Pediatr, 4:2.

16. Stellman JM (1979): The effect of toxic agents on reproduction. Occup Health Safety, 48:36-43.

17. Soyka LF, Jaffe JM (1980): Male-mediated drug effects on offspring. In: Drugs and Chemical Risks to the Fetus and Newborn. Alan R. Liss Inc., New York, 46-66.

18. Kilgore WW, Li MY (1980): Food additives and contaminants. In: Toxicology, Edited by J Doull, CD Klaasen, MO Amdur. MacMillan,, New York, 593-607.

19. Menzer RE, Nelson JO (1980): Water and soil pollutants. In: Toxicology, Edited by J Doull, C.D. Klaasen, M.O. Amdur. MacMillan, New York, 632-658.

20. Ad Hoc Committee on the effect of trace anesthetics on
    the health of operating room personnel (1974)
    Anesthesiology, 41:321.
21. Aviado DM (1982): Air pollution effects on the fetus.
    Perspectives Envir Health, (In Press)

MATERNITY CARE MONITORING: A NEW INFORMATION SYSTEM

E. Kessel

Founder and Senior Consultant
International Fertility Research Program
Research Triangle Park, North Carolina

INTRODUCTION

We are living in an age of dramatic changes in the
need for and provision of maternity care. It is estimated
that there were 130 million births in the world in 1980.
By the year 2000, the number will reach 163 million. The
increasing proportion of these births in developing
countries can be seen in Figure 1. As developed countries
approach stationary populations and near irreducible levels of maternal and perinatal mortality, it is clear that
the challenge to maternity care lies primarily in these
developing countries, where over 85 percent of births and
over 95 percent of maternal and perinatal mortality will
occur by the year 2000. The contrasts in extreme levels
of national maternal and child mortality rates of developed and developing countries are shown in Table 1. The
projected totals of these tragic losses in developing
countries for the last two decades of this century are
staggering: one million maternal and 40 million perinatal
deaths will occur, of which, by Western standards, 95
percent are preventable. These losses, in terms of
contribution to shorter life expectancy, surpass deaths
resulting from any specific disease category, such as all
infectious diseases, cardiovascular diseases, cancers or
accidents.

There is a common belief that improvements in maternity care are tied to general socio-economic development.
If we must wait for a rise in per capita income, then it
is easy to "prove" that only modest improvements in

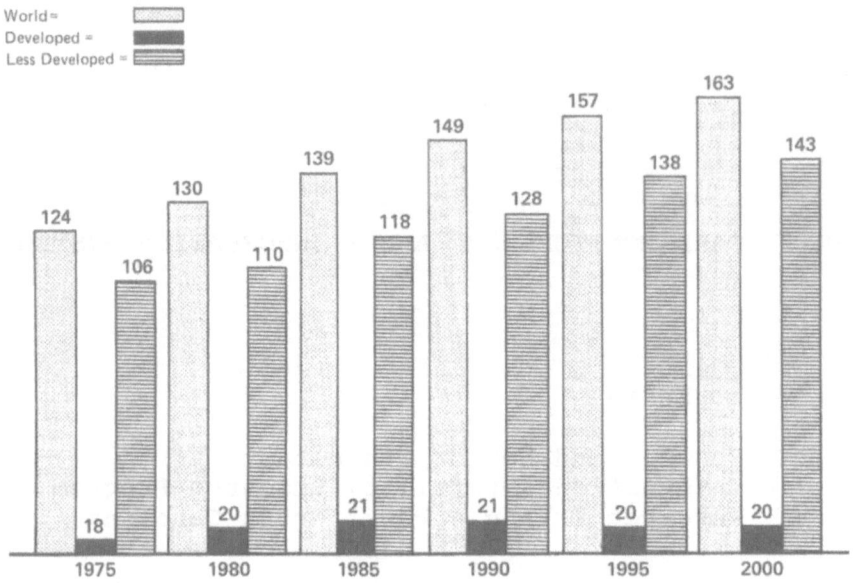

World =
Developed =
Less Developed =

Figure 1.   Births for the world and developed and less
            developed regions (1975 - 2000 in millions).
            [Source: US Census Bureau medium estimates]

maternity care can be expected by the end of the century,
especially for some of the largest and least urbanized
developing countries. These countries tend to have high
birth rates, high growth rates and a high proportion of
their population under 15 years of age. Their high dependency ratio necessitates large investments in schools
and health facilities and less investment available to
create jobs and higher productivity. The developing
countries are faced with marked increases in their working
age populations and inadequate capital to assure a Western
pattern of economic growth (1).

    Fortunately, there are examples of remarkable im-
provement in maternity care among the developing countries
that refute the necessity of socio-economic development as
a prerequisite. In the 1970s, maternal and perinatal
mortality in Sri Lanka fell to the level characteristic of
many developed countries with per capita incomes ten times
or more that of Sri Lanka. The impact of life expectancy
compared to the norm for developing countries can be seen
in Figure 2. Sri Lanka is, of course, an island country
with easy access to maternity care services that are
delivered in an efficient manner by a well-trained staff
of government health professionals. A long tradition of

Table 1.   Comparison of Extreme Levels of National
            Maternal and Child Mortality Rates.

	Highest levels (1)	Lowest levels (2)	Ratio of (1) / (2)
Perinatal mortality [b]	120	12 - 15	8 - 10
Infant mortality [b]	200	8 - 10	20 - 25
Childhood mortality [c]	45	0.4 - 1	45 - 75
Maternal mortality [d]	1 000	5 - 10	100 - 200

[a] WHO (Division of Family Health) estimates based on a variety of sources.

[b] Per 1000 live births.

[c] Per 1000 population.

[d] Per 100 000 live births.

midwifery training has also provided the personnel
necessary for maternity care.

     The example of the People's Republic of China is even
more impressive in view of its population size, predominantly rural residence of the population and very modest
per capita income. Since 1949, along with controlling
major epidemic and endemic diseases and overcoming widespread malnutrition, China has made remarkable progress in
reducing high-parity births through a birth planning
program and the provision of maternity care in community
health clinics.

     The emphasis on training of auxiliary personnel and
the ready availability of their services were certainly
important in the improvement of maternity care in China.
But, another factor is unique to the situation in China.
Maternity care and other health services are provided in a
milieu that assure utilization of the services. Service
providers are highly motivated to serve, and health education efforts fit into a more general educational program
with strong political support and acceptance. This
pattern has not been duplicated in other developing count-
tries, although a few are attempting a similar approach.

     In the majority of the developing world, much of
maternity care is still in the hands of traditional births
attendants (TBAs). Even where trained midwives are placed
in rural settings, their services may be little used. The
relationship between TBAs and the trained midwife is frequently one of mutual hostility that impedes referrals.
The TBA generally retains her standing in the community

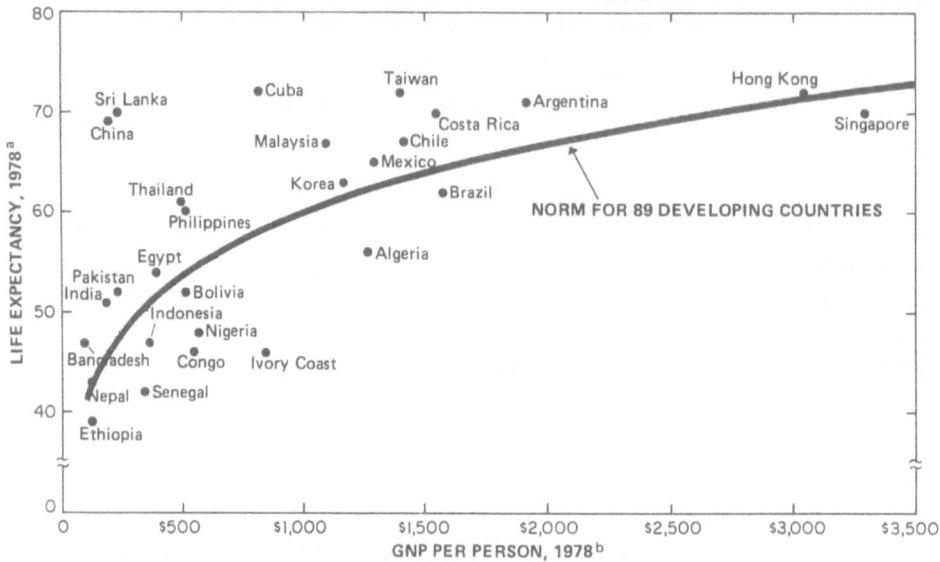

Figure 2.   Life expectancy in relation to income:
             Developing countries, 1978. [Source:
             Birdsall (3)]   Note: a = Life expectancy at
             birth is average number of years a newborn
             could be expected to live if current mortality
             conditions were to continue throughout its
             lifetime. b = GNP (gross national product) per
             person is the value of goods and services
             produced in a country, plus net income received
             from abroad from investments and citizens'
             earnings outside the country, per person
             residing in the country in a given year.

she serves. The trained midwife is all too often less
than enthusiastic about her work.

     How can other developing countries duplicate the
progress of Sri Lanka and the People's Republic of China?
Is it necessary to inherit a midwifery training tradition
or change one's political system to prevent a holocaust of
maternal and infant deaths? Or, can the resources of
successful experiences be incorporated into a universal
system that aids broader efforts to achieve primary health
care for all by the year 2000?

     To answer these questions, it is necessary first to
diagnose the defects in the organization of present
maternity services.

MONTH	1	2	3	4	5	6	TOTAL
Antenatal visits							
Iron tablets dispensed							
Maternal tetanus toxoid							
Infant DPT							
Deliveries							
Average age							
Average parity							
Low birth weight							
No. anemic							
Maternal deaths							
Perinatal deaths							
New FP acceptors							
Continuing FP visits							

Figure 3.   Illustration of a typical example of Report
Form from a peripheral center.

Let us look at the typical record keeping and
patterns of supervision of the trained midwife to see how
these contribute to low morale, lack of professional
interest and inadequate opportunities for improving
midwifery skills.

PRESENT REPORTING SYSTEMS AND SUPERVISION OF TRAINED
MIDWIVES

In Figure 3, an example of the usual reporting form
of a peripheral center regarding the activities of the
midwife is illustrated. This kind of reporting may indicate the general level of activity of the midwife, but
does not provide the information needed to create interest
in the service for either the midwife or her supervisor.
Traditionally, the trained midwife in a peripheral center
of developing countries, receives directions from a supervising nurse-midwife who makes infrequent and irregular
visits to a peripheral center. The directions generally
follow directives from higher levels of a health bureau-
cracy in limited contact with the life and work around a
peripheral health center. The midwife is evaluated
through summary service statistics, that is, counts of the
number of services she provided in a particular time
period. These totals of conducted deliveries, antenatal
visits or well-baby clinics, focus on the amount of
activity of the midwife and are generally of limited
interest or value to her. They are also of limited value
to the supervisor in judging either the value or quality
of services the midwife provides.

More interesting information might be, say for the
past six months, the number of antenatal visits by age,

ANTENATAL VISITS AMONG DELIVERIES, MONTHS 1-6

Variable		0 No. %	1-2 No. %	3-4 No. %	5+ No. %	All No. %
Age	20					
	20-30					
	30+	— —	— —	— —	— —	— —
	Total					
Previous parity	0					
	1-2					
	3+	— —	— —	— —	— —	— —
	Total					
Low birth weight		— —	— —	— —	— —	— —
Anemia at delivery		— —	— —	— —	— —	— —
Perinatal deaths		— —	— —	— —	— —	— —

Figure 4. Suggested recording of antenatal visits.

parity, low birth weight, anemia at delivery and perinatal
deaths expressed as rates per 100 deliveries. This information would highlight the importance of antenatal visits
in maternity care and could become a force to motivate the
midwife, through her community education work, to build up
her antenatal clinic. But to capture this information in
a manually produced report would require recording for
each grouping of antenatal visits and appropriate groupings
of all the other variables. For instance, if instead of
simply recording the totals of antenatal visits, the following information by number of antenatal visits were recorded: average age, average parity, number of women anemic and number of perinatal deaths among women delivered,
the recording would be like the illustration in Figure 4.
This kind of reporting high-lights the importance of the
activities of the midwife. Any further questions, such
as rate of anemia by previous parity would require an additional recording of the number of anemic women for each
chosen parity grouping. The task is obviously beyond
what can reasonably be asked of the already overburdened
midwife. But without this kind of information, the dialogue between supervisor and midwife is not likely to capture the interest of either, nor will there be created
useful information for establishing local norms of maternity care and comparisons between centers.

The end result of this lack of interesting information is a poor relationship betwen supervisor and midwife;
it will approximate that of a police investigator and
suspect. There is no hope that summary service statistics

can adequately serve the needs for training and professional development. It was this realization that led developing country leaders to apply modern methods of data collection and processing to this planet's greatest health problem.

FROM A MATERNITY RECORD TO A MONITORING SYSTEM

Maternity Care Monitoring (MCM) started as a request of the Sudan Fertility Control Association in 1975 for a coded record to study deliveries in major hospitals in Khartoum. The International Fertility Research Program (IFRP) responded to this request by developing their first Maternity Record. The computer-generated standard tables were found to be so useful that requests were received from additional centers in other countries to utilize the Maternity Record.

The International Federation of Gynecology and Obstetrics (FIGO) took a special interest in the Maternity Record studies. A cooperative trial between IFRP and FIGO of a revised Maternity Record developed in consultation with WHO was initiated in the spring of 1976. The Executive Board of FIGO officially endorsed the Maternity Record in 1978. In the five years since the cooperative trial of the Maternity Record was initiated, a total of over 400,000 records from more than 60 centers in 35 countries has been processed by IFRP, and additional records were processed by national centers that have acquired the computer program from IFRP.

At the urging of the Family Health Division of WHO, compatible records for peripheral maternity centers were further developed. The IFRP produced a Maternity Record Summary form useful for district hospitals. The International Federation for Family Health (IFFH) developed a Maternity Care Monitoring Record and Register for use in the most peripheral centers with a trained midwife. The IFRP has supported pretests of a pictorial record for the use of TBAs, and this has now been developed as a TBA Register. Finally, the IFFH developed a Referral Register to complete a record system for Monitoring Maternity Care on a provincial or national basis. The UNFPA supported the IFFH to provide consultation to developing country governments, on request, to formulate national projects for Maternity Care Monitoring. The complete scheme of MCM is illustrated schematically in Figure 5.

The MCM records are designed for the <u>monitoring</u>

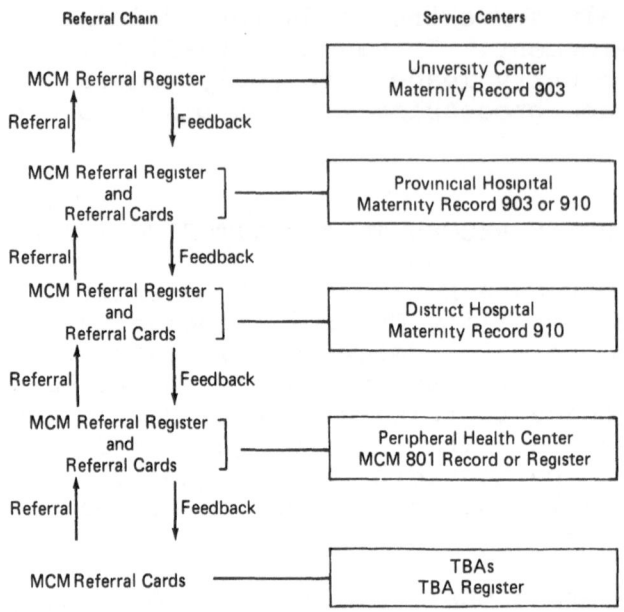

Figure 5.   Maternity Care Monitoring Records.

rather than the <u>provision</u> of maternity care. In this
respect they resemble an elaborately coded discharge summary or birth register. In register format they can be
substituted for the noncoded registers currently used.
The advantage, besides providing patient-specific information for analysis and feedback, is that a computer can
produce the maternity center's statistical report. This
report will be of far greater value to the midwife and her
supervisor and planning purposes at headquarters.

In record format, the MCM records can be integrated
into existing patient care records. The monitoring part
needs to be in duplicate so that coded section can be
transmitted for data processing.

Preprogramed computer generated standard tables are
available for the records used by trained personnel, that
is, the Maternity Record 903, Maternity Record Summary 910
or Maternity Care Monitoring 801 Record or Register. The
question of the 910 and 801 records are almost identical
to those appearing on the 903 record, but are fewer in
number. Essentially the same computer program is used for
the standard tables for each record and the tables are
comparable with few exceptions. The TBA Register is
manually analyzed by the TBA's supervisor and serves as a
guide to training and encourages appropriate referral.

MATERNITY CARE MONITORING: THE CONCEPT

Maternity Care Monitoring can serve three separate
but integrated purposes within a country. Through
continuous monitoring at major referral centers with the
Maternity Record 903 form, a process of <u>surveillance
research</u> can establish local norms of maternity care,
raise hypotheses for the improvement of maternity care and
evaluate changes in the provision of maternity care to
test the hypotheses. From an established data base,
important policy questions can be answered using local
data.

In defining what is normal in maternal health and
maternity care, there is a tendency to refer to textbooks
of developed countries. With a large data set from leading referral centers of a country, it is possible to
define local norms. For instance, expected rates of
pregnancy outcomes, such as low birth weight or perinatal
mortality, can be calculated for women without anemia or
other recorded antenatal condition. This approach will
provide norms that are relevant to each country. A key
policy question relating to the delivery of maternity care
services might be "How many antenatal visits give the
maximum improvement in pregnancy outcome?" This kind of
question can be easily answered from a surveillance
research data base.

A second broad function of MCM is to provide one
avenue for the <u>monitoring of progress of primary health
care</u>. The mother brings critical information to the
maternity center regarding her own health, the survival
pattern of her children and the outcome of her current
pregnancy. If MCM is operational in sentinel centers that
are reasonably reflective of cultural patterns of the
country, the progress of improved primary health care
should be reflected in MCM patterns over time.

By far the most important purpose of MCM, however, is
the <u>professional development</u> of providers of maternity
care. To use this resource to develop pride and a sense
of responsibility, that is, professionalism among maternity care providers, the feedback from MCM must mirror their
performance. Professionalism does not evolve in isolation, but as a group process among peers. The feedback of
MCM should be studied in peer review sessions involving
service providers in each geographic area. To be effective, the data studied must be interesting and presented
in a manner that ranks the performance of the centers
participating in the review process.

This concept of <u>epidemilogical surveillance and peer review</u> is not new. All modern medical facilities of developed countries have their various committees of peers to review many aspects of medical care. The result of their work is a consensus concerning standards of practice and a concerted effort by all involved practitioners to live up to these standards. What is new about MCM is its application of this well-established process to consensus formation in developing countries, where it has been largely lacking.

The absense of professional development through epidemiological surveillance and peer review has left much of the developing world to turn to a top-down pattern of supervision and targets of performance, with little involvement of providers of service in formation of such targets. The failure of this approach has stimulated thought for reasonable alternatives.

In a way, the poor quality of maternity care in the majority of developing countries can be viewed as part of a crisis in consensus formation. The pattern of consensus formation varies in different cultural and political settings. In China, the political process is dominant. In Indonesia, there is an effective village organization, typified by the Banjar system on Bali. Sri Lanka has a tradition of professional education extending to midwifery that contributes to a consensus concerning standards of maternity care. All aspects of the process of consensus formation - political, traditional and educational - are at work in every country in varying degrees. Unfortunately, in many of the most populous and the poorest of developing countries, political will is lacking, traditional patterns have been largely lost in a colonial period, and professional education has become degree-rather than content-oriented. These are the countries where there is no choice but to rebuild from below. MCM offers only one facet of a complex process of community consensus formation; but it is one focused on a most important health problem of developing countries. In this respect, MCM is part of a larger process of community development and consistent with other efforts to broaden communiy participation in the development process.

CONCLUSION

We are living through a remarkable explosion of new information and revolutionary ways of storing and processing information. The microchip and microcomputers have made this possible. An impressive array of software programs has been written for these relatively inexpensive computers that focus on both management and scientific tasks. Most of these programs are designed for developed country markets, and little thought has gone into how this development can be used to solve the poor health, poverty and social disorganization of the Third World.

MCM is one model application of the potential of new information technology to one of the world's most serious problems. Although MCM was developed with the use of large computers, the programs can now be run on a micro-computer. Such a computer and software program would be adequate for the monitoring of maternity care in almost any developing country. It is no longer merely a research tool for "studies"; MCM is a practical option for today.

International health statistics are simply summary data that can rarely be used to produce indices useful for the health care challenge of the balance of this century. The progress of declining infant and child mortality is slowing (2) as maximum benefits of disease control pro-grams, based on environmental efforts, are realized. Further progress will require changes in individual beha-vior, especially as control of disease in the future will increasingly depend on immunization. To accelerate behavior change efforts, client-specific information that can be readily processed to identify high-risk groups in a population will be needed. The model of MCM might point the way to a new international information system for health statistics through a scheme of continuous surveil-lance reporting at sentinel centers with occasional community health surveys to calibrate the routine recording of MCM.

The present endorsement of the Maternity Record by FIGO and support of the UNFPA for design of country projects for Maternity Care Monitoring are important landmarks in the internationalization of this new informa-tion system. The logic of need, declining cost and the keen interest of the health profession make one optimistic that this important goal will be reached.

REFERENCES

1. Demeny P (1981): The North-South income gap: A
       demographic perspective, New York. The Population
       Council, Center for Policy Studies, Working Paper
       No. 69, January.

2. Gwatkin D (1979): <u>The end of an era?</u> Recent
        evidence indicates unexpectedly early slowing of
        mortality declines in many developing countries.
        Paper prepared for the Overseas Development
        Council, Washington, July, p. 18.
3. Birdsall N: Population and Poverty in Developing
        Countries. <u>World Bank Staff Working Paper</u> No.
        404, Washington.

MATERNITY CARE AND PERINATAL MORTALITY IN INDONESIA

R. P. Bernard and S. Sastrawinata

International Federation for Family Health
(IFFH) Geneva, Switzerland; and Coordinating
Board of Indonesian Fertility Research
(BKS PENFIN), Bandung, Indonesia

INTRODUCTION

Pregnant women and neonates remain the most vulnerable group in any population and many risk factors during pregnancy affect the birth outcome. Crowded and unhygienic living conditions and lack of access to primary maternal care are risk factors known to influence pregnancy outcome. Since formal education and literacy are linked with these conditions, a statistical analysis is mandatory. Furthermore the provision of prenatal care is a direct short-term health intervention requiring quantitative assessment with pregnancy outcome. Since education and prenatal care often exists together, both variables need adequate epidemiologic control when assessing pregnancy outcome. Sufficient prenatal care for low education women (LED) might lead to a more favorable pregnancy outcome than insufficient prenatal care for high education women (HED). If this hypothesis can be substantiated with adequately collected epidemiologic data, the implication would be commanding. High priority deployment of maternity care programs independent of the development of the educational system would be highly desirable.

This report addresses this subject by using data collected with a Standard Maternity Record at the time of parturition (1). The results of examining risk factors that were present during pregnancy as they relate to pregnancy outcome are discussed below.

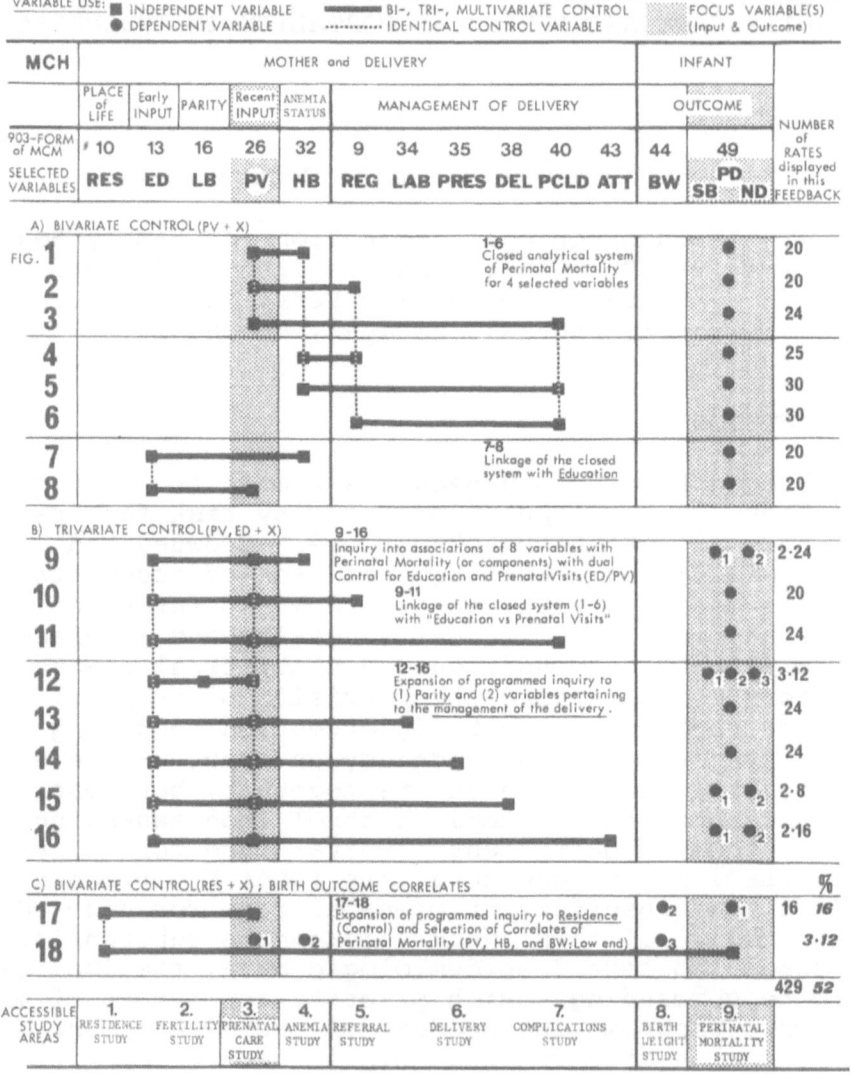

Strategy of Data Analysis with Standard Computer Outputs (SCOs). Focus on Prenatal Visits and Perinatal Mortality. Access to Display of both Format and Findings in 18 consecutive Figures. BKS PENFIN, INDONESIA, 1978-1980. 11-Center Pool with 36,802 Women with single birth.

Diagram 1.

Anatomy of Analysis and Synthesis performed with Standard Computer Outputs (SCOs). Numbers refer to the 24 Figures. BKS PENFIN, INDONESIA, 1978-1980. 11-Center Pool with 36,802 Women with single birth.

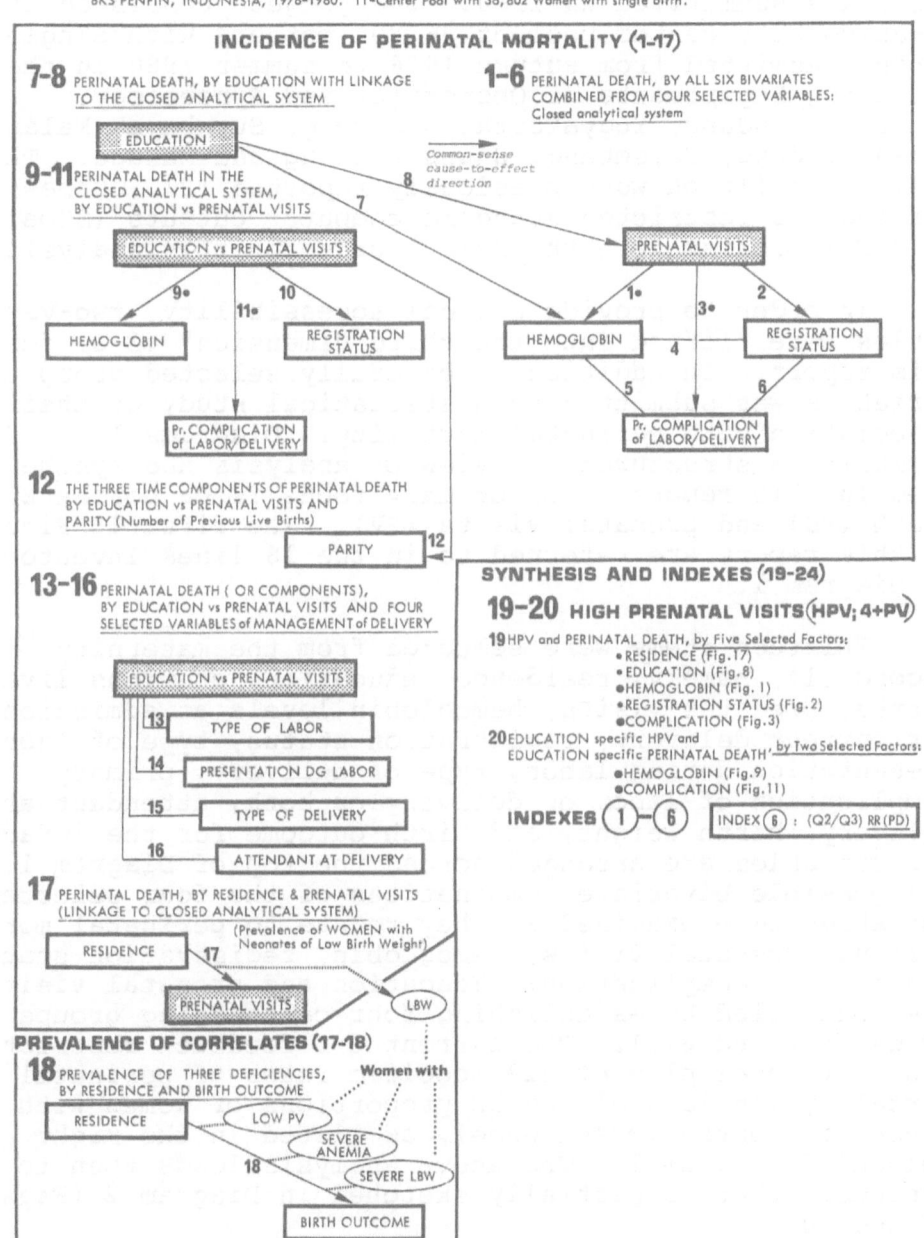

Diagram 2.

MATERIALS AND METHOD

The Indonesian project of Maternity Care Monitoring (MCM) was summarized in 1980. The project consisted of 11-university center pool of 36,802 mothers with single births, admitted from autumn 1978 to summer 1980 in the following Departments of Obstetrics and Gynecology: Jakarta, Bandung, Yogyakarta, Semarang, Surabaya, Malang, Medan, Padang, Palembang, Ujung Pandang and Manado. This pool was built on work previously reported (2). Unrestricted and restricted standard computer outputs (SCOs) of this MCM program were the sole source for this analysis.

In order to provide optical accessibility, two-way tables were "lifted into the third dimension" (3-D) for this report. In addition, a carefully selected group of variables was submitted to a statistical study of their association with perinatal mortality. Diagrams 1 and 2 summarize a structured overview of analysis and synthesis used in this report. The primary focus is on perinatal death (PD) and prenatal visits (PV). The first 18 Figures of this report are referred to in the 18 lines Inventory in Diagram 1.

Thirteen items were selected from the maternity record (1), namely, residence, education, previous live births, prenatal visits, hemoglobin levels at admission for current delivery, registration status, type of labor, presentation during labor, type of delivery, primary complication of labor or delivery or both, attendant at delivery, birth weight, and birth outcome for the infant. The variables are arranged across the top of Diagram 1. All possible bivariate combinations of the four selected variables were examined as they relate to perinatal mortality: prenatal visits, hemoglobin, registration status, and primary complication. Education and prenatal visits are controlled by establishing four contrasting groups (Figs. 8.2 and 8.3). The current 3-D feedback restricts itself to a display of 429 specific rates of perinatal mortality (incidence) and 52 proportions of women with given attributes (prevalence), as listed in the right column of Diagram 1. The above analysis leads then to a synthesis that is partially sketched in Diagram 2 (Figs. 19 and 20).

The prevalence of high (four or more) prenatal visits (HPV;4+) is studied by residence, education and the variables of perinatal mortality (Fig. 19). Specificity in education is introduced and three indices of relative prevalence (RP) of high prenatal visits defined (Fig.

20.1). This leads to the four-quadrant ED/PV system and associated risks of perinatal mortality by selected maternal conditions (Fig. 20.2). The findings lead to the definition of three indices of relative risk (RR) of perinatal mortality.

Each 3-D bar diagram carries both the rate or proportion together with the cell size. This enables any interested reader to select specific factors to test a hypothesis and apply appropriate statistical tests. Hence the baseline aspect of the first collection of 3-D illustrations. Also, this approach is the beginning of a quantitated prognostic matrix of perinatal survival for Indonesia's university referral network of maternity centers.

RESULTS

The major portion of this report includes eighteen self-contained figures that may be accessed individually (multiple entry) or in a programmed sequence by the two diagrams. This first pictorial report should lead to the development of teaching and reference manuals for the obstetrical profession in Indonesia. The current description cannot be more than an introduction to a new approach to analysis and interpretation of research data relating to provision of reproductive health care.

Prenatal Visits

Figures 1 to 6 display the risk of perinatal mortality for the four variables under review (prenatal visits, hemoglobin, registration status, and primary complication of labor and/or delivery). The reader should become familiar with the first six figures since they contain many answers to previously formulated hypotheses.

Two great divides delineate the low risk of perinatal mortality when controlling for prenatal visits and hemoglobin level (Fig. 1). The eight cells defined by both high prenatal visits (HPV;4+) and mild (8 and 9 g HB/100 ml) or no anemia (10+ g HB/100 ml) are associated with perinatal mortality rates below 30/1000. Of these, the four cells with 7+ prenatal visits are associated with perinatal mortality rates below 20/1000, despite two cells being linked with mild anemia. Furthermore, the bivariate study of perinatal mortality associated with the remaining 12 cells of higher risk shows that the number of prenatal visits to exert a greater mortality reducing effect than

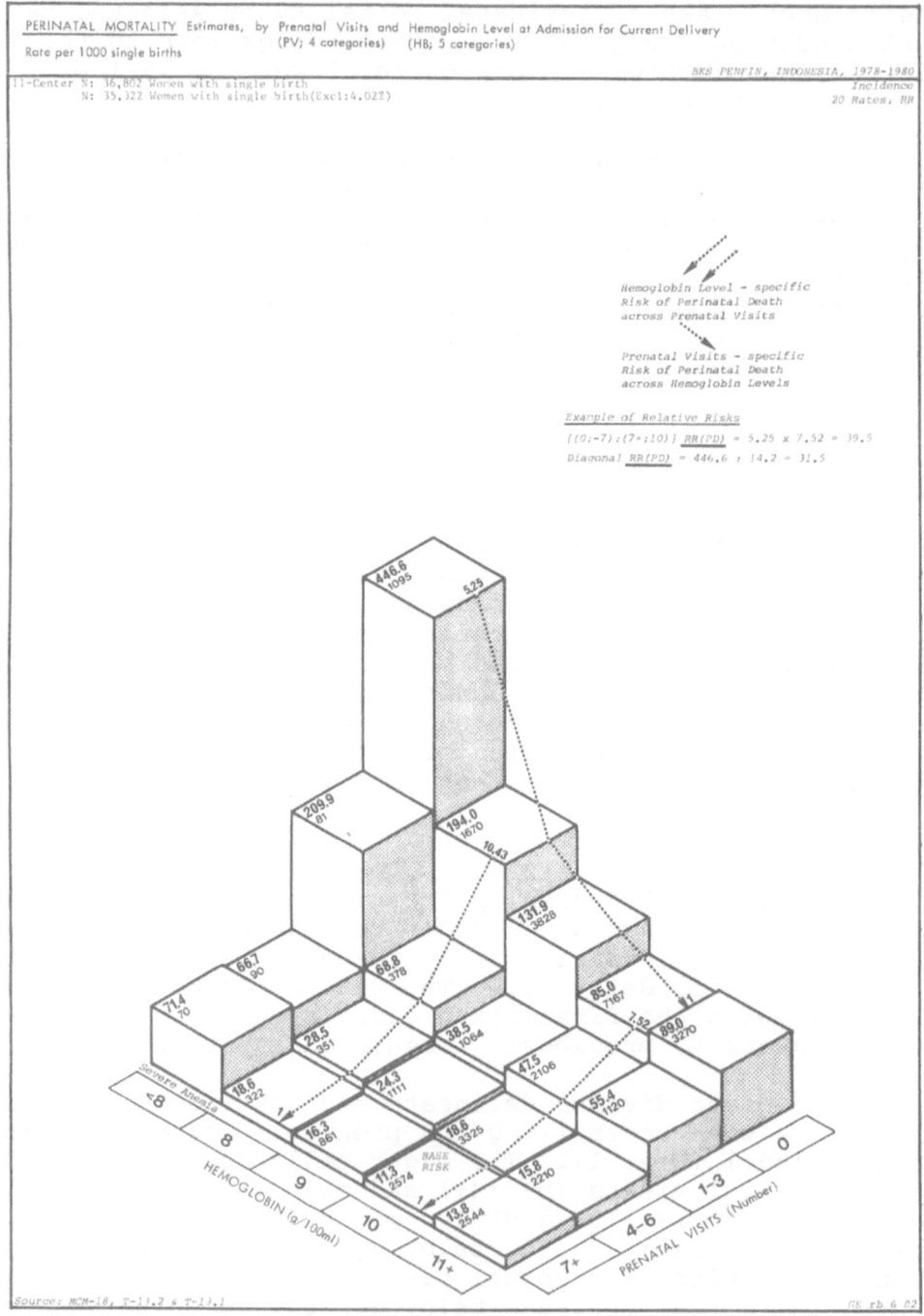

Figure 1: Perinatal mortality, by prenatal visits and hemogloblin.

hemoglobin level. Nevertheless, for severe anemia (<8 g
HB/100 ml) perinatal mortality rates remain multiples of
those associated with the next higher level of hemoglobin
(8 g Hb/100 ml) at each level of prenatal visits. This
would suggest a causal factor to be involved with perinatal mortality for women admitted with severe anemia. The
hypothesis imposes itself: perinatal mortality among
women with severe anemia delivering at these referral centers is preponderantly linked with a causal factor rather
than with a status of maternal morbidity, such as malnutrition anemia. This hypothesis may in turn be examined
by delineating specific risk groups and producing the
respective standard computer outputs.

By controlling for number of prenatal visits and
registration status (Fig. 2), the risk of perinatal mortality show only one imposing divide. At all levels of
prenatal visits, emergency admissions exhibit a multiple
risk of perinatal mortality as compared with the next lower risk categories: the referrals by either physician or
midwife. Nevertheless, a persistent prenatal visits
effect is noted across all categories of registration
status. For instance, among referrals by midwives, the
rate of perinatal mortality drops from 154.0/1000 for
women with no prenatal visits to 40.0/1000 for women with
7+ prenatal visits and a similar gradient is noted for
physician referrals (201.0 to 51.6). The lowest rate of
perinatal mortality (11.4/1000) was calculated for women
with 7+ prenatal vists and whose delivery had been booked
(PV;REG Base Risk). This finding is unexpected since it
applies to 6032 women delivering in 11 university departments from 1978 to 1980 in key centers of major provincial
agglomerations across Java, Sumatra and the Celebes. The
16.4 percent of all deliveries associated with perinatal
deaths is comparable to perinatal mortality recorded during the same period in most developed countries. Another
18.5 percent of all deliveries generated the next lowest
rate of perinatal mortality (16.0/1000): the women who
were booked and had 4 to 6 prenatal visits. Both factors
- prenatal visits and booking - are short range input
variables that apparently become the most important
discriminators of perinatal mortality.

By controlling for number of prenatal visits and
primary complication of labor and/or delivery (Fig. 3),
the rates of perinatal mortality show two important divides. The 6 cells defined by both high number of prenatal
visits (HPV;4+) and complications other than hemorrhage
(none, hypotonic uterine contractions, and prolonged/
obstructed labor) are the combinations of lowest perinatal

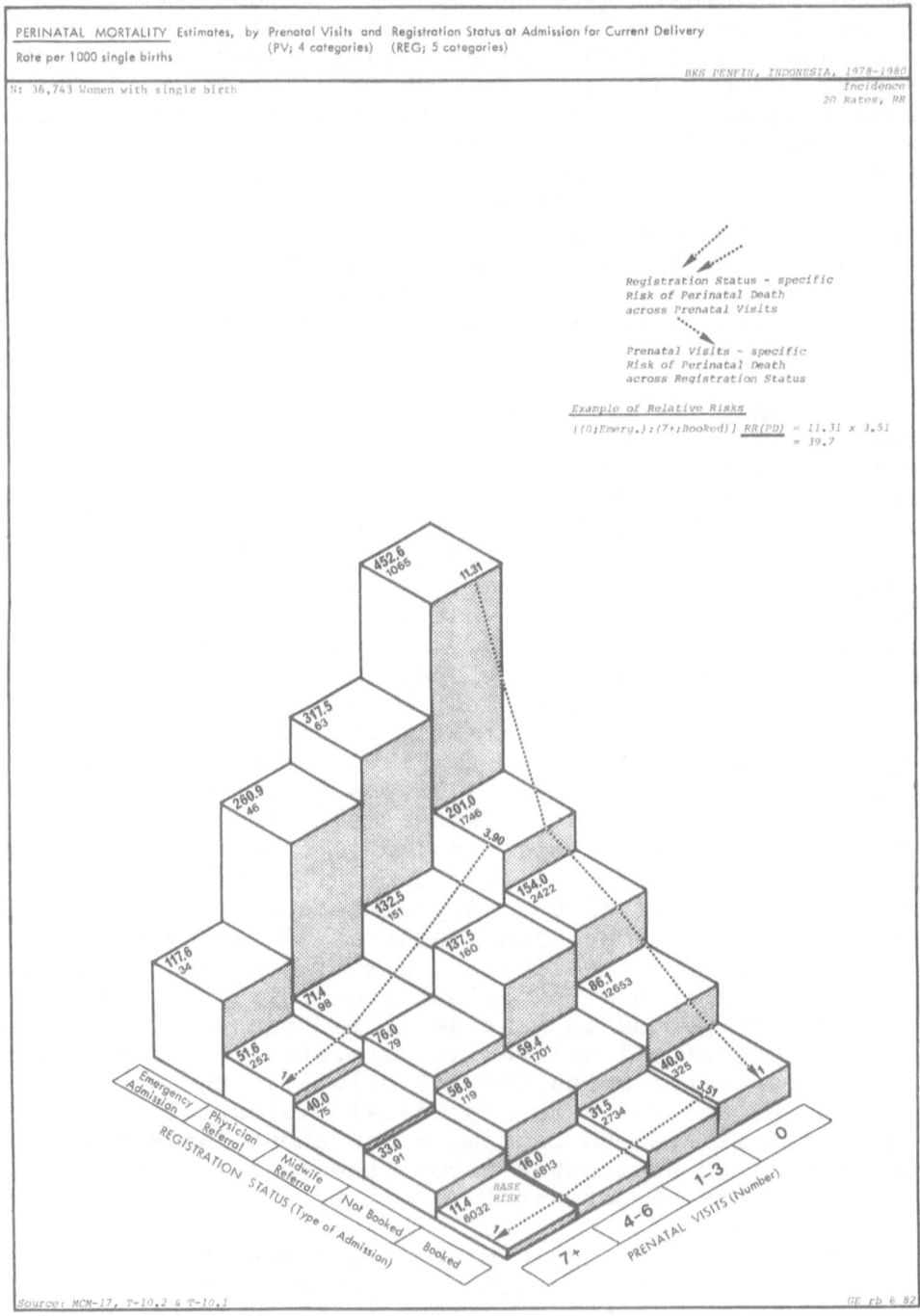

Figure 2:   Perinatal mortality, prenatal visits and
            registration status.

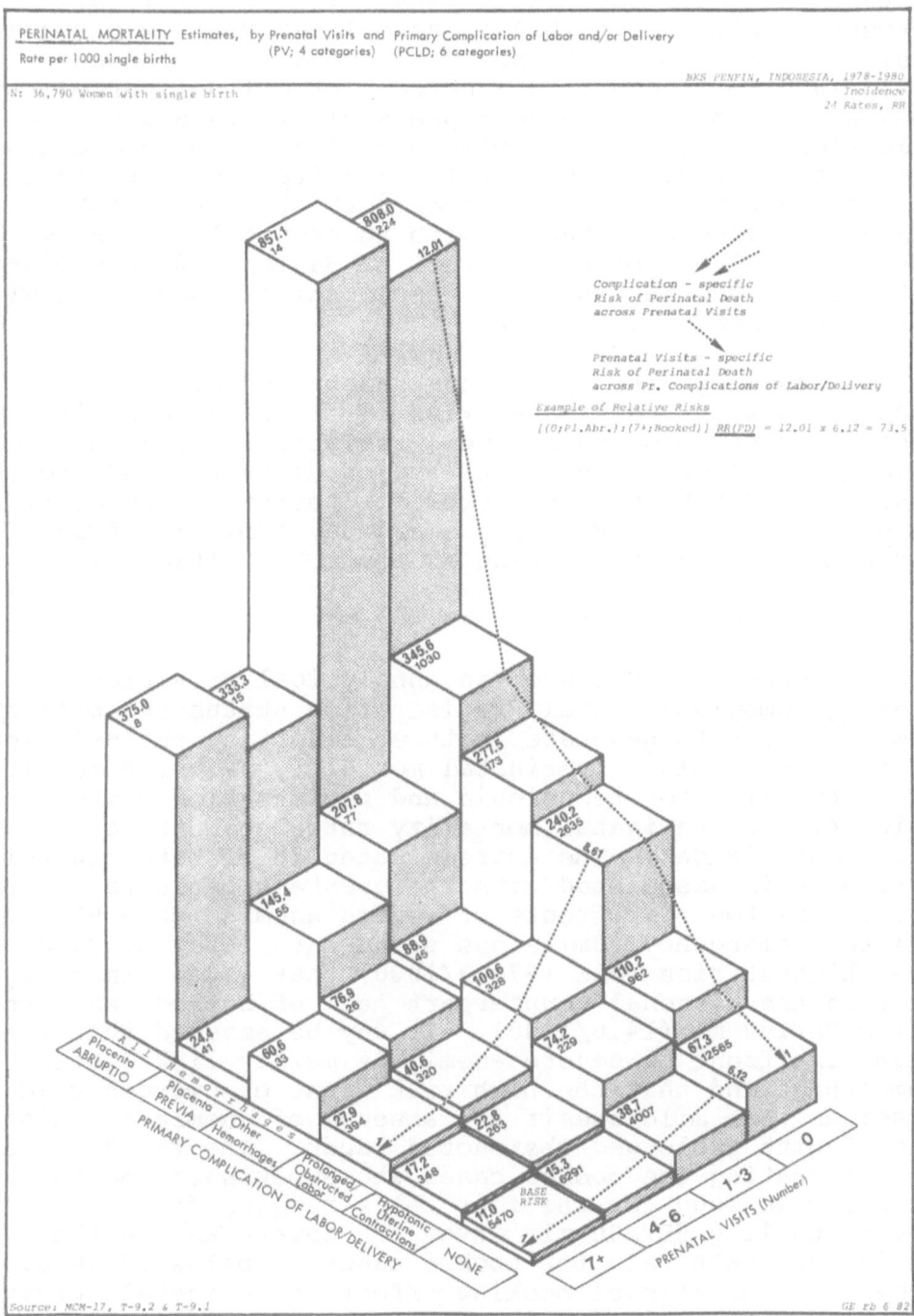

Figure 3:   Perinatal mortality by prenatal visits and primary complication.

mortality rates. The lowest rate (11.0/1000 for 14.9
percent of all deliveries) is associated with 7+ prenatal
visits and no complications, the second lowest rate
(15.3/1000 for another 17.1 percent of all deliveries)
applies to women with 4 to 6 prenatal visits and no complications. Placenta abruptio and placenta previa exhibit
the highest risks of perinatal mortality. Nevertheless,
an important "prenatal visits effect" persists. For
instance, placenta abruptio with no prenatal visits is
associated with a mortality rate of 345.6/1000 as compared
with 145.4/1000 for the same complication among women with
4 to 6 prenatal visits.

In summary, the number of prenatal visits is
associated with a decreased risk of perinatal mortality
regardless of hemoglobin level, registration status, and
primary complication of labor and/or delivery, and the
most discriminating risk factor for perinatal mortality
were severe anemia (Fig. 1), emergency admission (Fig. 2),
and complications pertaining to hemorrhage (Fig. 3).

Blood Hemoglobin

Diagrams 1 and 2 show an annalytical provision for
linking hemoglobin level, registration status and primary
complications to generate in three bivariate analysis specific risk levels of perinatal mortality (Figs. 4 to 6).
By controlling for hemoglobin and registration status
(Fig. 4), the perinatal mortality rates show three
important divides. The extreme category of both control
variables is associated with the greatest perinatal death
rate. The two risk fronts of severe anemia (<8 g HB/100
ml) and emergency admissions stand out. They converge in
the highest risk cell (672.7/1000) that is 45 times higher than the diagonal counterpart cell of booked cases and
11+ g HB/100 ml (14.8/1000). It may be assumed that the
high risk front of severe anemia is mainly linked with
hemorrhage and that the high risk front of emergency admissions with mild anemia and absence of anemia is mainly
linked with prolonged/obstructed labor. The third divide
is delineating the booked cases whose perinatal death rate
is below 20/1000 for the four cells ranging from 8 g HB
100 ml to 11 g HB/100 ml. Even for severe anemia the
perinatal death rate for booked cases is below 50/1000.
Clearly, a beneficial booking effect on perinatal survival
emerges across all levels of hemoglobin. Since booking
and prenatal visits go together, the favorable pregnancy
outcome is linked with this dual short-term input.

By controlling for hemoglobin level and primary

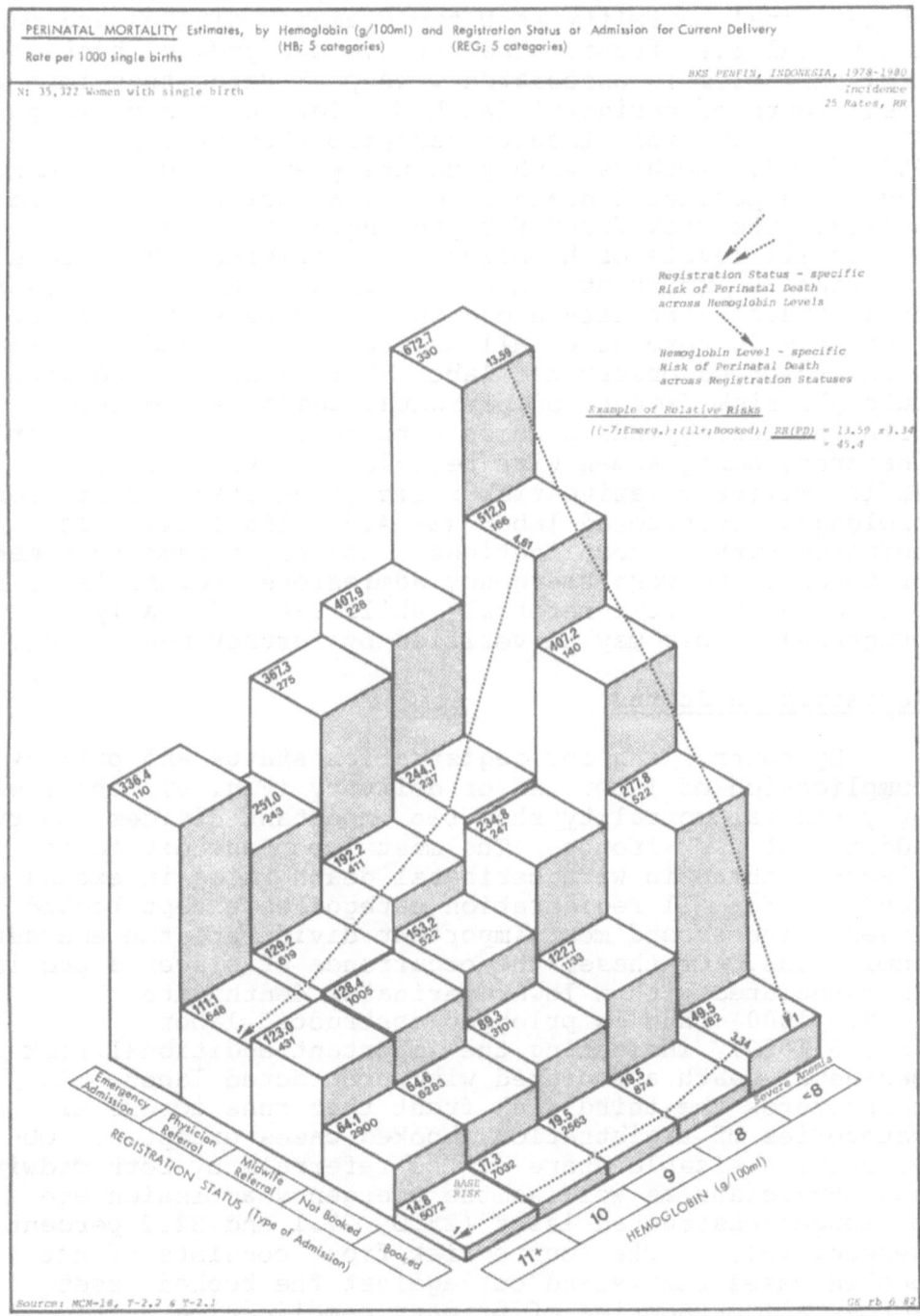

Figure 4: Perinatal mortality by hemoglobin and registration status.

complication of labor and/or delivery (Fig. 5), the risks
of perinatal mortality show two dramatic divides and one
additional risk front. The extreme category of both control variables is associated with peak rates that form two
risk fronts of perinatal death for severe anemia (<8 g
HB/100 ml) and for placenta abruptio that meet at
937.0/1000. Mothers with placenta previa show much more
favorable perinatal death rates if associated with mild
anemia. The risk front for prolonged obstructed labor
across all levels of hemoglobin is striking. This identification is important since it points to a major problem
of perinatal mortality among the 11 university centers.
Precisely 10 percent of all deliveries occurred in women
with prolonged/obstructed labor that is associated with
multiple risk factors of perinatal death as compared
with the corresponding women with no complication. For
instance, among women with hemoglobin levels of 10 g
HB/100 ml the relative risk ratio of perinatal death for
prolonged/ obstructed labor was 4.83 (165.1/34.2) as
compared with no complications. One may assume that many
of these cases were emergency admissions, referrals or not
booked cases ("self-referral" while labor in early
progress). This may be verified by further monitoring.

Registration Status

By controlling for registration status and primary
complication of labor and/or delivery (Fig. 6), the risks
of perinatal mortality show two important divides and two
additional risk fronts. The most important divide is
placenta abruptio with perinatal death rates in excess of
700/1000 for all registration categories except booked
cases. The second most important divide are the emergency
admissions. Of these, the occurrence of placenta previa
is associated with a lower perinatal death rate
(368.0/1000) than is prlonged/obstructed labor
(531.5/1000), indicating the important additional risk of
perinatal death associated with protracted labor. It
constitutes the third risk front that runs across all
categories of registration, booked cases excepted. Obviously, a sizable share of the referrals by both midwives
and physicians as well as the emergency admission are
prolonged/obstructed labor (25.3, 27.1 and 22.2 percent
respectively). The fourth risk front consists of not
booked cases that stand out against the booked cases
across all categories of primary complication. This
observation is important since it suggests a necessary
programmatic input: booking of delivery during pregnancy.
Even among women with no complications of labor and/or
delivery, the risk of perinatal death is 3.8 fold for

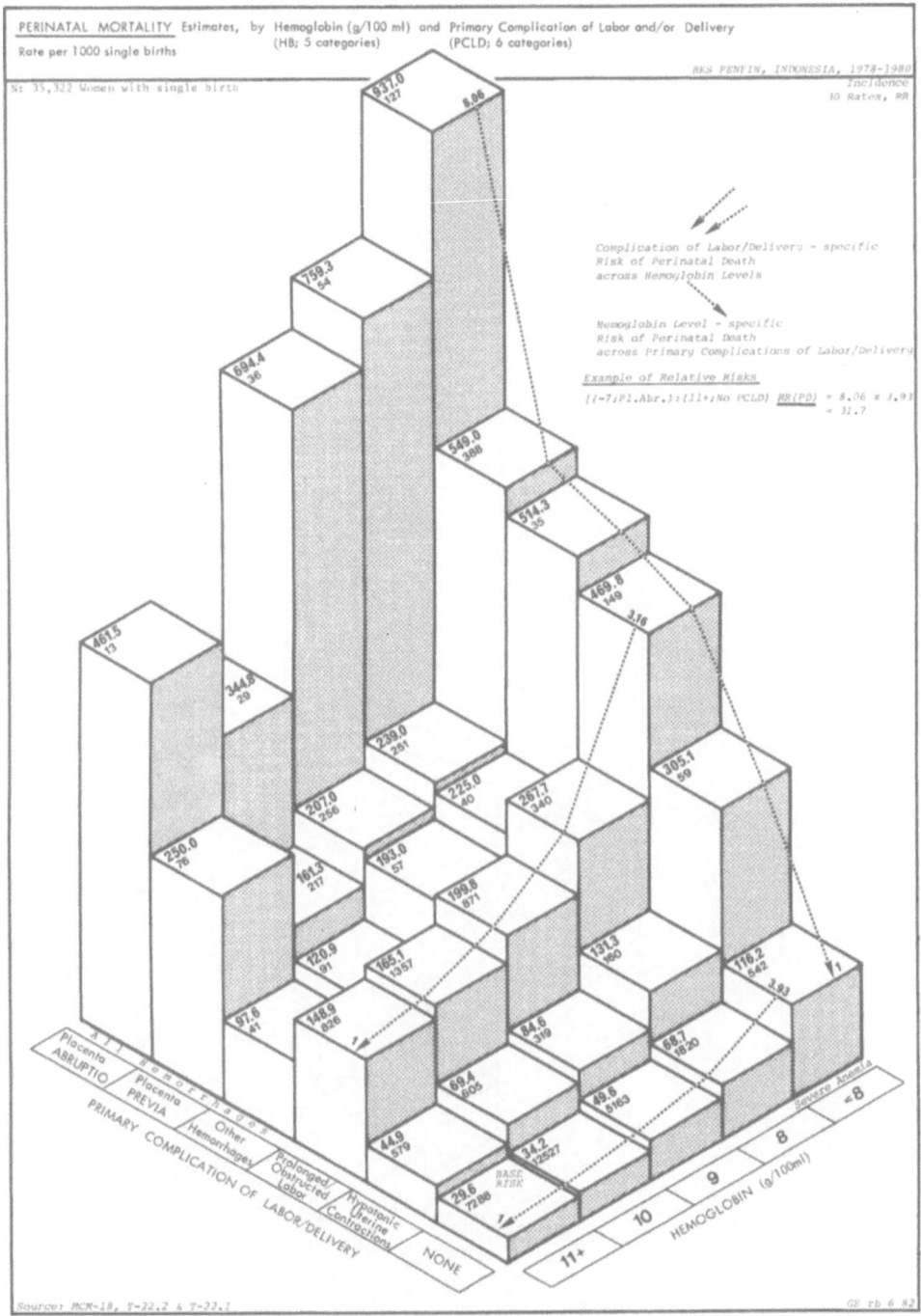

Figure 5: Perinatal mortality by hemoglobin and primary complication.

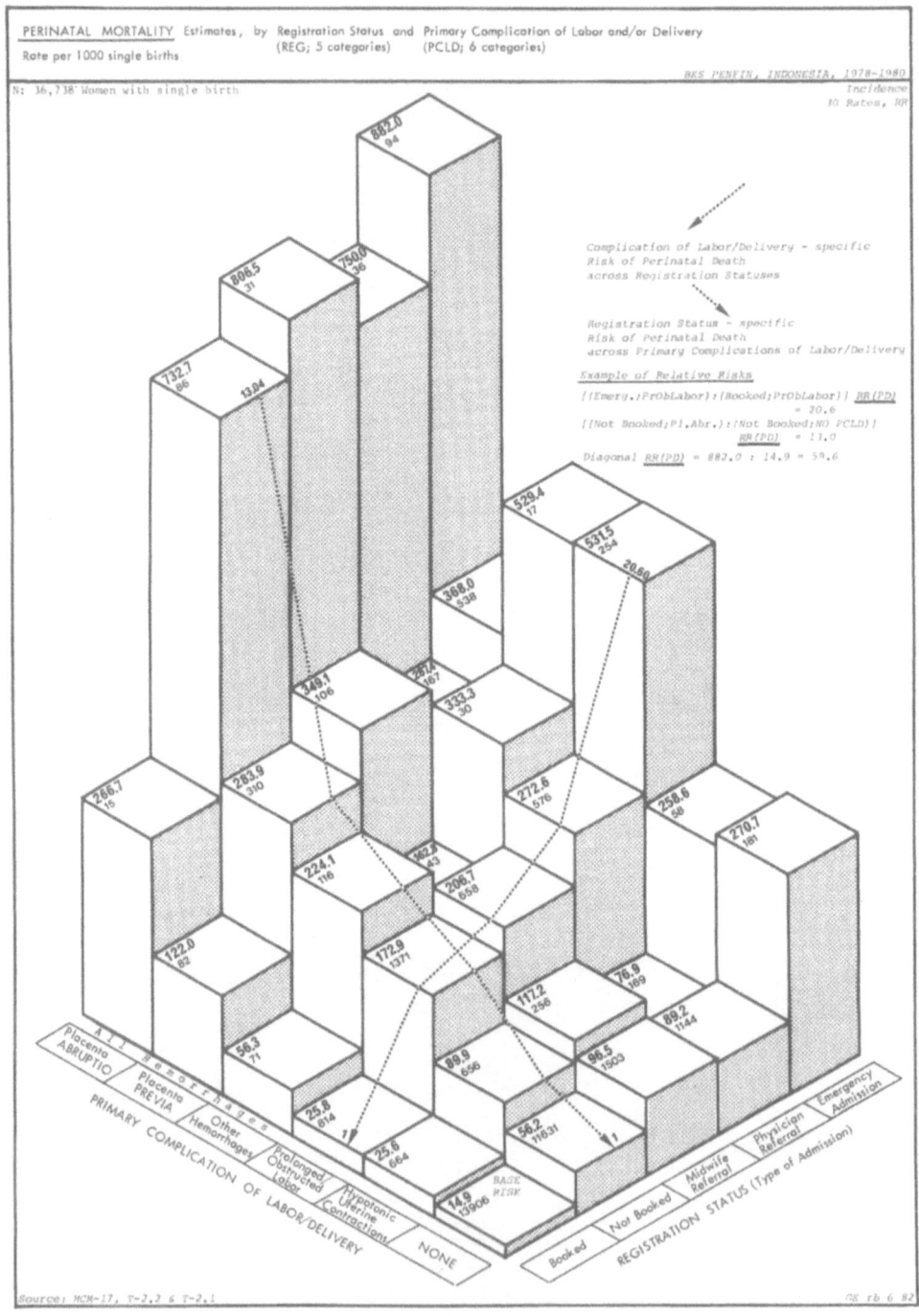

Figure 6:   Perinatal mortality by registration status and
            primary complication.

unbooked cases as compared with booked cases (56.2/4.9). The limitation of this multifold risk is easy to understand since it applies to 31.7 percent of all deliveries.

In summary, high excess perinatal death is linked with severe anemia across all categories of registration status (Fig. 4) and across all categories of existing primary complication (Fig. 5) suggesting that hemorrhage is a major cause of excess mortality in the perinatal period. Finally, the analysis by control for registration status and primary complication identifies not booked cases and prolonged/obstructed labor as high risk groups.

Education

As displayed in Figure 7, the risk of perinatal mortality recorded at the referral institutions is less affected by formal school education than by the parturient's hemoglobin level. A significant change occurs at 8 g HB/100 ml. At all education levels, the risk of perinatal mortality increases multifold when comparing mothers with more than 8 g HB/100 ml and those with less than 8 g HB/100 ml. For instance, for women with 3 to 6 years education, the corresponding rates of perinatal mortality are 156.5/1000 and 411.9/1000 respectively. Even among mothers with formal school education of 11+ years, the difference is impressive: 56.2/1000 and 188.7/1000 are the corresponding perinatal mortality rates. Nevertheless, the education effect exists, and Figure 7 indicates that 6 years of education is a significantly important dividing level for perinatal mortality regardless of all hemoglobin levels. Among women with the lowest risk of perinatal mortality when controlling for hemoglobin level (10 g HB/100 mg), a comparison of mothers with 3 to 6 years education and those with 7 to 10 years reveals significent decrease in perinatal mortality rate (from 63.8/1000 to 38.7/1000). But an additional effect emerges among mothers with 10 g HB/100 ml or 11+ g HB/100 ml and with low education attainment (0 to 2 and 3 to 6 years). The increased perinatal mortality rate at the upper end of the hemoglobin scale for women with low education suggests the importance of factors other than education and hemoglobin that influence perinatal mortality. Most likely, two standard computer runs comparing low education women (0 to 6 years) with 10 g HB/100 ml against those with 11 g HB/100 ml would suggest a problem linked with registration status and primary complications other than hemorrhage. Prolonged or obstructed labor deserves additional attention.

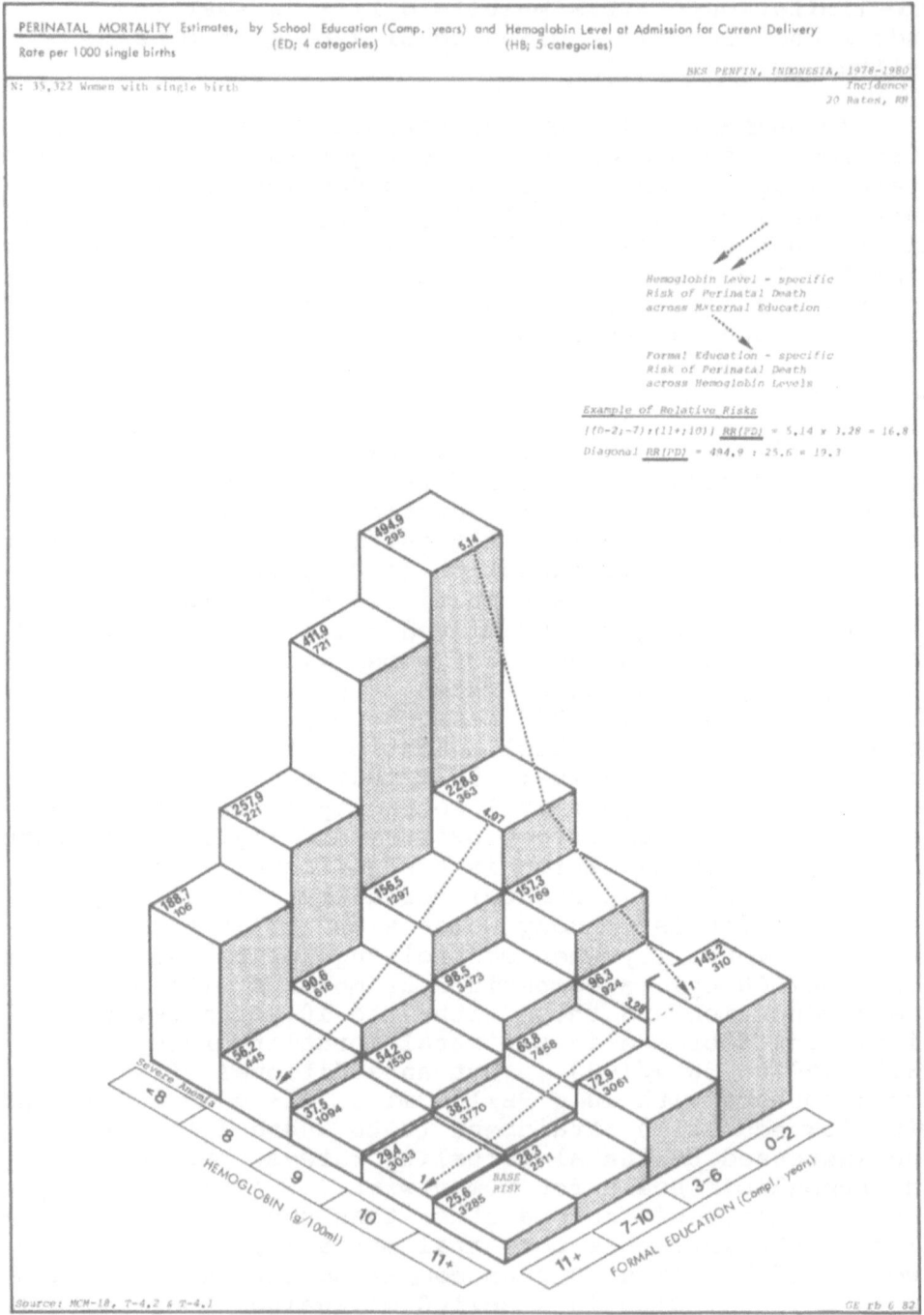

Figure 7: Perinatal mortality by formal education and
            hemoglobin.

As shown in Figure 8.1, perinatal mortality rate recorded at the referral institutions is less affected by education than by prenatal visits. The education effect is virtually erased if the women had sufficient number of prenatal visits (4+PV). Indeed, a significant difference in perinatal mortality rates occur independent of education between mothers with 1 to 3 prenatal visits (over 40/1000) and women with 4+ prenatal visits (around 20/1000). Furthermore, among mothers with 1 to 3 prenatal visits, a plateau of perinatal mortality emerges across all levels of education. However, among women with no prenatal visits education matters since an impressive gradient of perinatal mortality rate is observed across education that spans from 60.7/1000 for mothers with 11+ education to 226.8/1000 for 0 to 2 years education. From the research point of view, one may want to generate two standard computer outputs and study the differential profiles of low education women (LED; 0 to 6 years) with no prenatal visits (the two cells with risk of perinatal mortality in excess of 100/1000) versus all other women (2 cells vs 14 cells). It is likely that registration status and complications will emerge as major problem areas. Figure 8.1 also suggests another comparison scheme: a harmonious four-quadrant classification that is executed in Figure 8.2. As noted in Figure 8.1, each of the four risks of perinatal mortality for women with low education (0 to 6 years) but high number of prenatal visits (4+ PV) is by a multiple smaller than the four risks associated with high education (7+ years) but low prenatal visits (0 to 3 PV). The two sets of four quadrants each may be contracted into 2 single quadrants as shown in Figure 8.2. The corresponding summary of perinatal mortality rates are then 21.1/1000 for LED/HPV women against 66.8/1000 for HED/LPV women, a relative risk of 3.17. This observation influenced the entire analysis, since Figures 9 to 16 then explore specific risks of perinatal mortality according to this four-quadrant ED/PV classification and a series of selected variables pertaining to maternal conditions (hemoglobin and complications) and obstetrical management (type of labor, presentation during labor, type of delivery and attendant at delivery.

Education Versus Prenatal Visits

The trivariate control of the two major components of perinatal deaths (stillbirth and neonatal death) with education, prenatal visits and hemoglobin in Figure 9 shows the following ranking in decreasing importance of both risks: perinatal visits, hemoglobin level and education. This sequence is particularly striking for stillbirths.

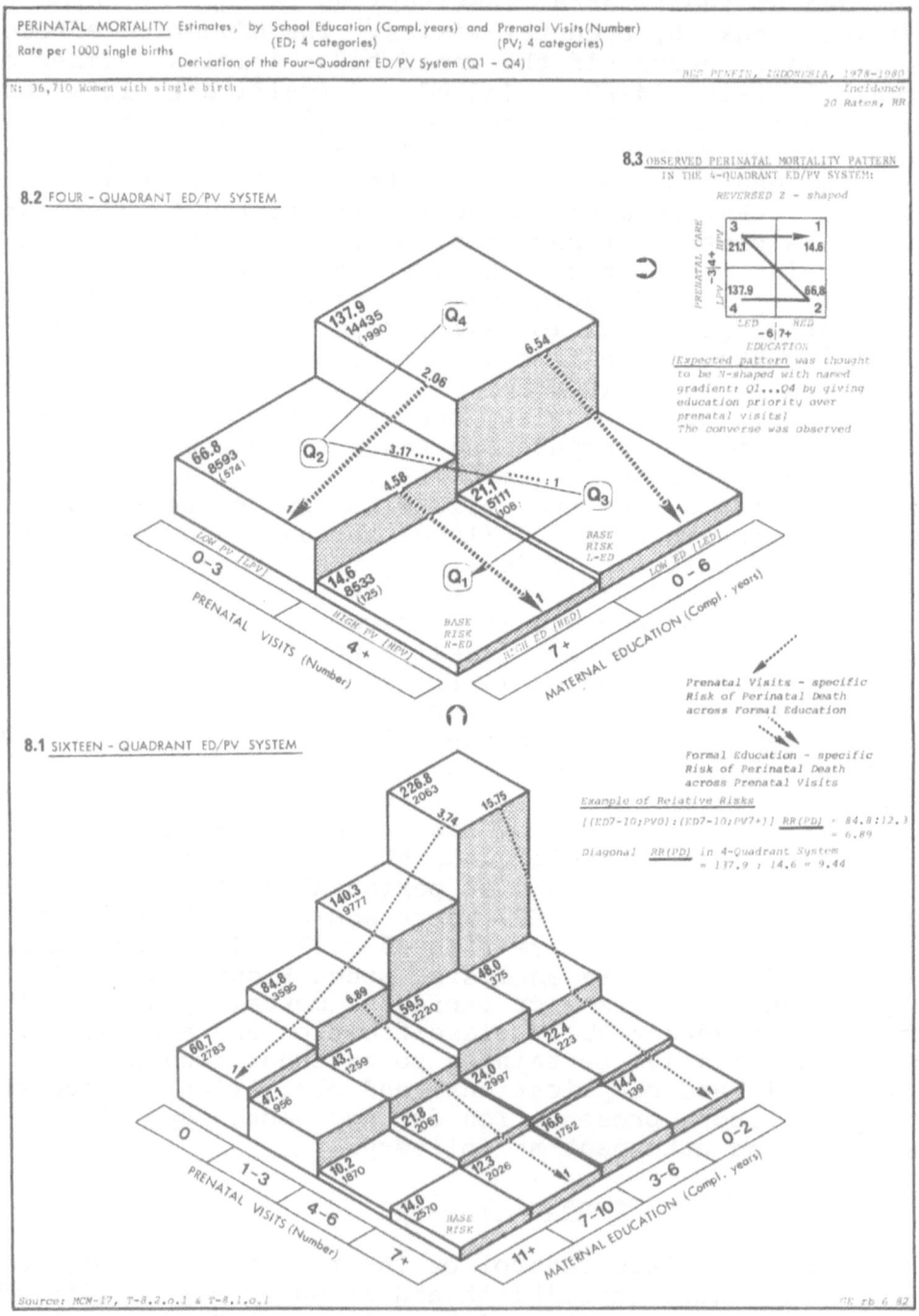

Figure 8: Perinatal mortality by formal education and prenatal visits.

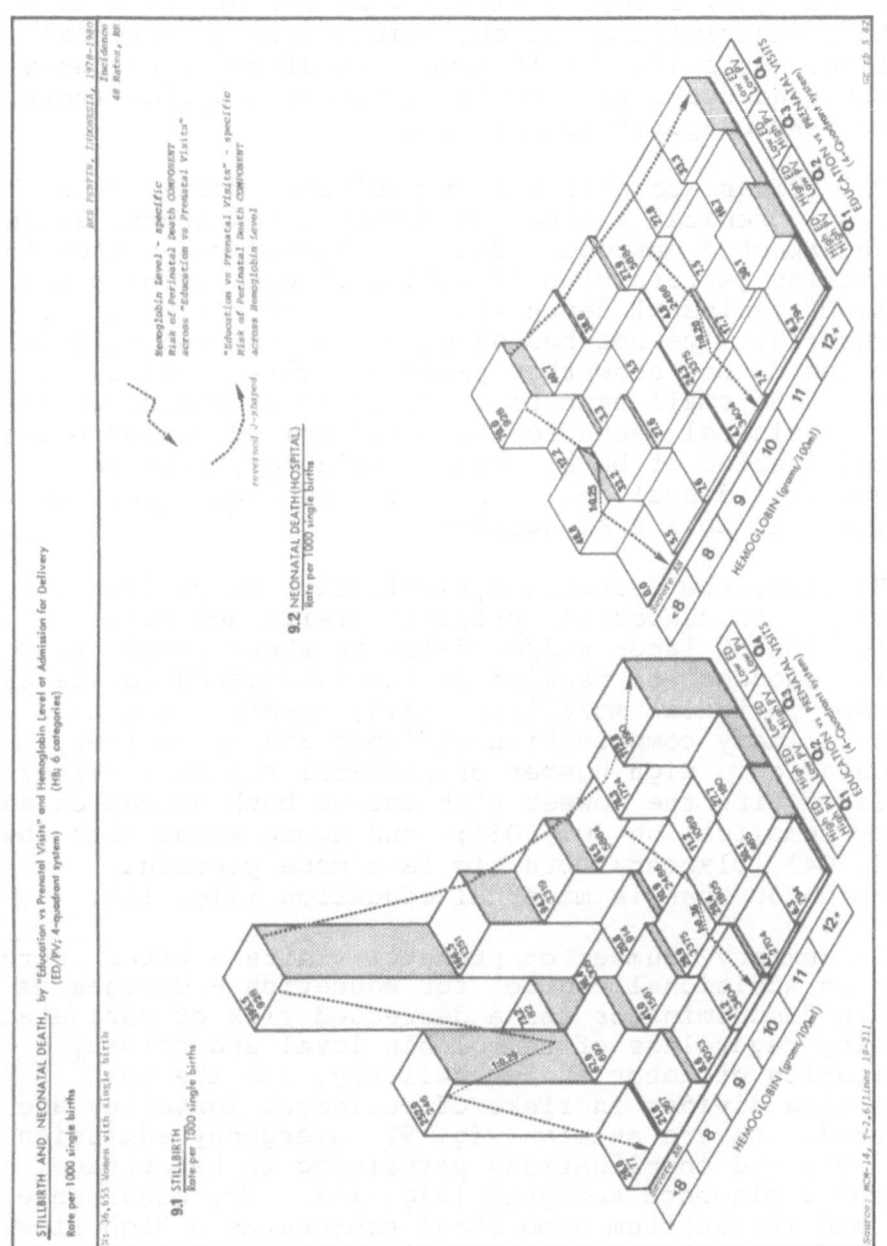

Figure 9: Stillbirth and neonatal death by education vs prenatal vists and hemoblogin level.

High prenatal visits (HPV;4+) is asociated with the lowest
risk of both components of perinatal death across both
education and hemoglobin (Q1; Q3). But among women with
low PV (Q2, Q4), severe anemia (<8 HB/100 ml) is a more
important discriminator of stillbirth than is maternal
education. This insight is important since it suggests
the increased death rate during antepartum period (note
the two "skyscrapers" in Fig. 9.1).

The trivariate analysis of perinatal mortality with
education, prenatal visits and registration status leads
to an unexpected outcome. Only the booked cases show the
now familiar pattern with Q3 (LED;HPV) exhibiting a smaller risk of perinatal death than Q2 (HED;LPV), as displayed
in Figure 10. The not booked cases and the two referral
categories do not show this pattern. This could be due
either to the small numbers in Q3 or to a genuine greater
risk of perinatal death for selected low education women,
or a combination of both. Other variables, such as
distance (residence) and transportation facilities may
contribute to this risk pattern.

Finally, the trivariate examination of perinatal
mortality with education, prenatal visits and primary
complication of labor and/or delivery shows again the
familiar sequence of ranking of the associated levels of
decreased perinatal mortality risks, namely: prenatal
visits, primary complication of labor and/or delivery;
and education. High number of prenatal visits (HPV;4+) is
associated with the lowest risk across both education and
primary complication (Q1, Q3); and among women with low
PV (Q2, Q4), placenta abruptio is a more powerful
discriminator than is maternal education (Fig. 11).

In summary, number of prenatal visits - after introducing an additional control for education - emerges as
the main discriminator for a decreased risk of perinatal
mortality regardless of hemoglobin level and primary
complication of labor and/or delivery, and the most
contrasting divides in risks of perinatal mortality are
unaltered: severe anemia (Fig. 9), emergency admission
(Fig. 10), and complications pertaining to hemorrhage, in
particular placenta abruptio (Fig. 11). The occurrence of
ante- and intrapartum hemorrhage emerges as a high risk
factor of perinatal death.

Parity

As shown in Figure 12, the risk of each of the three
components of perinatal mortality (antepartum, intrapar-

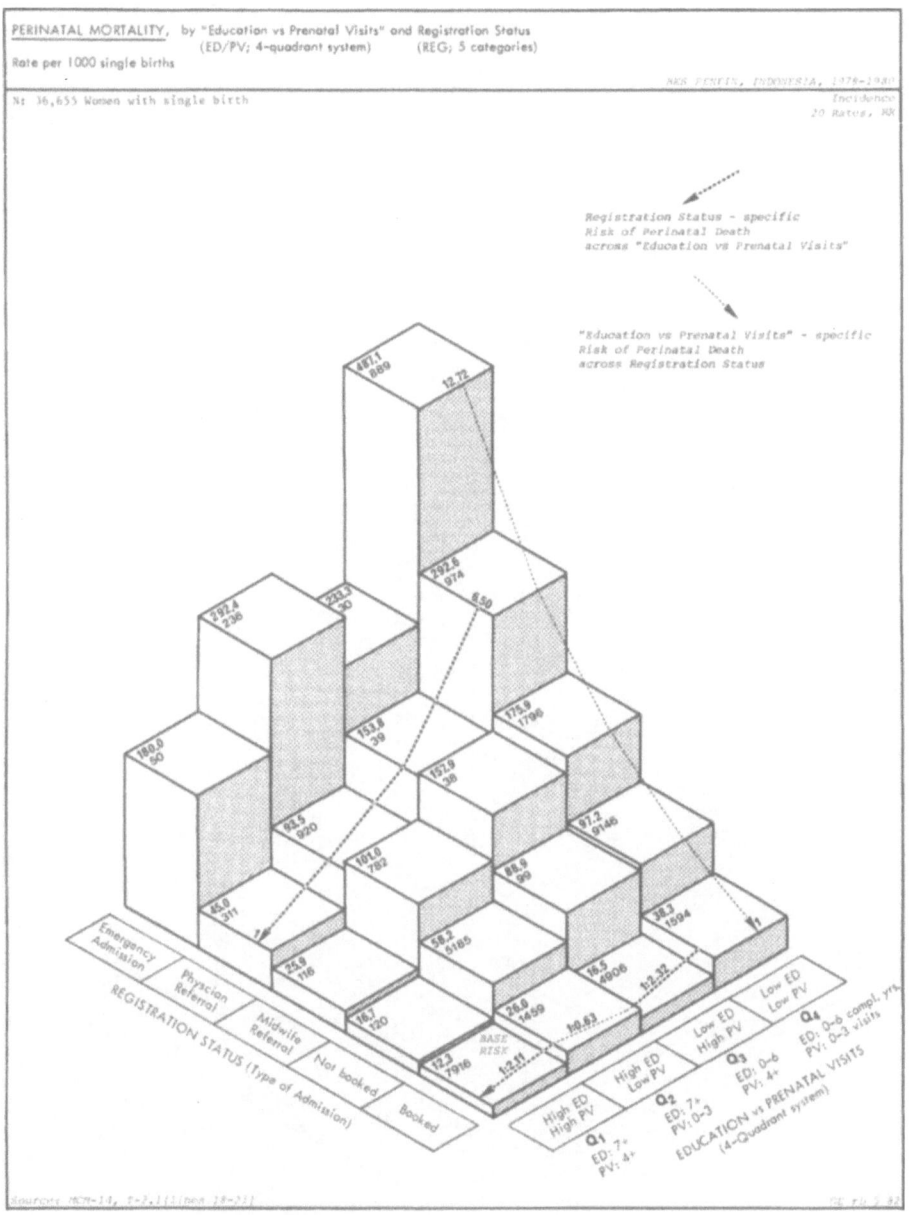

Figure 10:   Perinatal mortality by education vs prenatal
              visits and registration status.

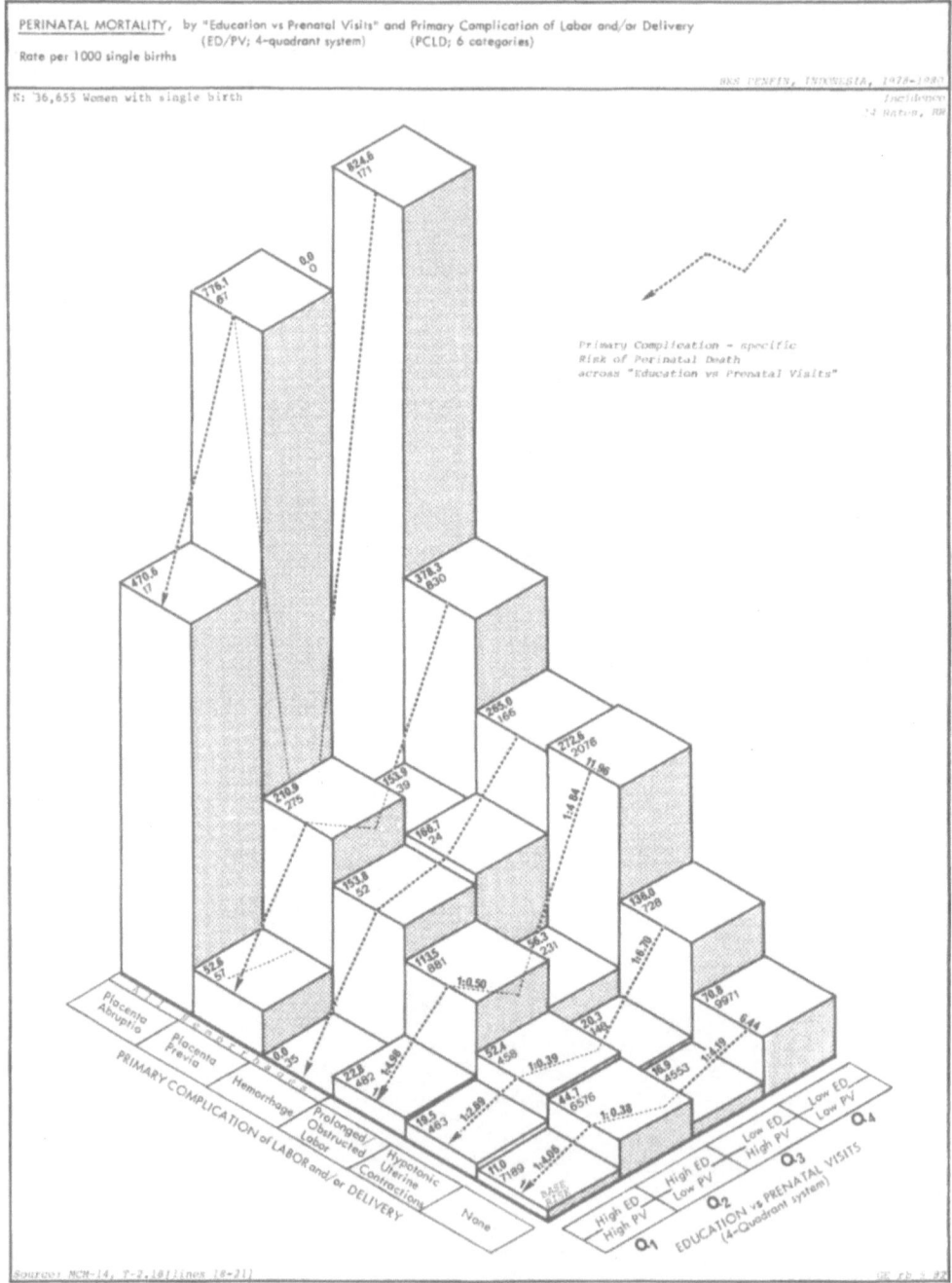

Figure 11:   Perinatal mortality by education vs prenatal
             visits and primary complication.

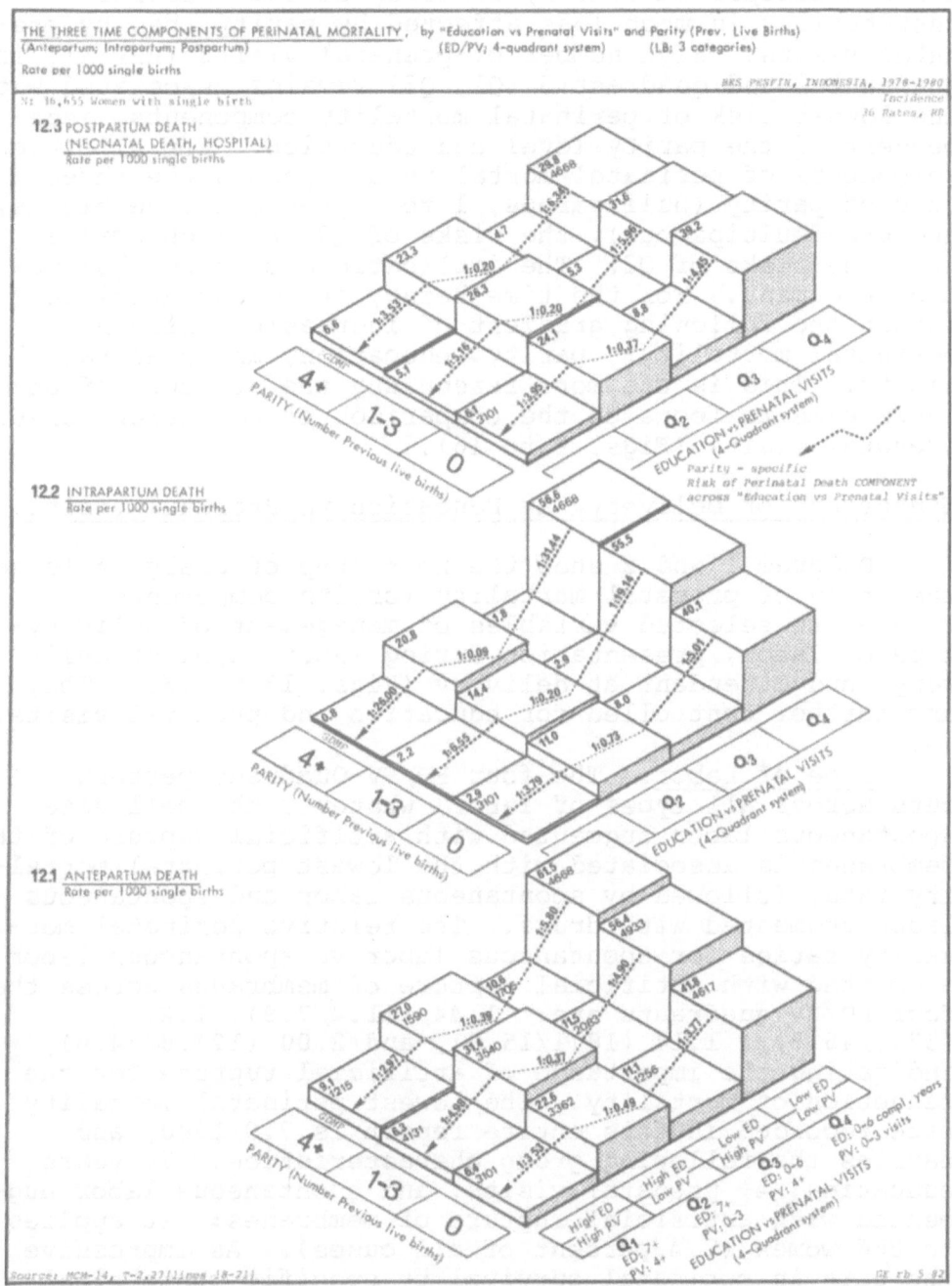

Figure 12. The three time components of perinatal mortality by education vs prenatal visits and parity (previous live births).

tum and postpartum deaths) recorded at the referral
institutions is much less affected by parity than by prenatal visits. High number of prenatal visits (HPV;4+) in
quadrant 1 and quadrant 3 (Q1, Q3) remains associated with
the lowest risk of perinatal mortality components, independent of the parity level and education. For all three
components of perinatal mortality and across the three levels of parity (nulliparous, 1 to 3 previous live births,
and grandmultiparous), the risks of Q3 are much smaller
than the risks of Q2. The implications of this observation are many. For the time being, it is essential to
retain the following gradient of increasing influence of
perinatal mortality: parity, education, and prenatal
visits. This is one more reason why the strategy of analysis came to focus on the comparison of education versus
prenatal visits (Figs. 9 to 16).

Management of Delivery, By Education vs Prenatal Visits

Diagram 1 and 2 show the next step of analysis to be
the study of prenatal mortality (or its components)
related to selected variables of management of delivery:
type of labor, presentation during labor, type of delivery, and attendant at delivery (Figs. 13 to 16). They
are further controlled for education and prenatal visits.

Type of Labor. The four ED/PV-Quadrant pattern
cuts across all types of labor, whatever the cell size.
Spontaneous labor augmented with artificial rupture of the
membranes is associated with the lowest perinatal mortality rate, followed by spontaneous labor and spontaneous
labor augmented with drugs. The relative perinatal mortality ratios for spontaneous labor vs spontaneous labor
augmented with artificial rupture of membranes across the
four ED/PV quadrants are: 1.44 (11.4/7.9), 1.27
(57.6/45.5); 1.14 (18.1/15.9), and 2.00 (127.8/64.0),
indicating the importance of artificial rupture for the
reduction of mortality. The lowest perinatal mortality
rate recorded in this entire report is 7.9/1000, and
carries the following group characteristics: 7+ years
education, 4+ prenatal visits, and spontaneous labor augmented with artificial rupture of membranes; it applies
to 886 women (2.4 percent of all cases). As impressive is
the gain in perinatal survival by specific obstetrical
intervention for women with low education levels and low
number of prenatal visits (Q4): the perinatal death rate
was reduced into half and applies to 1687 women (4.6 percent). This observation merits immediate feedback to the
sponsoring university departments. In addition, two
standard computer outputs (SCOs) should be run for the Q4

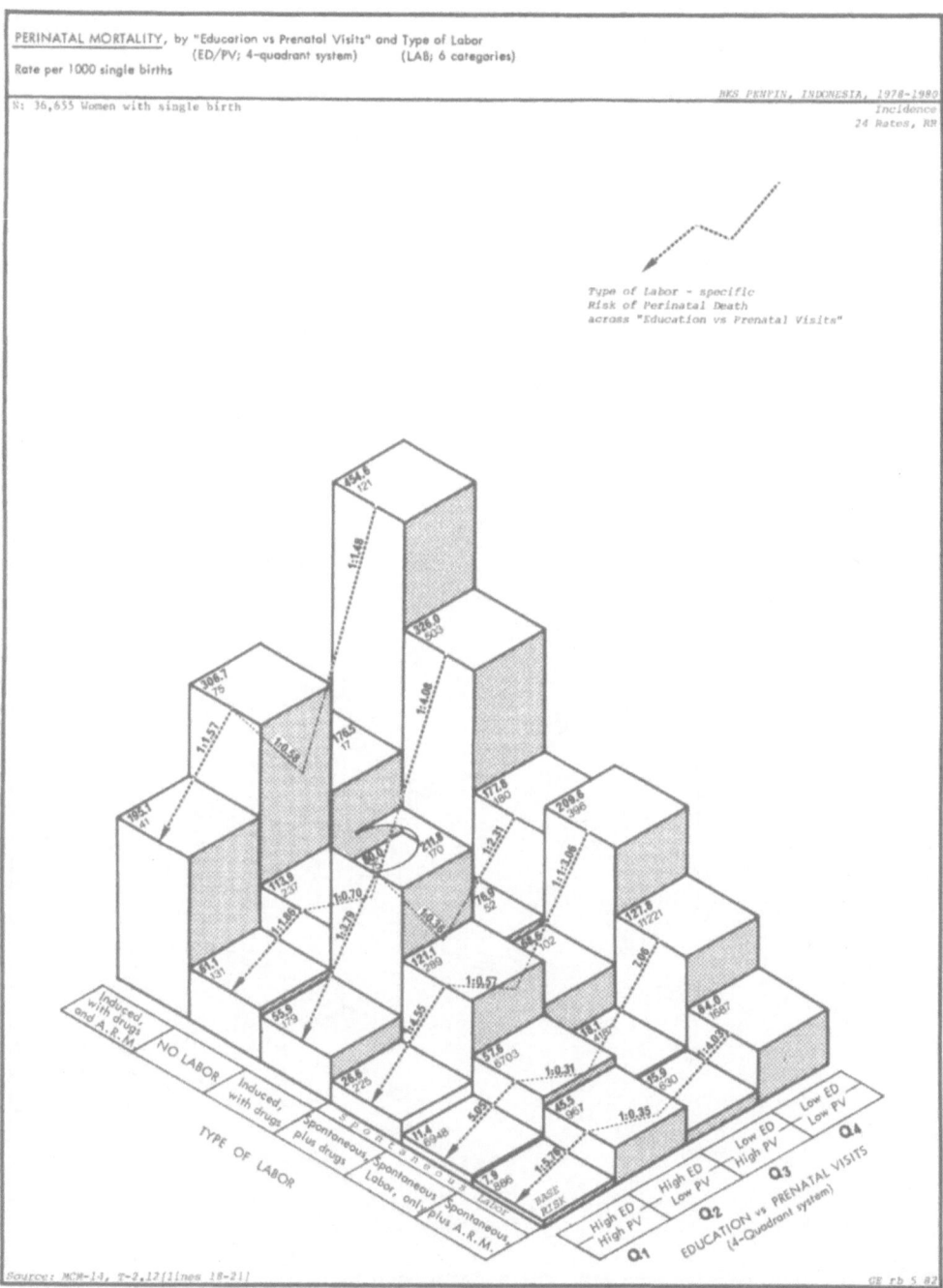

Figure 13. Perinatal mortality by education vs prenatal visits and type of labor.

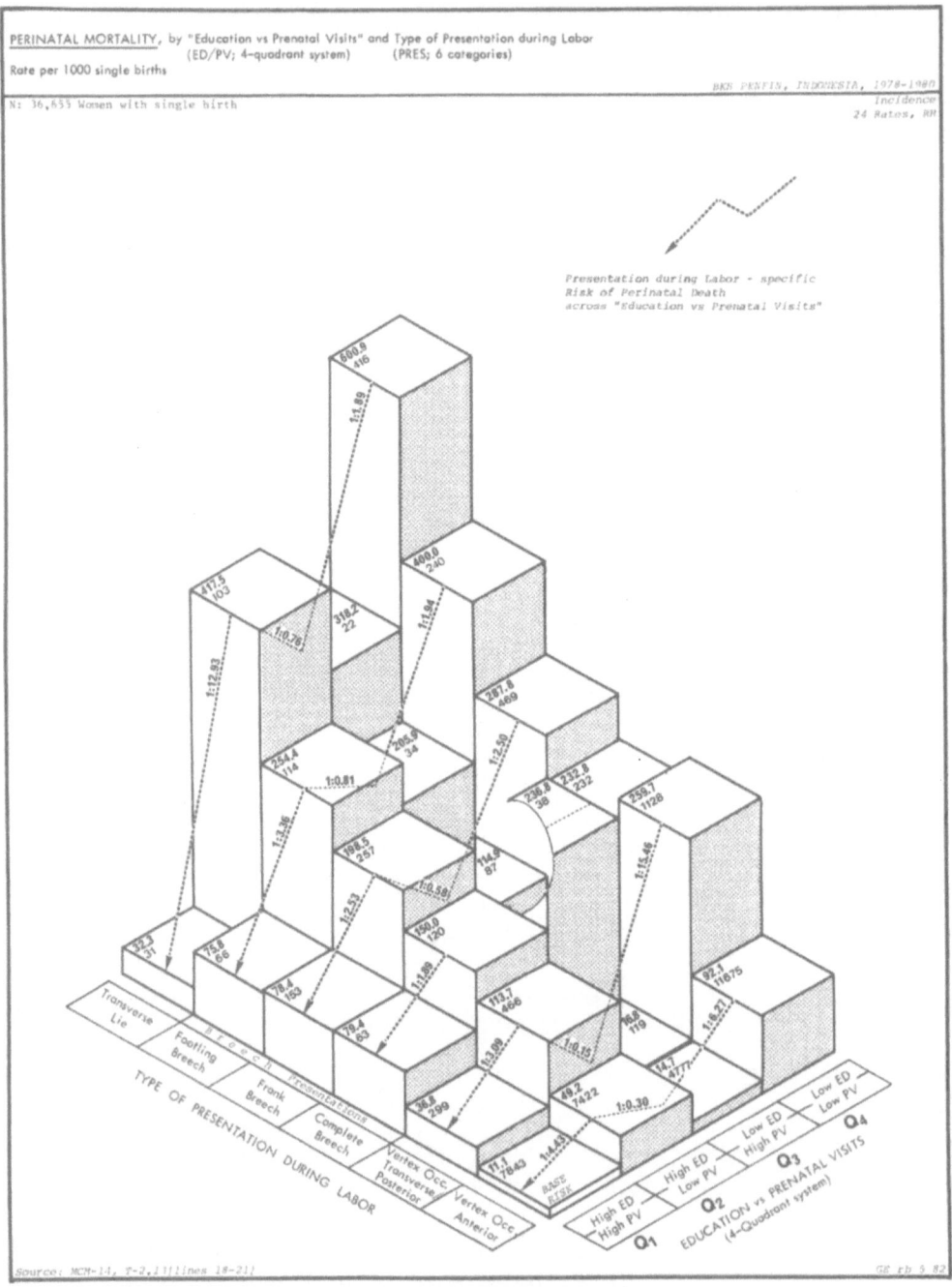

Figure 14.   Perinatal mortality by education vs prenatal visits and type of presentation during labor.

specificites of spontaneous labor (N=11,221) and spontaneous labor augmented with artificial rupture of membranes (N=1687). The two cells contain 35.2 percent of all women.

Type of presentation during labor. Except for one cell with small number (N=38), the four ED/PV-Quadrant pattern cuts across all types of presentation during labor. Newborns with vertex occiput anterior show the lowest rate of perinatal mortality, followed by vertex occiput transverse or posterior, the three types of breech presentation, and finally, transverse lie. Among breeches, the footling group carries the highest risk of perinatal death among women with low number of prenatal visits (Q2, Q4); and complete breech the lowest. Transverse lie among women with low education and low prenatal visits (Q4) is associated with a perinatal death rate of 600.9/1000 and applies to 1.13 percent of all women. A standard computer output restricted to these 416 women may provide new insights for the improvement of this excessively high risk. Finally, it should be noted that the lowest risk cell (N=7843) of 11.1/1000 applies to 21.4 percent of all women under review, an impressive share.

Type of delivery. The four ED/PV-Quadrant pattern of risk applies to both components of perinatal mortality (stillbirth and neonatal death) as well as to the two selected types of delivery (spontaneous delivery and cesarean section), as shown in Figure 15. The display of differential rates suggests the development of two companion thesis, the common cell being Q4/spontaneous delivery carrying risks of stillbirth of 64.8/1000 and of neonatal death of 21.4/1000 that apply to 10,552 (28.8 percent) women under review. The work can be performed with standard computer outputs. An impressive observation is that number of prenatal visits is associated with decreased risks of both stillbirth and neonatal death for the two extremes of delivery: spontaneous and cesarean section. This would indicate the paramount importance of prenatal visits since its operation affects the risks of all subsequent interventions by obstetricians. Future active reduction of perinatal mortality suggests a programmatic combination of prenatal visits, booking for delivery in appropriate institutions along the referral chain and professional intervention at the time of delivery by training of traditional birth attendants, nurse/midwives, trained midwives, physicians, and obstetricians/gynecologists, in this order. From a preventive medicine point of view, it is to be stressed that a programmatic deployment of prenatal visits with professional linkage to

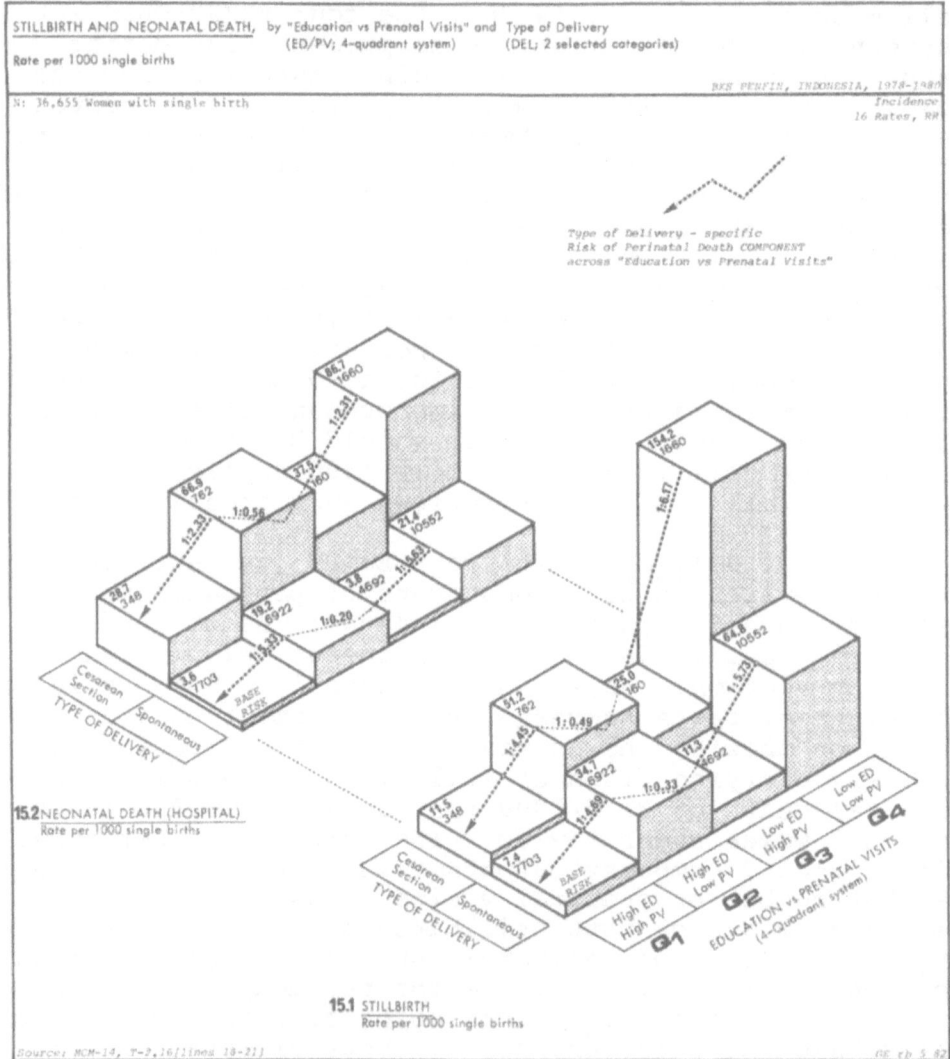

Figure 15. Stillbirth and neonatal death by education vs prenatal visits and type of delivery.

the referral chain will likely achieve the greatest impact for early national reduction of perinatal deaths. The appropriate level of specialized birth attendance, however, cannot erase the more fundamental input to be made during pregnancy: prenatal vists. This is emphasized in the next section.

Attendant at delivery. The four ED/PV-Quadrant pattern of risks applies to both components of perinatal mortality (stillbirth and neonatal death) as well as to the four selected categories of specialized birth attendants: obestetrician/gynecologist physician, qualified midwife, medical student and student nurse/midwife. This is a significant finding. Specialized manpower of birth attendance is powerless vis-a-vis the risk associated with absence or insufficient prenatal care. Whatever obstetrical risk pattern is to be encountered by specialized birth attendants: the birth outcome remains greatly affected by pregnancy care efforts. This is the major conclusion to emerge from Figure 16.

In summary, birth outcome by specialized management of delivery is significantly affected by health care input prior to confinement. This was demonstrated for the following four variables of management of delivery: type of labor, type of presentation during labor, type of delivery and type of birth attendant. It appears that surveillance research at the referral institutions gives access to a systematic identification of factors that will have to be programmatically controlled across the entire catchment area of that referral center, if indeed the regional rate of perinatal mortality is to be reduced. The referral institution is in a position to calculate reference standards for prenatal visits and associated risk of perinatal mortality.

Residence

As shown in Figure 17.1, the risk of perinatal mortality recorded at the top referral institutions is less influenced by residence than by prenatal visits. The slum effect for urban women is erased if they had some (1+) prenatal visit. There is a significant reduction of the risk of perinatal mortality at 4+ prenatal visits from around 45/1000 to around 17/1000. For rural women, the same reduction is noted with a drop from 91.6/1000 to 30.8/1000. However, among women with no prenatal visits (PVO), residence matters. The risk of perinatal mortality for urban women is 79.9/1000 as compared with 303.6/1000 for rural slum women. Clearly, rural women

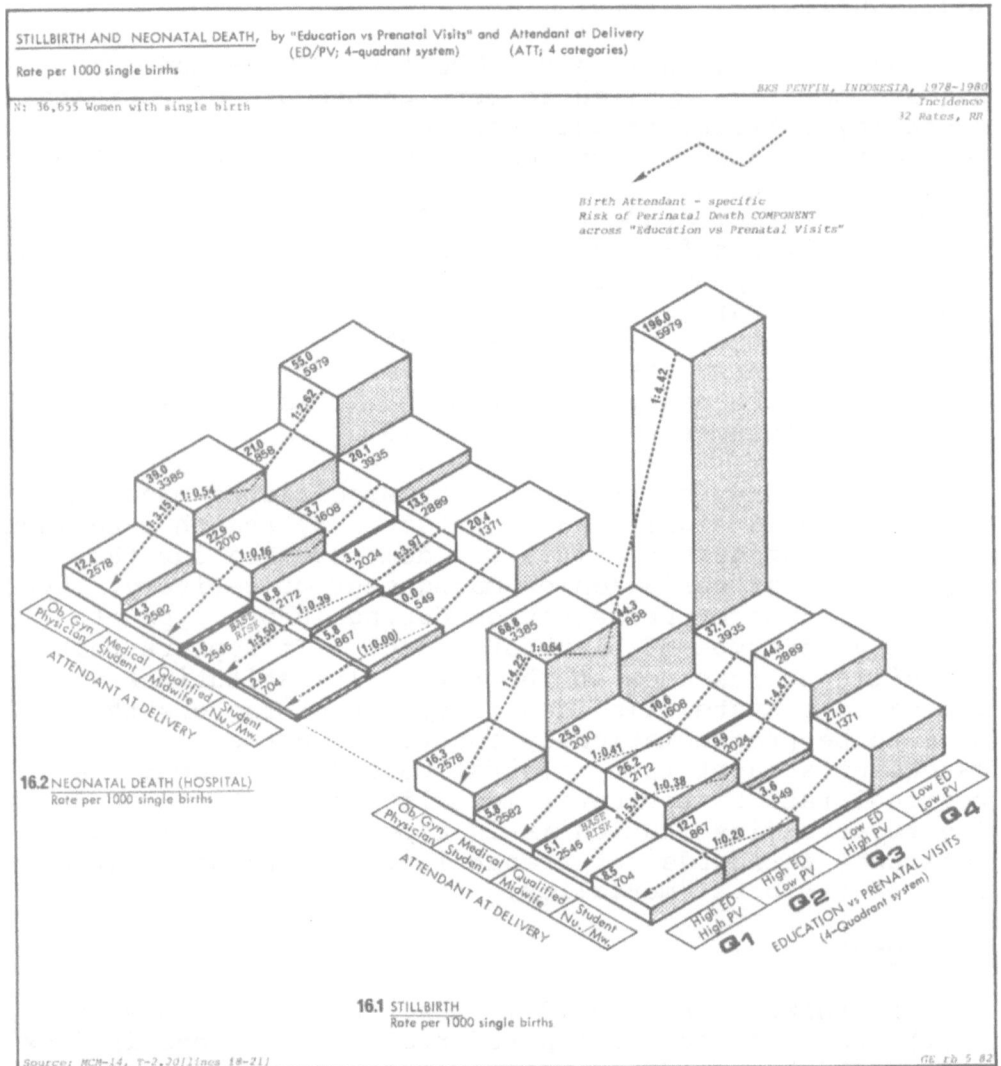

Figure 16.   Stillbirth and neonatal death by attendant at
delivery.

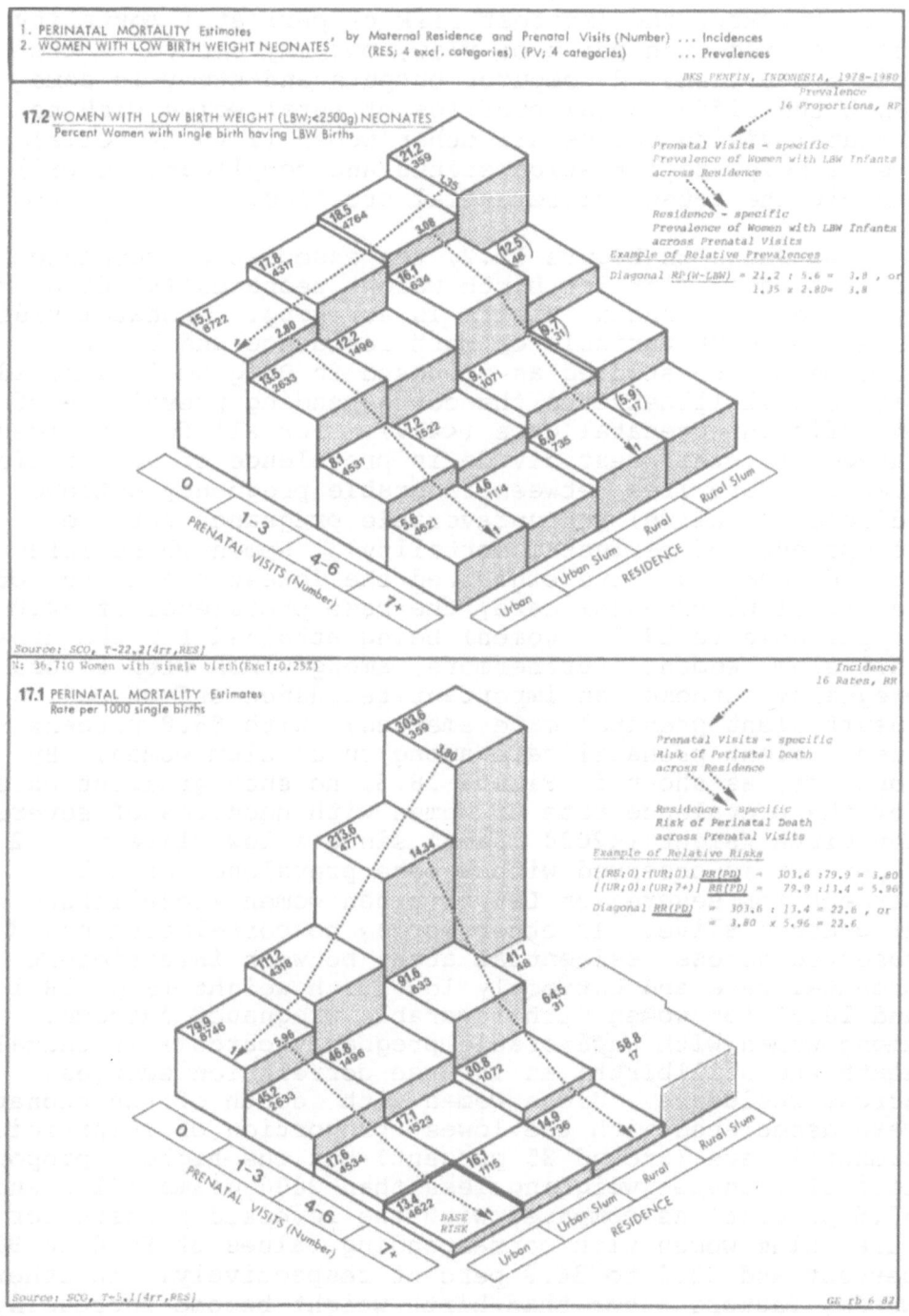

Figure 17. Perinatal mortality and percent of women with low birth weignt neonates by maternal residence and prenatal visits.

with no prenatal visits who deliver at the referral institution carry the greatest risk of perinatal mortality.
From the research point of view, one may create in the
future two standard computer outputs and study in some
depth the differential profiles of rural women with no
prenatal visits versus all other women (2 vs 14 cells).
Most likely, registration status and complications will
exhibit the retest differential profiles.

As shown in Figure 17.2, the associated prevalence
rate of women with low birth weight neonates (<2500 grams)
by number of prenatal visits is striking. Prenatal visits
as a dependent variable of both residence and birth
outcome may be studied as proposed in Diagram 1, line 18.
Figure 18.1 illustrates the corresponding prevalence of
insufficient prenatal care (<4PV). For all four residence
categories, the great divide in prevalence of insufficient
prenatal care lies between favorable pregnancy outcome
(discharged alive) and unfavorable pregnancy outcome
(components of perinatal mortality). Women whose infants
were discharged alive exhibited the lowest prevalence of
insufficient prenatal care, the base prevalence of 54.0
(applicable to 19,575 women) being attained for the urban
(non slum) women. Furthermore, among women with favorable
pregnancy outcome, an important residence effect on
insufficient prenatal care emerges; with 86.8 percent
insufficient prenatal care among rural slum women. By
contrast, as shown in Figure 18.3, no such gradient exists
for the prevalence rate of women with neonates of severe
low birth weight (<2000 grams) since a low plateau of 2 to
3 percent is observed with a base prevalence of 2.1
percent for severe for LBW of urban women whose infant was
discharged alive. In other words, no correlation could be
observed across residential areas between insufficient
prenatal care and extremely low birth weight (Fig. 18.1
and 18.3) for women with favorable pregnancy outcome.
Among women with unfavorable pregnancy outcome (neonatal
death and stillbirth) an inverse correlation emerges
across residence. Urban women with death of the neonate
were associated with the lowest proportion of insufficient
prenatal care (around 85 percent) but the highest proportion of neonates weighing less than 2000 grams (41.2 and
57.6 percent) as compared with the reversed pattern for
rural slum women with corresponding values of 96.0 to 98.0
percent and 23.1 to 34.8 percent respectively. In other
words, factors other than birth weight become increasingly
associated with perinatal mortality across residence of
women who delivered at the university centers. Most
likely, studies of registration status and complications
would clarify the effects of emergency admission and

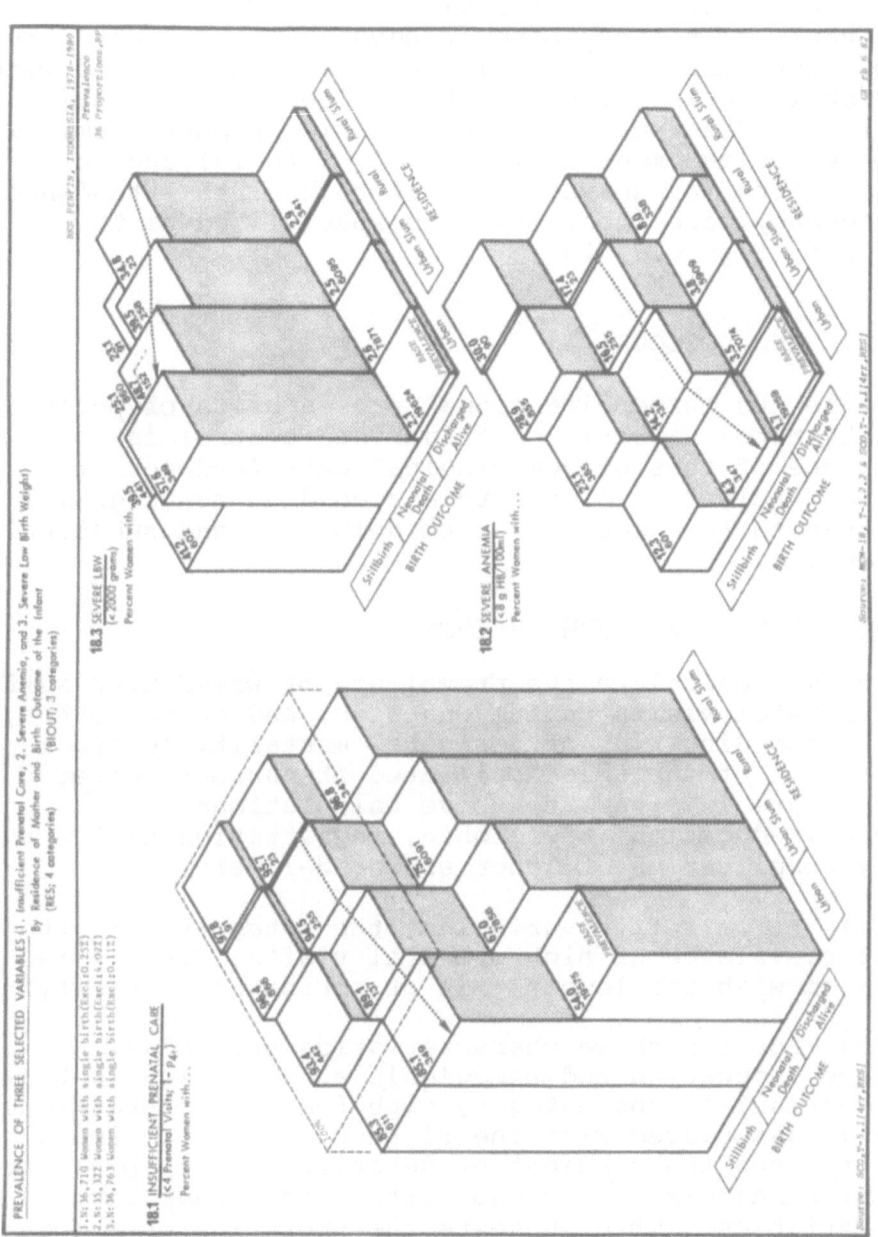

Figure 18. Prevalence of three selected variables (insufficient prenatal visits, severe anemia, and severe low birth weight) by maternal residence and birth outcome.

referrals on the one hand, and on the other, complications
such as prolonged or obstructed labor and ante- and
intrapartum hemorrhage. As shown on Figure 18.2, severe
anemia (<8 g HB/100 ml) increases with distance, indicating that emergency and referral admissions from remote
places carry a greater share of hemorrhage (placenta previa, placenta abruptio, etc.) known to be associated with
high risk of perinatal mortality (aside from maternal
mortality). The remaining part of this report examines
some observations made so far (Figs. 1 to 18) and tests
new indicators for surveillance of both birth attendance
and pregnancy care input prior to specialized birth
attendance (Figs. 19, 20).

SYNTHESIS AND OUTLOOK

     While the three-dimensional presentation of perinatal
mortality rates with bi- or trivariate control is the
centerpiece of this epidemiological data feedback, the
programmed selection of controls according to Diagram 1
leads then to two groups of methodological and substantive
implications.

Correlation of Input and Outcome

     One may calculate the prevalence of women with suffi-
cient prenatal visits on the one side, and on the other,
the corresponding risk of perinatal mortality across a
selected set of variables collected at current center
stay. Figure 19 gives the above calculations for
residence, education, hemoglobin, registration status and
primary complication of labor and/or delivery.

     (a) For all five variables, the category with the
highest prevalence of high prenatal visits (HPV;4+) is
associated with the lowest risk of perinatal mortality.

     (b) For the three characteristics variables,
residence, education and hemoglobin at admission (a health
status variable), the category with the lowest prevalence
of HPV is associated with the highest risk of perinatal
mortality, and the gradient of deterioration in perinatal
survival parallels the categorization continuum for the
three variables. This suggests the operation of a dose-
response mechanism across three variables that
characterize the mother at admission for delivery.

     (c) Excepting cells with small numbers (other
hemorrhage and placenta abruptio) a similar dose-response

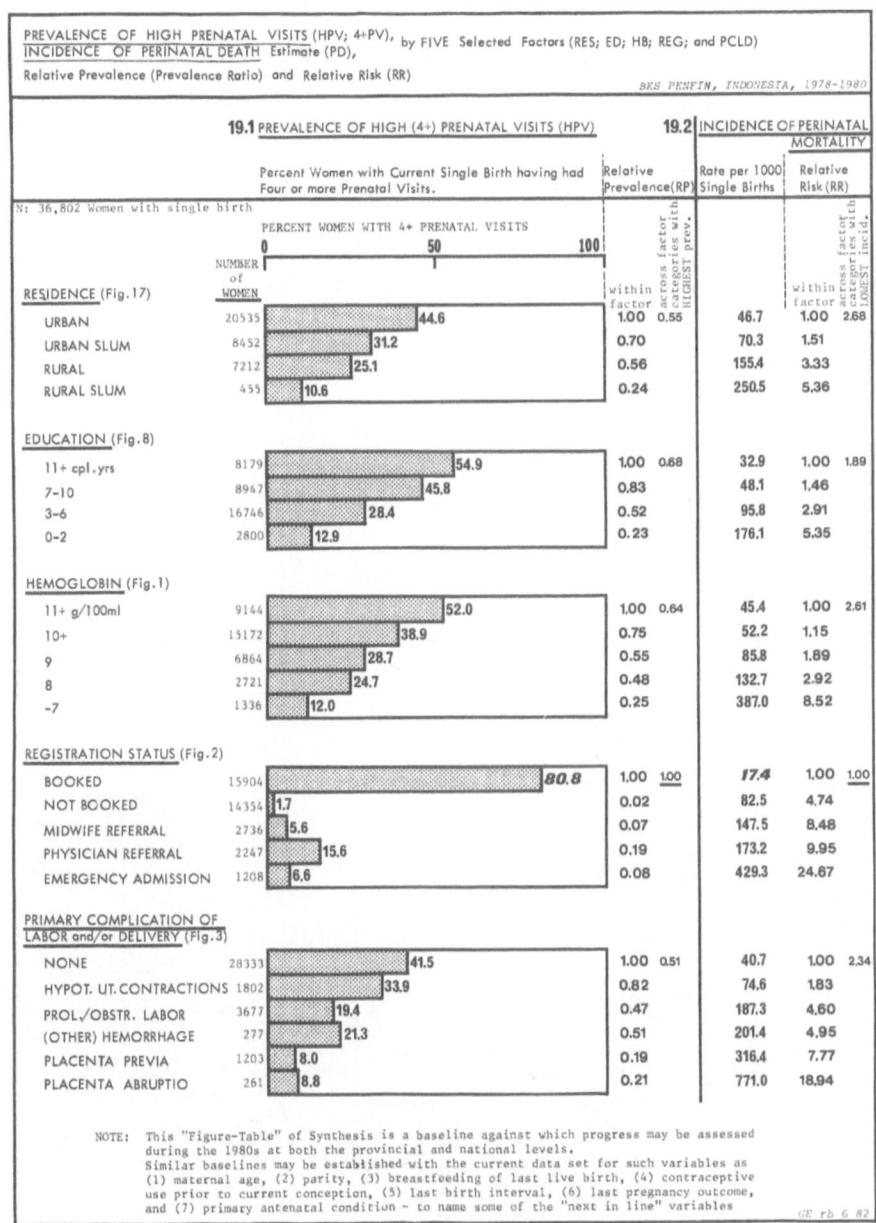

PREVALENCE OF HIGH PRENATAL VISITS (HPV; 4+PV), by FIVE Selected Factors (RES; ED; HB; REG; and PCLD)
INCIDENCE OF PERINATAL DEATH Estimate (PD),
Relative Prevalence (Prevalence Ratio) and Relative Risk (RR)

BKS PENFIN, INDONESIA, 1978-1980

	NUMBER of WOMEN	PERCENT WOMEN WITH 4+ PRENATAL VISITS	Relative Prevalence(RP) within factor	across factor categories with HIGHEST prev.	Rate per 1000 Single Births	Relative Risk (RR) within factor	across factor categories with LOWEST incid.
19.1 PREVALENCE OF HIGH (4+) PRENATAL VISITS (HPV)					**19.2** INCIDENCE OF PERINATAL MORTALITY		
N: 36,802 Women with single birth							
RESIDENCE (Fig.17)							
URBAN	20535	44.6	1.00	0.55	46.7	1.00	2.68
URBAN SLUM	8452	31.2	0.70		70.3	1.51	
RURAL	7212	25.1	0.56		155.4	3.33	
RURAL SLUM	455	10.6	0.24		250.5	5.36	
EDUCATION (Fig.8)							
11+ cpl.yrs	8179	54.9	1.00	0.68	32.9	1.00	1.89
7-10	8947	45.8	0.83		48.1	1.46	
3-6	16746	28.4	0.52		95.8	2.91	
0-2	2800	12.9	0.23		176.1	5.35	
HEMOGLOBIN (Fig.1)							
11+ g/100ml	9144	52.0	1.00	0.64	45.4	1.00	2.61
10+	15172	38.9	0.75		52.2	1.15	
9	6864	28.7	0.55		85.8	1.89	
8	2721	24.7	0.48		132.7	2.92	
-7	1336	12.0	0.25		387.0	8.52	
REGISTRATION STATUS (Fig.2)							
BOOKED	15904	80.8	1.00	1.00	17.4	1.00	1.00
NOT BOOKED	14354	1.7	0.02		82.5	4.74	
MIDWIFE REFERRAL	2736	5.6	0.07		147.5	8.48	
PHYSICIAN REFERRAL	2247	15.6	0.19		173.2	9.95	
EMERGENCY ADMISSION	1208	6.6	0.08		429.3	24.67	
PRIMARY COMPLICATION OF LABOR and/or DELIVERY (Fig.3)							
NONE	28333	41.5	1.00	0.51	40.7	1.00	2.34
HYPOT. UT. CONTRACTIONS	1802	33.9	0.82		74.6	1.83	
PROL./OBSTR. LABOR	3677	19.4	0.47		187.3	4.60	
(OTHER) HEMORRHAGE	277	21.3	0.51		201.4	4.95	
PLACENTA PREVIA	1203	8.0	0.19		316.4	7.77	
PLACENTA ABRUPTIO	261	8.8	0.21		771.0	18.94	

Column header note: Percent Women with Current Single Birth having had Four or more Prenatal Visits

NOTE: This "Figure-Table" of Synthesis is a baseline against which progress may be assessed
during the 1980s at both the provincial and national levels.
Similar baselines may be established with the current data set for such variables as
(1) maternal age, (2) parity, (3) breastfeeding of last live birth, (4) contraceptive
use prior to current conception, (5) last birth interval, (6) last pregnancy outcome,
and (7) primary antenatal condition - to name some of the "next in line" variables

GE rh 6 82

Figure 19. Prevalence of high prenatal visits and
incidence of prenatal death by five selected
factors (residence, education, hemoglobin,
registration status, and primary complication.

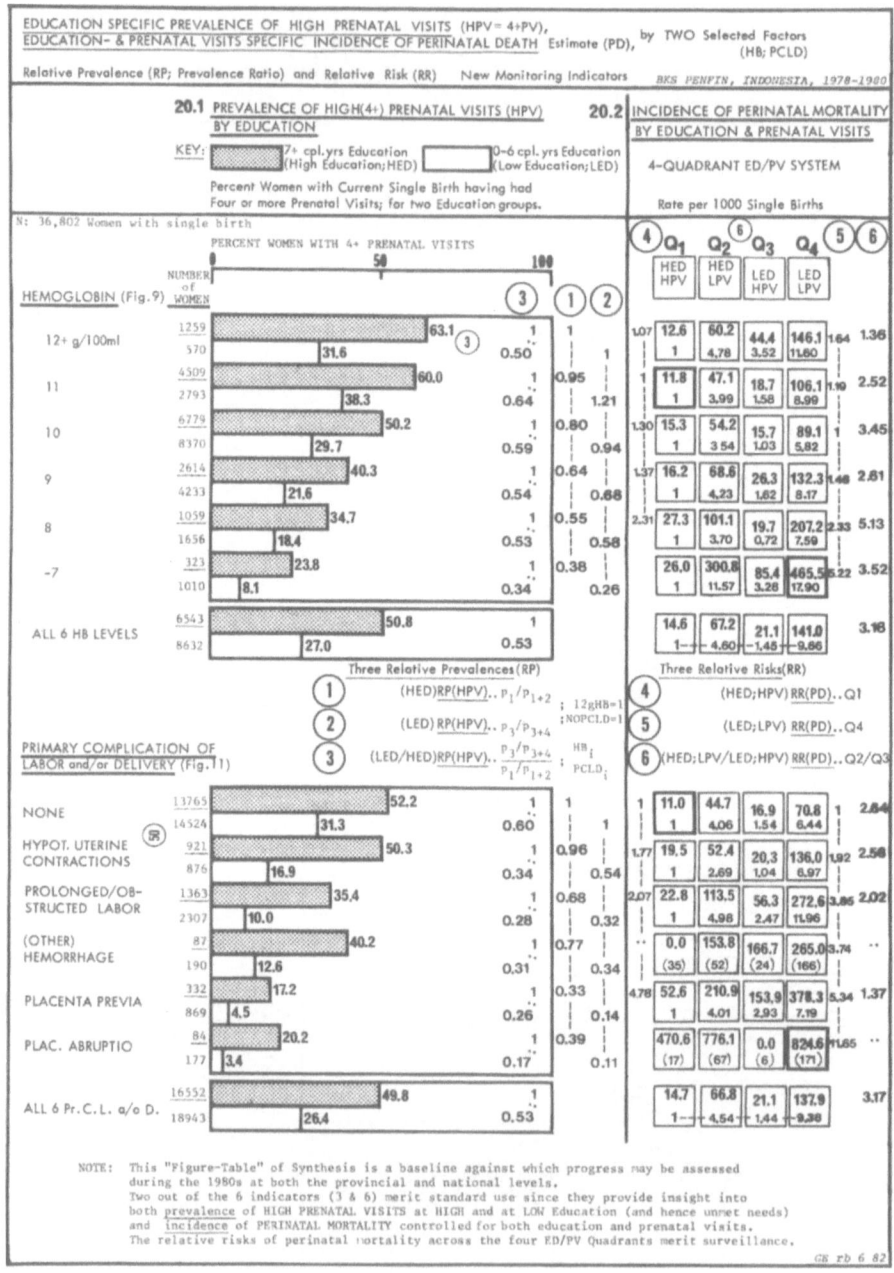

Figure 20. Education specific prevalence of high prenatal visits, education and prenatal visits specific perinatal death by two selected factors (hemoglobin and primary complication). Definition and application of 6 indexes for monitoring.

pattern of HPV and perinatal mortality is noted across
primary complication of labor and/or delivery.

(d) No such dose-response pattern may be observed
across registration status. This is understandable, since
it is the variable par excellence that introduces bias of
selection - the key feature of referrals and emergency
admission.

(e) Comparison of prevalence of HPV and incidence of
perinatal death across the factor categories with the
highest HPV each, reveals again a dose-response pattern.
Booked cases exhibit the highest (at large) prevalence of
HPV (80.8 percent) and the lowest risk (at large) of
perinatal death (17.4/1000). This points to a very strong
association between booking and prenatal visits - a truism
that translates another kind of cause-to-effect relationship. Generally, prenatal visits is the prerequisite for
booking. Pregnancy care shoud lead to preventive behavior
of the mother for the infant to enter this world: booking
of the delivery is an extension of prenatal care.

As proposed in Figure 20, the observation of a dose-
response relationship between input at the stages of both
pregnancy and delivery, and outcome of birth may be controlled further, by introducing education. The analysis
restricts itself to two important variables: hemoglobin
and complication of labor and/or delivery. The following
two additional observations merit consideration:

(f) Within all categories of both hemoglobin and
complications, the prevalence of HPV is much higher for
women with high education (HED;7+) than for women with low
education (LED;0-6), pointing to a strong correlation of
education and prenatal visits. Since future programmatic
intervention in national reproductive health care is to
advance via primary health care, into the broad segments
of low education, it is desirable to monitor the prevalence of HPV at both low and high education levels. Indices
1 and 2 in Figure 20.1 give these prevalences relative to
the base prevalence obtained for the most favorable category (HB; 12+ g/100 ml and PCLD; None). Then, the two
ED-spec. proportions may be put to ratio, leading to Index
3. If HED (HPV) is taken as base (denominator), the Index
3 becomes a measure of the currently attained prevalence
of HPV among low education women as compared with high
education women, the latter taken as reference unit.
Thus, and overall, Index 3 is 0.53, as shown at the bottom
of both variables in Figure 20.1. It should become a
priority to narrow the gap of the ED-spec. proportions

that is, Index 3 should be approaching 1.00. This Index
of Relative Prevalence of HPV for LED may be introduced
for routine surveillance at any institution of maternity
care, that is at the primary health care center
(PUSKESMAS) that could monitor home deliveries, at the
rural maternity center, at the regency department of
obstetrics, at urban maternity centers, and top referral
institutions. Since reference prevalence is thereby care
level specific, each level of maternity care can evaluate
the progress in prevalence of HPV. Obviously, coordination of these calculations for uniformity in methodology
will lead to a vertical cross section of HPV prevalence.
Repeated or continued monitoring gives them access to
quantitated progress in prenatal care penetration along
the vertical axis of health care provision.

(g) The introduction of a twofold specificity in input (education and prenatal visits) leads necessarily to a
minimum of 4 specific rates of outcome. Figure 20.2 gives
these rate quartets of perinatal mortality for the categories of hemoglobin and complication. Indices 4 and 5 are
the incidences of perinatal death (or its components) for
HED/HPV (Q1) and LED/LPV (Q4) relative to the base risk.
The latter is not necessarily coinciding with the base
prevalence, neither are base risks of Q1 and Q4 necessarily coinciding. Since education and prenatal visits
co-affect perinatal survival, it is particularly desirable
to monitor the incidence of perinatal death for the counterpart quadrants 2 and 3 and to express them as ratio.
If the risk for Q3 is taken as base (denominator), then
Index 6 becomes a measure of the currently obtained risk
of perinatal death for HED/LPV relative to the op- posite
combination LED/HPV. Overall, Index 6 is 3.2, which is a
more provocative Index of Relative Risk of Perinatal
Death, since its routine calculation and feedback at all
levels of specialized maternity care constitutes a constant reminder of the paramount importance of pregnancy
care.

Controlled Birth Outcome Correlates

Finally, this report has barely touched upon an
impressive versality of standard computer output analysis.
Any variable can be displayed either as independent or
dependent variable. Diagrams 1 and 2 show for Figures 17
and 18 the independent and dependent treatment of prenatal
visits. In other words, one may establish ad libidum prevalence baselines for any variable that is used as control
variable. Currently, such baselines are growing for prenatal visits, anemia and severe anemia, and referrals and

emergency admissions. Plannned are the following
additional variables: breast feeding or last live birth,
prior contraceptive use, birth interval, last pregnancy
outcome and blood transfusion during current delivery.

CONCLUSION AND RECOMMENDATION

     During the early and mid-eighties, microcomputers may
introduce a revolution in information gathering and result
feedback for the programmed improvement of health care
systems. A significant benefit may be expected for the
early improvement of reproductive health care provision
since completed trials with maternity care monitoring have
prepared the way for early implementation. The current
report was built upon standard computer outputs (SCOs).
But new software packages addressing specific issues are
additionally needed in order to make uniformly treated
information available to all participants of surveillance
research.

     Analysis and feedback must be guided by an epidemio-
logical outlook. Diagrams 1 and 2 show the focus taken
for this analysis: pregnancy outcome and number of
prenatal visits are emphasized, but a careful selection of
additional variables enabled the framing with a mutually
linked control system. The transparency was fully maintained for professionals who serve the women. ·Additional
regression-type techniques may be needed.

     The 3-D display of controlled risk of perinatal
mortality and correlates is an innovation. Perusal of the
figures gives immediate access to "risk fronts" and neatly
delineated "risk valleys" that are immediately intelligi-
ble to the entire profession of reproductive health care,
both medical and paramedical. This transparency in
risks will profit professional dialogue.

     Correlation of input and outcome has become possible
with surveillance research data of maternity care
monitoring. Special statistical techniques may generate
equations of dose-response (specific for region, institutions, health personnel, etc.) that could lead to the
identification of the minimum number of prenatal visits
needed to achieve the most cost effective and optimal
reduction of perinatal mortality, as well as maternal
mortality.

     Pointed creation of prevalence baselines will uncover
weaknesses of management. High priority areas are:

referral and emergency admissions, blood transfusion and
fetal distress during labor. The time is nearing when
Indonesia can initiate intrauterine growth studies with
controlled MCM information (4). Also, management of
delivery is ready for a more careful review (5). Prenatal
visits emerges as a more important variable for high
perinatal survival than education, the major finding of
this analysis. Severe anemia due to hemorrhage is a key
cause of perinatal death. Prolonged/obstructed labor is
another high risk of perinatal mortality.

Maternity Care Monitoring is ready for broad general
use in Indonesia and other countries. Variables
pertaining to family size should be treated in a similar
manner as proposed in Diagrams 1 and 2. Likely, the need
for family planning may be derived from these health care
data. Variables pertaining to Birth Interval Behavior
(breast feeding, contraceptive use, and prenatal visits)
should be included among future strategies of analysis.

ACKNOWLEDGMENTS

We would wish to thank His Excellency, Dr.
Suwardjono, Minister of Health of Indonesia, for his
personal and continued interest and encouragement for the
professional deployment of Maternity Care Monitoring.
Gratitude goes also to the heads and involved staff of the
11 university departments of obstetrics and gynecology who
carried out this project sponsored by BKS PENFIN. Initial
help of IFRP and transfer of appropriate technology is
acknowledged. Dr. T. Agoestina's indefatigable efforts at
coordination and the office of BKS PENFIN were critical to
the success of this multi-center cooperative venture.
Special thanks is due to Dr. Elton Kessel whose untiring
promotion of MCM has provided inspiration and tenacity to
dozens of program persons as well as to the current
analyst. The latter thanks IFRP for according time and
means to develop methodology with standard computer outputs for broader use in Asia, Africa and Latin America.
E.M. Kendall, long-time assistant to the analyst has also
been instrumental in various phases of the Indonesia project. In Geneva, thanks are also owed to Professor H. De
Watteville, whose continued interest in prenatal visits
has led to the closed analysis system. The current
analysis has also profited from two consultations with
Professor S. Sureau, Paris, during the Congress of
IAMANEH.

REFERENCES

1. FIGO News (1980): Int J Gyn Obstet, 15:476-477.
2. Bernard RP, Sulaiman S, Agoestina T, Kendall EM (1980):
    Maternity care monitoring (MCM) in Indonesia:
    early findings and implications for the 1980s.
    Indonesian J Obstet Gyn, 6:191-290.
3. Ariawan S, Hanafiah MJ, Kendall EM, Kessel E, Bernard
    RP (1980): Social and biological aspects of
    stillbirth: and Indonesian study of residence and
    referral. In: Proceedings, Third International
    Seminar on Maternal and Perinatal Mortality, New
    Delhi, India. FOGSI/AIIMS, Bombay and Delhi, India.
4. Bernard RP, Kendall EM, Manton KG (1980):
    International maternity care monitoring (MCM-3). A
    beginning. In: Clinical Perinatology, A. Aladjem,
    A. Brown, C. Sureau, (Editors), C. V. Mosby Co., St.
    Louis, Chapter 23:521-559.
5. Bernard RP, de Watteville H, Kessel E, Ravenholt RT,
    Kendall EM (1979): International maternity care
    monitoring (MCM-2): Results of a pretest. Int J
    Gyn Obstet, 17:24-39.

ANALYSIS OF DATA AND ITS IMPACT ON STRATEGIES

FOR MATERNAL AND NEONATAL CARE

S. Sastrawinata

Chairman, Department of Obstetrics and Gynecology
Hasan Sadikum Hospital
Bandung, Indonesia

INTRODUCTION

Family health has a high priority in national health programs, especially in developing countries due to the fact that mothers and children constitute more than 60 percent of the population (1). Furthermore, the majority of disorders affecting mother and child are preventable so that efforts to improve maternal and child health (MCH) must receive high priority. In general, MCH in developing countries is still unsatisfactory and measures to improve it is urgently needed. To design an effective and efficient health program for mother and child, reliable and relevant data on human reproduction and child health care are of prime importance but unfortunately this is seldom available in developing countries. To assist the government in collecting data on human reproduction, obstetricians of 12 teaching hospitals in Indonesia founded the Coordinating Board of Indonesian Fertility Research (BKS PENFIN) in 1977. One of the important project launched by this organization is the Maternity Care Monitoring (MCM) initially sponsored by IFRP.

MATERIALS AND METHODS

Monitoring of maternity care is carried out by completing forms designed by IFRP and FIGO. This activity started in 1978 and by the end of 1980, about 37,000 deliveries were recorded. This single sheet form collects information relating to four main themes:

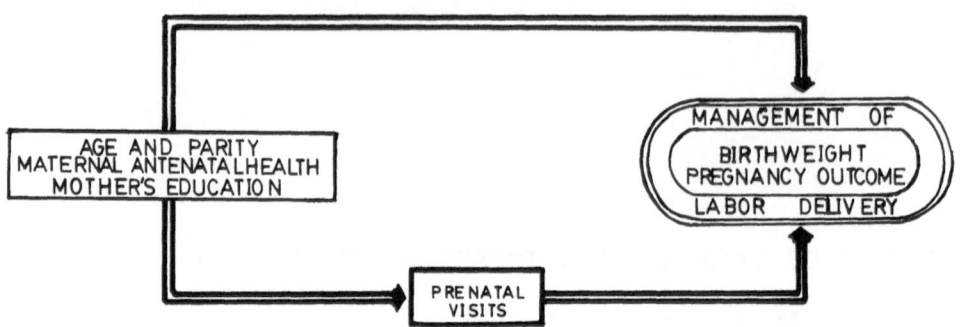

Figure 1.   Maternity care monitoring.

        (a)   Family formation and reproductive history.
General patient characteristics and reproductive history
are assessed.   The impact of family planning programs
should be apparent from information relating to patient
characteristics and reproductive history.   Of course this
section also provides us with information to identify
subgroups that are at higher risk.

        (b)   Family health and reproduction.   Data pertaining
to the health of the mother (like antenatal condition and
pregnancy duration) and to the health of the infant (as
birth weight and Apgar score) is collected.   The data is
important because it has a cause and effect relationship.

        (c)   Management of pregnancy and delivery.   One of
the objectives of MCM is to correlate methods of
management with pregnancy outcome with the ultmate goal of
reducing maternal as well as infant mortality and
morbidity.

        (d)   Desired family size and family planning
practices.   This section enables us to assess trends in
family size desired and the quality of postpartum
contraceptive services.

        This paper focuses mainly on maternal charac-
teristics, antenatal conditions, prenatal visits and
pregnancy outcome;   it will discuss the linkage between
the above-mentioned variables in order to improve
strategies for maternal and neonatal care (Fig. 1).

        Table 1 shows that 14.3 percent of the women were 35
years or older and that 25.4 percent of the patients had
already four or more children.

RESULTS

Age and Parity

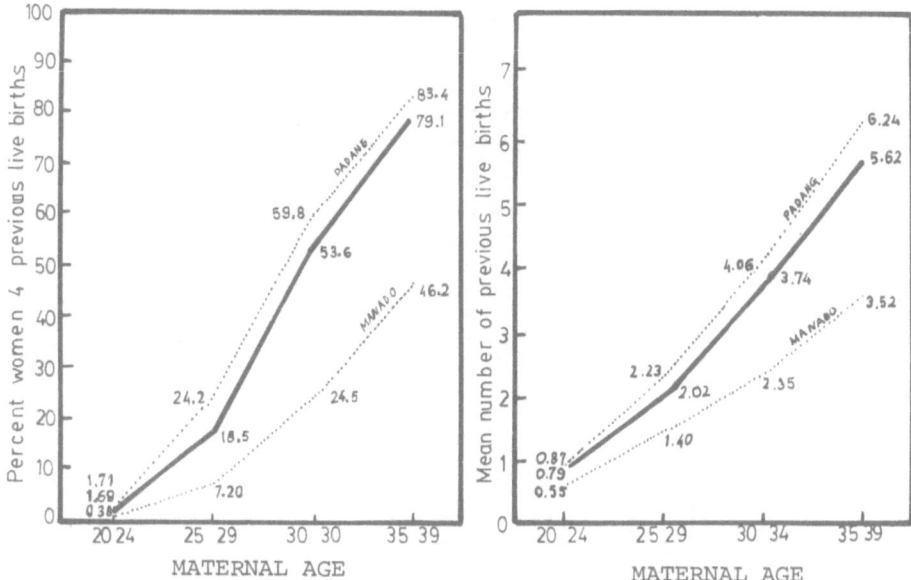

Figure 2.   (Left)   Percent of women being grandmultiparous
             (GDMP) by maternal age at current birth.
             (Right)   Mean number of previous live births by
             maternal age at current birth.

         Figure 2 (left) shows that in the 25 to 29 age
group, 18.5 percent of the women had already four or more
previous live births; 30 percent in this group had three
or more previous live births. The mean number of previous
live births of this age group is 2.01 (Fig. 2, right).
This means that to approach the 5 member family concept,

Table 1. Maternal Age and Parity Included in Study.

	MATERNAL AGE		PARITY
(Years)	Parity	Parity	Percent
19	10.82	0	34.06
20 - 24	33.52	1	18.20
25 - 29	25.73	2	12.93
30 - 34	15.64	3	9.45
35+	14.29	4+	25.36

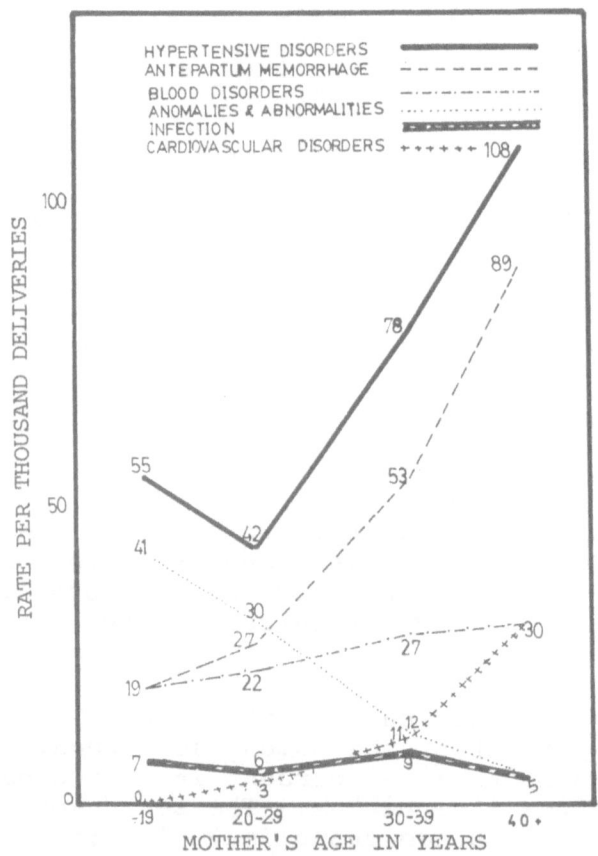

Figure 3.   Six most frequent primary antenatal conditions
            by mother's age at admission for current
            delivery.

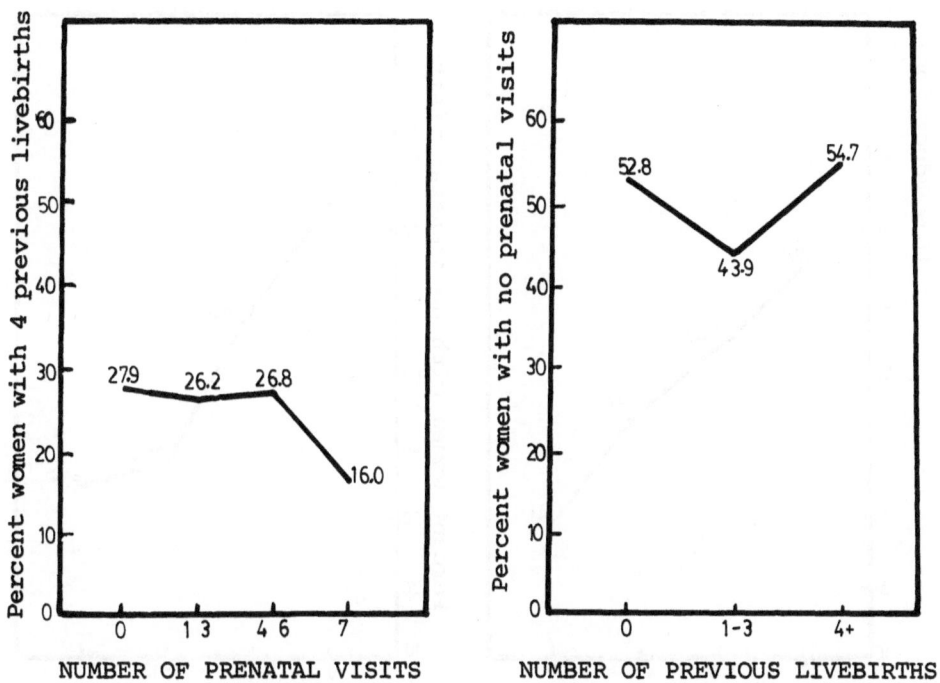

Figure 4. (Left) Percent of women with 4 or more
previous live births (GDMP), by prenatal
visits.
(Right) Percent of women with no prenatal
visits (NOPV), by previous live births.

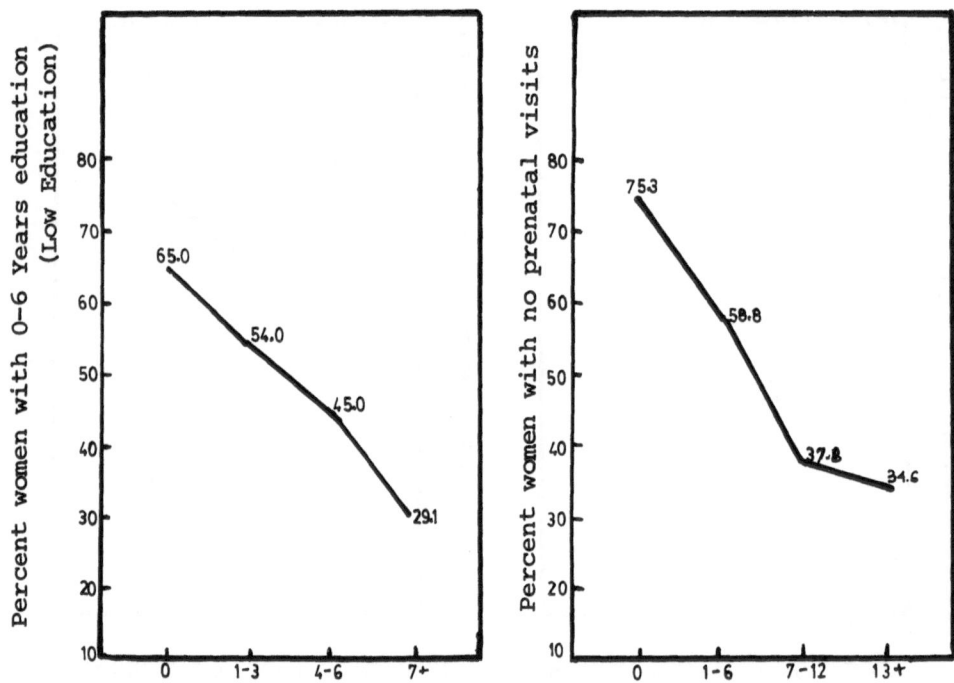

Figure 5.   (Left)   Percent of women with 0 to 6 years
             education by number of prenatal visits. High
             priority index.
             (Right)   Percent of women with no prenatal
             visits, by maternal education. High priority
             index.

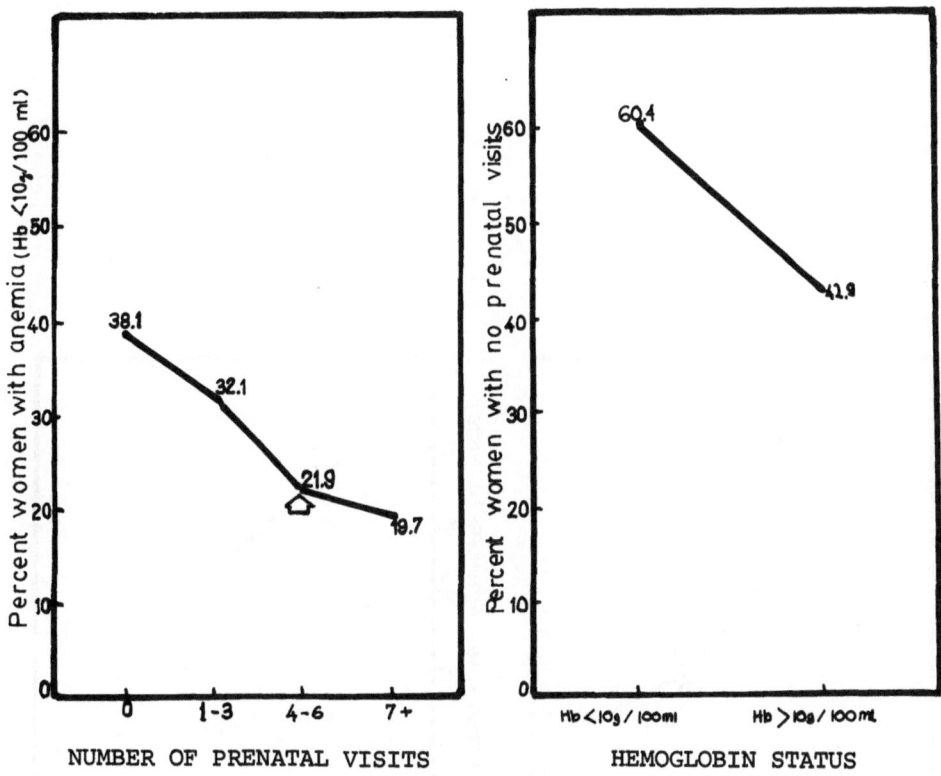

Figure 6. (Left) Percent of women with anemia at current
birth, by prenatal visits. One index.
(Right) Percent of women with no prenatal
visits, by hemoglobin status. One index.

women at the age of thirty or over should be advised to
terminate their fertility.

Primary Antenatal Condition

        Data from five centers revealed the six most fre-
quent antenatal conditions as shown in Figure 3. The data
also clearly show age dependency of these six most
prevalent complications. After age 30, the prevalences of
hypertensive disorders and of antepartum hemorrhage rise
sharply.

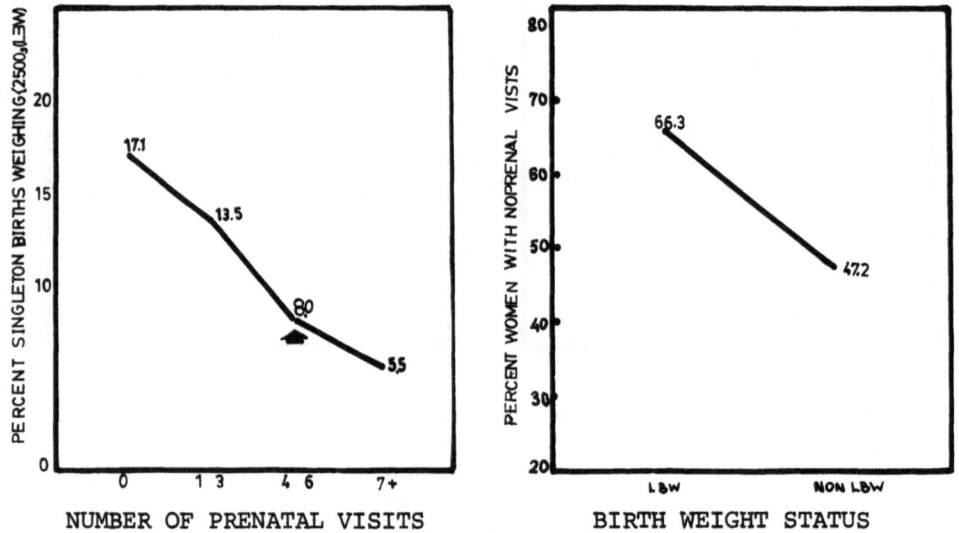

Figure 7. (Left) Percent of women with singleton birth weighing less than 2500 grams (LBW), by prenatal visits.
(Right) Percent of women with no prenatal visits (NOPV), by birth weight status. Two indexes.

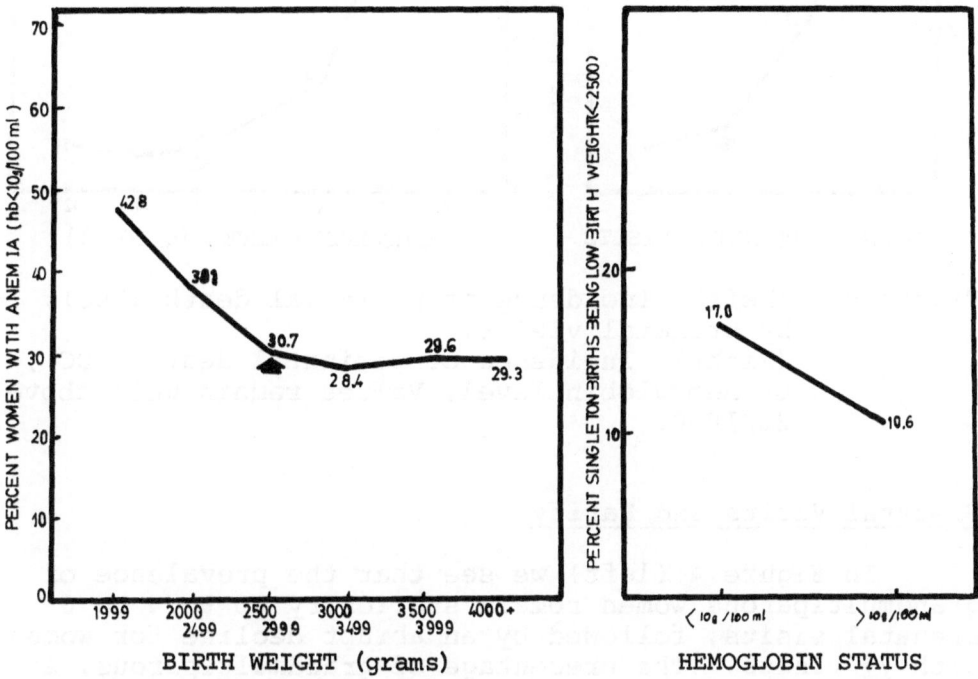

Figure 8.   (Left)   Percent of women with anemia at
            current singleton birth, by birth weight.
            (Right)   Percent of women with singleton
            birth weight below 2500 (LBW), by hemo-
            globin status.

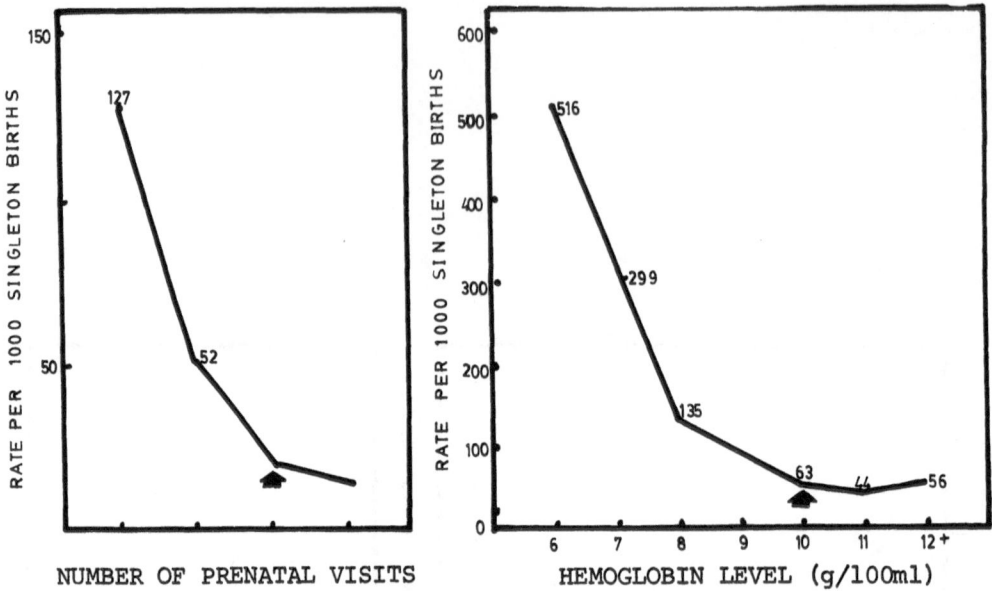

Figure 9.   (Left) Incidence of perinatal death (PDC),
            by prenatal visits.
            (Right) Incidence of perinatal death (PDC),
            by hemoglobin level. Values remain well above
            25/1000.

Prenatal Visits and Parity

In Figure 4 (left) we see that the prevalence of
grandmultiparous women remain stationary up to 4 to 6
prenatal visits, followed by an abrupt decline for women
with 7+ visits. The precentage of grandmultiparous, as
well as nulliparous women should decrease (Fig. 4, right).

Prenatal Visits and Education

Figure 5 illustrates that education has an important effect on prenatal visits. The percentage of low
education among women with no prenatal visits amount to 65
percent; that of women with no education delivered, without prenatal visits is 75 percent. Increased attention to
this high-risk category should result in a significant
improvement of maternal and child health.

Prenatal Visits and Hemoglobin Level

A marked decline in anemic prevalence associated
with an increase in prenatal visits as shown on Figure 6.

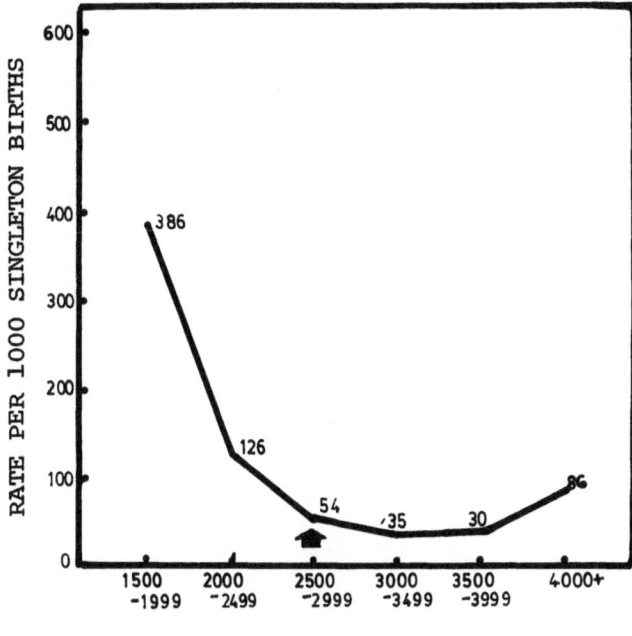

Figure 10. Incidence of perinatal death (PDC), by birth
          weight.

Prenatal Visits and Birth Weight

A sharp decline of low birth weight infants is
associated with increasing number of prenatal visits up to
4 to 6 visits, after which the decline is more gradual
(Fig. 7). Five prenatal visits may appear to be a target
number for MCH programs.

Hemoglobin Level and Birth Weight

For infants weighing 2500 g or more, the curve of
anemia prevalence forms a plateau, but for infants weighing less than 2500 g, the plateau changes into an
ascending curve, as shown on Figure 8.

Prenatal Visits and Perinatal Death

There is a nine-fold decrease of perinatal death
when moving from total absence of prenatal visits to 7+
prenatal visits (Fig. 9). The greatest gain in perinatal
mortality decline with the smallest number of prenatal
visits is achieved at 5 visits. It appears that with 4 to
6 prenatal visits, a perinatal death rate of less than 20

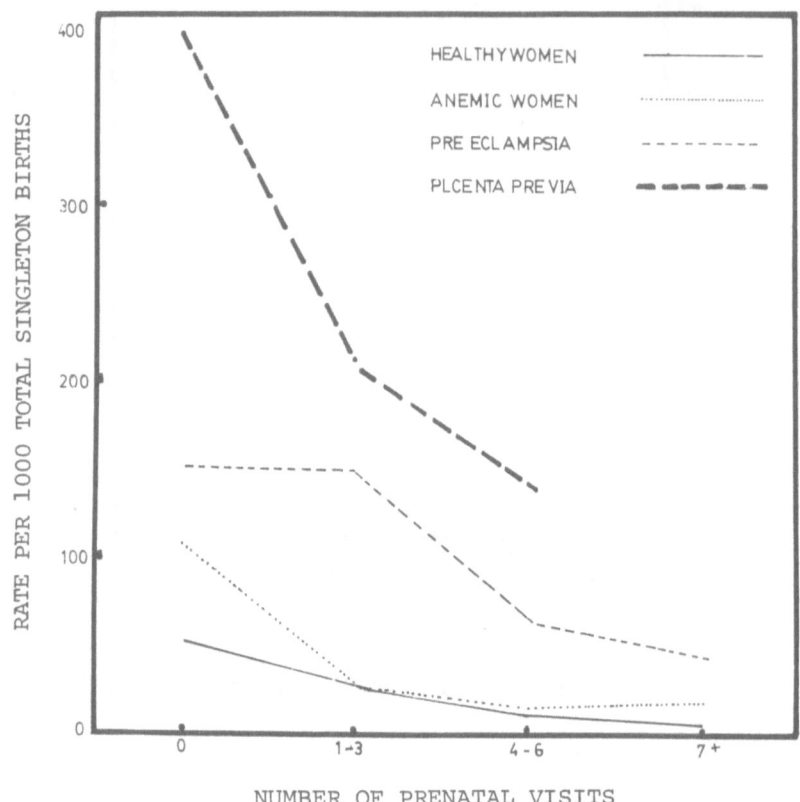

Figure 11. Perinatal deaths, by prenatal visits.

per 1000 and a 6.5-fold decrease of perinatal mortality could be achieved.

Hemoglobin Level and Perinatal Death.

Figure 9 (right) shows that a hemoglobin blood level below 8 g per 100 ml raises perinatal death rate beyond 500 per 1000 singleton births. The lowest rate of peri-natal death is associated with hemoglobin levels of 11 g per 100 ml (44 per 1000). An important observation is that 4 to 6 prenatal visits are associated with a much lower perinatal death rate (20 per 1000) than 11 g Hb/100 ml, the difference being over twofold.

Birth Weight and Perinatal Death.

With birth weights below 2500 g, the perinatal death rate rises sharply. The lowest rate of perinatal death

(35.2 per 1000) is linked to the birth weight category of 3000 to 3499 g, which is still 1.8 times higher than the perinatal death rate for women with 4 to 6 prenatal visits (Fig. 10). This suggests that prenatal visits are an important method of intervention that reduces perinatal death rate directly as well as indirectly by increasing birth weight.

Maternal Antenatal Condition and Perinatal Death.

Figure 11 shows that placenta previa is the most important cause of perinatal death followed by pre-eclampsia and anemia. All three causes though are significantly affected by prenatal visits. Even for healthy women, there is an eight-fold decrease of perinatal deaths from none to 7+ prenatal visits.

DISCUSSION

The data collected in 12 teaching hospitals clearly show:

(a) An unfavorable age and parity structure: 14.3 percent of the women delivering in above mentioned hospitals are 35 years or over, and 25.4 percent are of parity 4+.

(b) Fifty three percent of the women have low educational attainment (0 to 6 years).

(c) The most important antenatal complications are, according to order of prevalence, hypertensive disorders, antepartum hemorrhage and blood disorders (specifically anemia); ranked according to their effect on perinatal deaths, they are antepartum hemorrhage, preeclampsia and anemia. These antenatal complications are age-dependent.

The unfavorable age parity structure does not only affect pregnancy outcome in a direct way but also indirectly by underusage of prenatal care services as shown in Figures 4 and 5. It seems that the small family concept is not fully apprecated; therefore health education should be intensified and directed especially to young people, in order to prepare them for their future responsibilities as parents. This parent craft education should include family planning, nutrition, home economics, child rearing, environmental sanitation, etc.

The women organizations in Indonesia are already

involved in these important activities and it is hoped
that the effect will become apparent in the near future.
In fact, cohort studies in Indonesia indicate that the
desired family size is becoming smaller (2). Considering
the fact that the 25 to 29 age group has already a mean
parity of 2, sterilization might be considered for mothers
in the late twenties.

Improvement of the age parity structure should also
affect the most prevalent antenatal complications which
are clearly age-dependent. MCM has shown again that prenatal care is the most important method of intervention to
improve maternal and child health as shown in Figures 6 to
11. Other Maternal Care Monitoring studies have shown
that its effect is greater than education and that the
lowest perinatal mortality is achieved by sufficient
number of prenatal visits. Increase in hemoglobin levels
or birth weight were not able to reach this low figure of
perinatal mortality.

Data revealed that 5 prenatal visits is the optimal
number linked with a perinatal mortality of 20 per 1000.
Unfortunately, about 50 percent of all women deliver without prenatal care; 52.8 percent of the multiparous, 54.7
percent of the grandmultiparous, and 65 percent of the low
education group had no prenatal visits. Again the
importance of availability, accessibility and quality of
prenatal services is felt. It is apparent that maternal
and child health services should increase their coverage
and should in particular reach risk groups such as the
multiparous, the grandmultiparous and low educational
groups and the women with antenatal complications; in
other words, the center effect should have greater impact
on the number of prenatal visits than patient characteristics or social conditions. The "health passport" idea
could be tested in Indonesia.

Measures to improve nutrition in general and in
particular of pregnant mothers should also improve
maternal and child health. One of its indicators, the
hemoglobin blood level, would monitor this improvement.

CONCLUSION

An integrated maternal and child health service
(Fig. 12) is proposed for the improvement of maternal and
neonatal care. Health education, maternal and child care,
family planning and nutrition should be the main components of the MCH package. In the premarital period, young

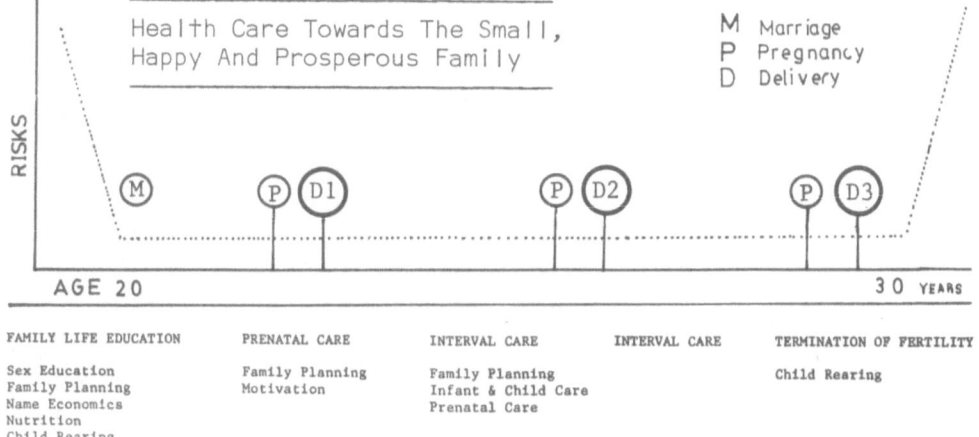

Figure 12. Integrated MCH services.

people should prepare themselves for their future
responsibilities by receiving the necessary knowledge to
become able parents.

During the first pregnancy, the mother-to-be should
have the benefit of prenatal care and should be counseled
to decide on a method for spacing children. All procedures of pregnancy and delivery care should promote the
acceptance of breast feeding. After delivery, the woman
should be exposed to birth interval care consisting of
obstetrical follow-up, family planning and neonatal care;
the importance of continuing breast feeding and regular
checkups for her child at least up to 5 years should be
stressed. Preferably, during her second or third pregnancy after the following delivery, termination of fertility
should be offered. Hospitals should be equipped and
staffed to provide therapeutic care for identified
high-risk mothers and children.

REFERENCES

1. Biro Pusat Statistik (1979): Profil statistik anak
      dan ibu di Indonesia. Jakarta.
2. Bernard RP, Sulaiman S, Agoestina I (1980): Maternity
      care monitoring in Indonesia. Majalah Obstetri
      dan Ginekologi Indonesia, 6:191.

MATERNITY CARE MONITORING IN TWENTY-TWO

HOSPITALS IN WEST JAVA

S. Sastrawinata

Chairman, Coordinating Board of
Indonesian Fertility Research (BKS PENFIN)
Bandung, Indonesia

INTRODUCTION

Since late 1979, Maternity Care Monitoring (MCM) has been carried out in 12 teaching hospitals scattered throughout the Indonesian archipelago (1). Through this network, data have been collected, processed and analyzed which could be very useful in determining strategies on maternal and child health care (1). The limitation of these data, however, is that they were collected in large selected hospitals and therefore cannot be called representative of the country. To obtain more representative data, the BKS PENFIN proposed to the government to implement MCM in 22 hospitals (mostly regency hospitals and some military hospitals), which participated in the hospital family planning program in West Java. This proposal was accepted and necessary preparations were made which included designing of a register form for MCM as well as Child Care Monitoring (CCM)., referral forms and maternity death forms; and the training of medical and paramedical personnel in completing the various forms used. Another important factor was the occurrence of a health organization at various institutions such as the BKS PENFIN, the BKKBN, the Department of Health, and the health division of the Indonesian Armed Forces.

MATERIALS AND METHOD

In contrast with the conventional MCM forms, the register forms included information relating to abortions,

Table 1. Incidence of Abortion, Ectopic
and Molar Pregnancies.

Hospital Group	Number of Pregnancy	Abortion		Ectopic		Hyd. Mole		Pregnancy Wastage
		No.	%	No.	%	No.	%	
Hasan Sadikin	1336	300	22.5	32	2.4	36	2.7	27.5
Bandung & Suburbs	2506	384	15.3	21	0.8	21	0.8	17.0
Outside Bandung	4336	754	17.4	32	0.7	56	1.3	19.4
Total	8178	1438	17.6	85	1.0	113	1.4	20.3

molar pregnancies, ectopic pregnancies and postpartum
complications.

For comparison, the 22 hospitals in West Java were
divided into three groups:

(a) Hasan Sadikin Hospital (the top referral hospital)
represented by 1336 patients;
(b) Seven hospitals in and around Bandung, consisting of
hospitals covering a predominantly urban area,
contributing 2500 cases;
(c) Fourteen hospitals outside Bandung, scattered over
West Java, contributing 433 cases.

RESULTS

Considering the importance of prenatal care, nutrition (monitored by blood hemoglobin level) and family
planning, this report will focus the factors discussed
below.

Pregnancy Wastage

Table 1 shows that 20 percent of all pregnancies in
the hospitals terminated by abortion, ectopic pregnancy or
hydatidiform mole. The prevalence of hydatidiform mole is
of the same magnitude as ectopic pregnancy.

Age, Parity and Education

Figure 1 reveals that a large number of women in the
25 to 29 age group are already grandmultiparous and that

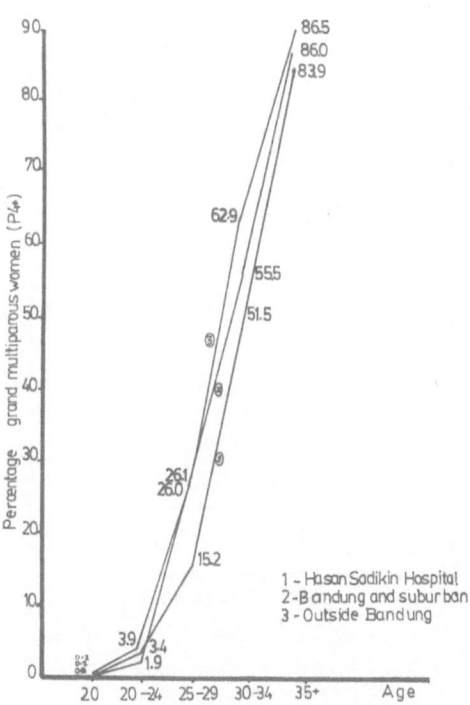

Figure 1. Prevalence of grandmultiparous women.

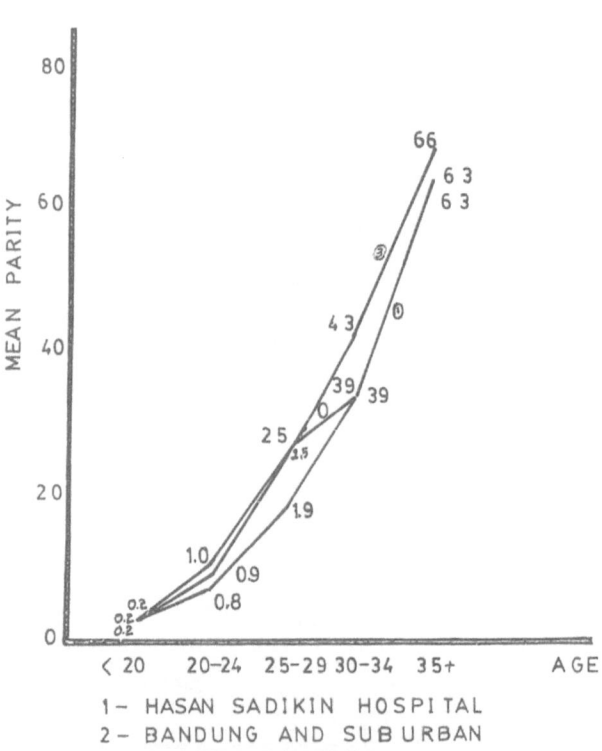

Figure 2. Mean parity by maternal age.

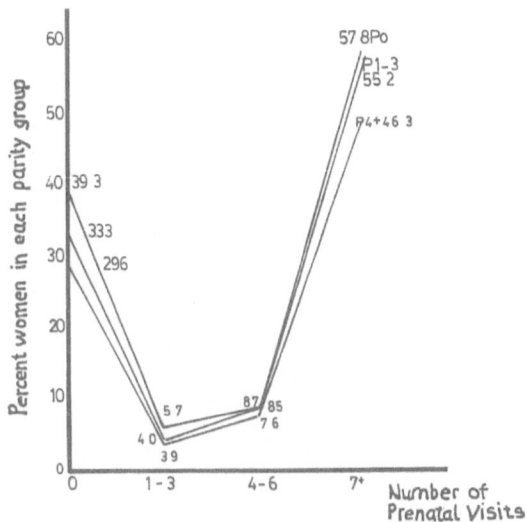

Figure 3.   Parity and prenatal visits: Hasan Sadikin.

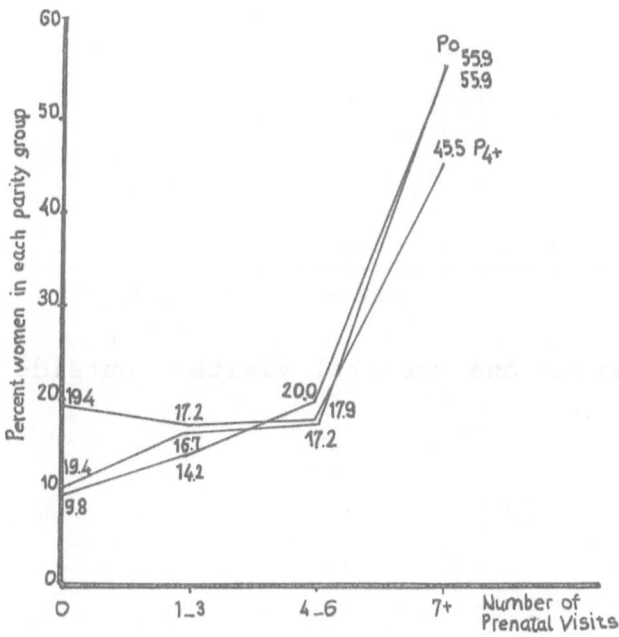

Figure 4.   Parity and prenatal visits: Bandung.

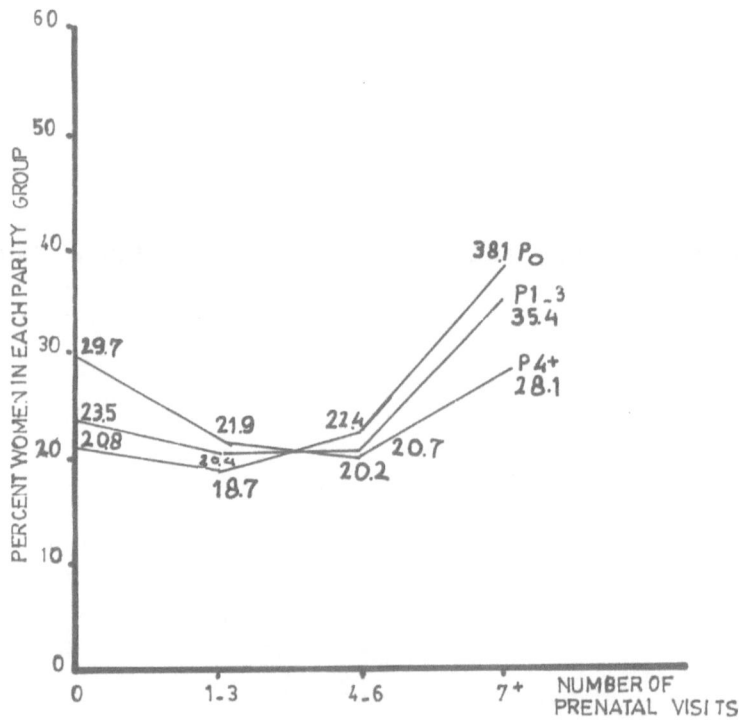

Figure 5. Parity and prenatal visits: outside Bandung.

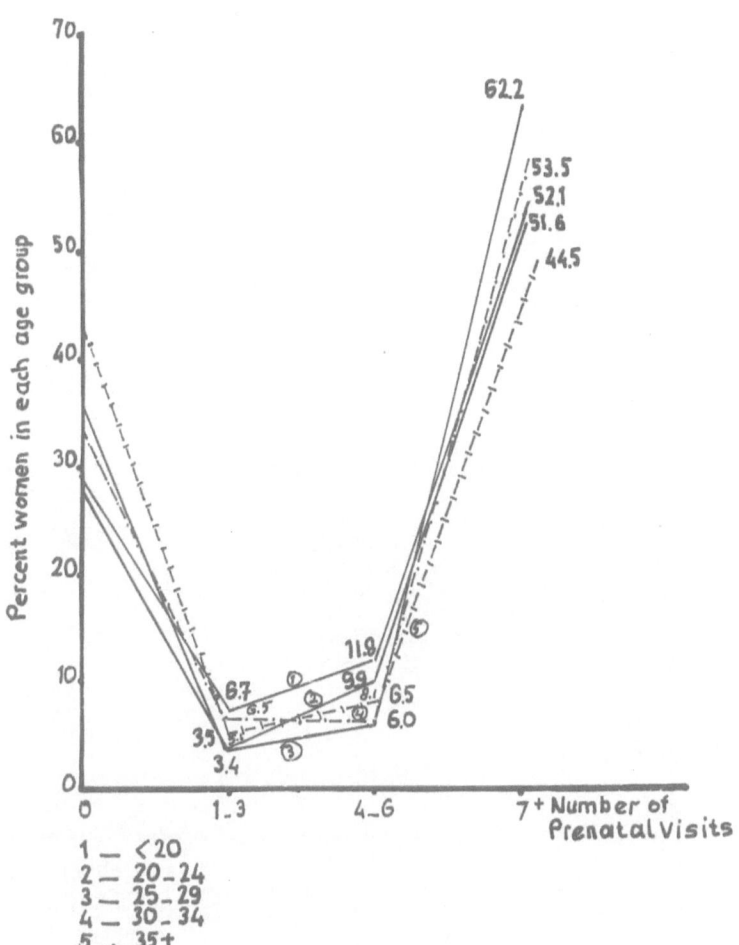

Figure 6. Age and prenatal visits: Hasan Sadikin Hospital.

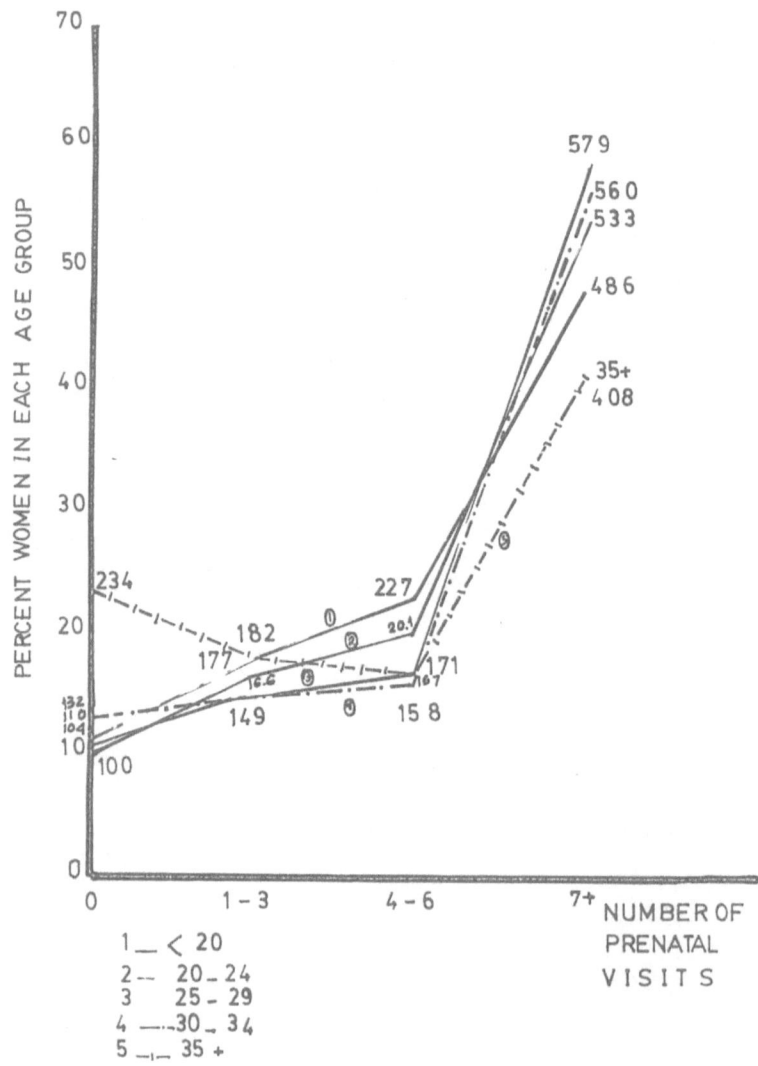

Figure 7.   Age and prenatal visits: Bandung and suburbs.

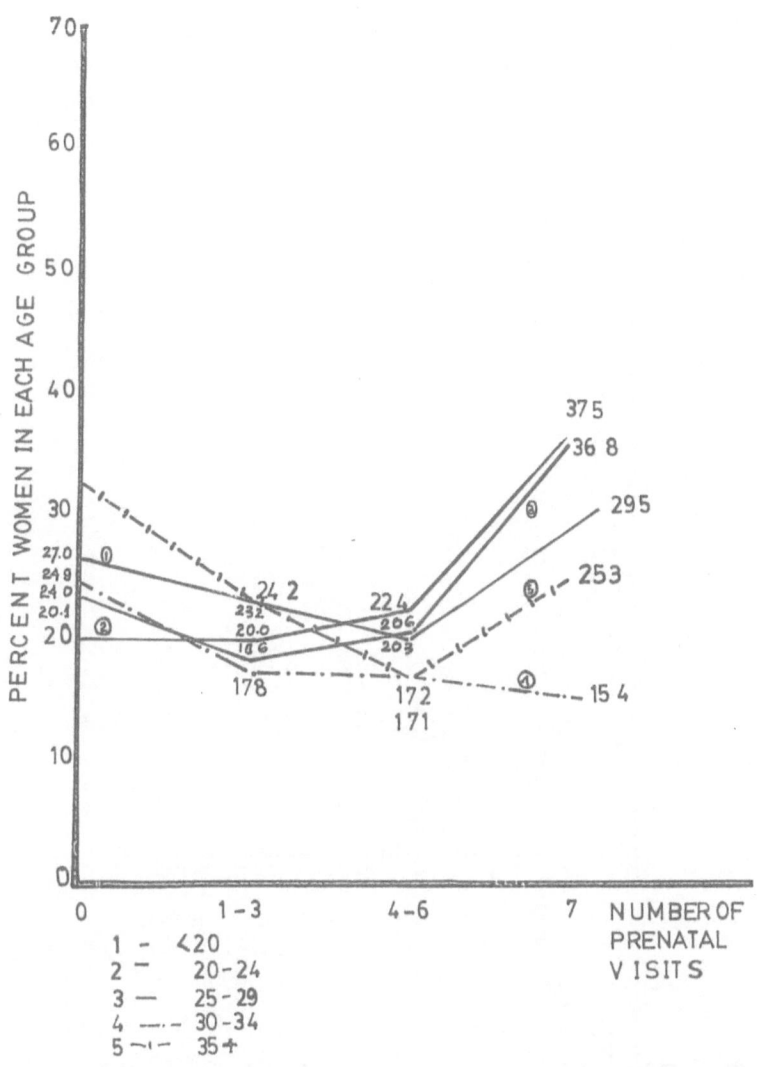

Figure 8. Age and prenatal visits: outside Bandung.

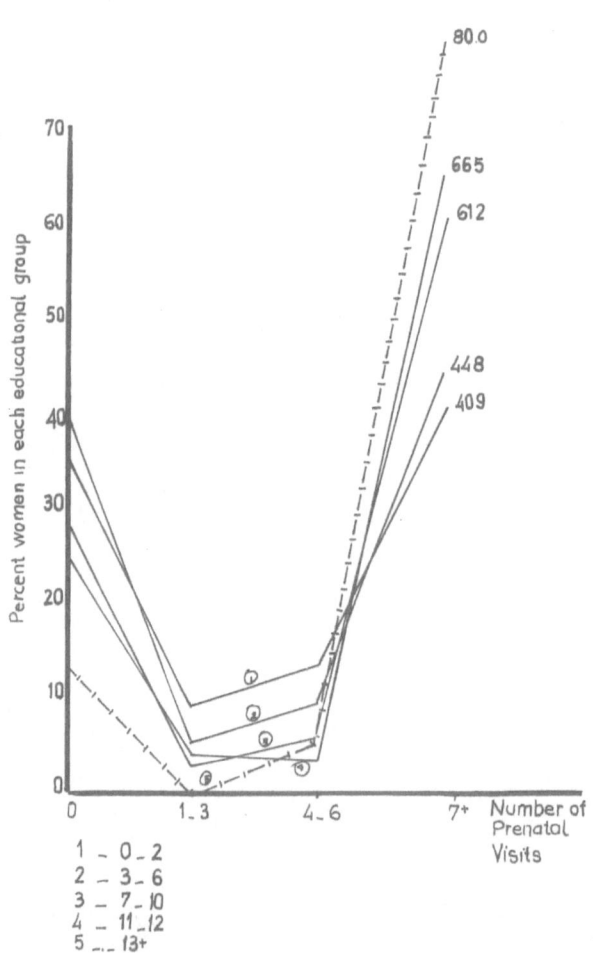

Figure 9.   Education and prenatal visits: Hasan Sadikin.

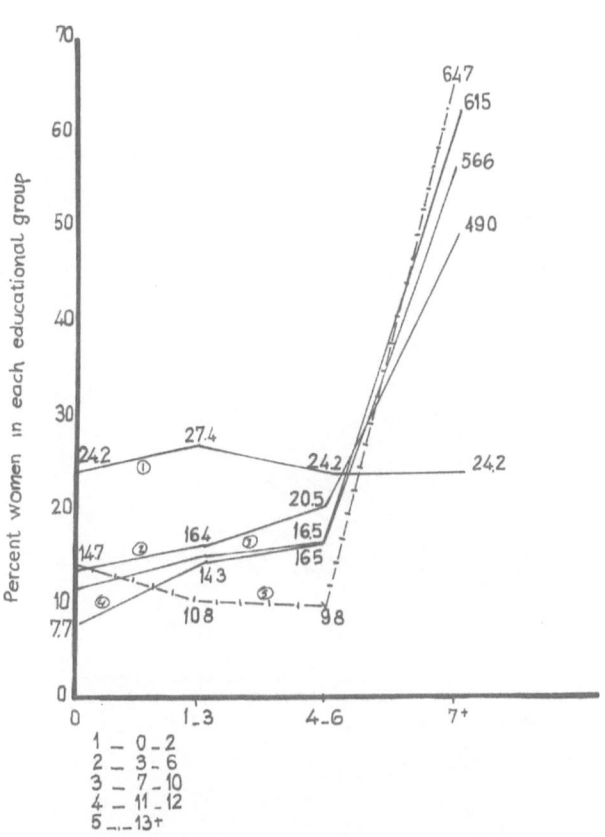

Figure 10. Education and prenatal visits: Bandung and suburbs.

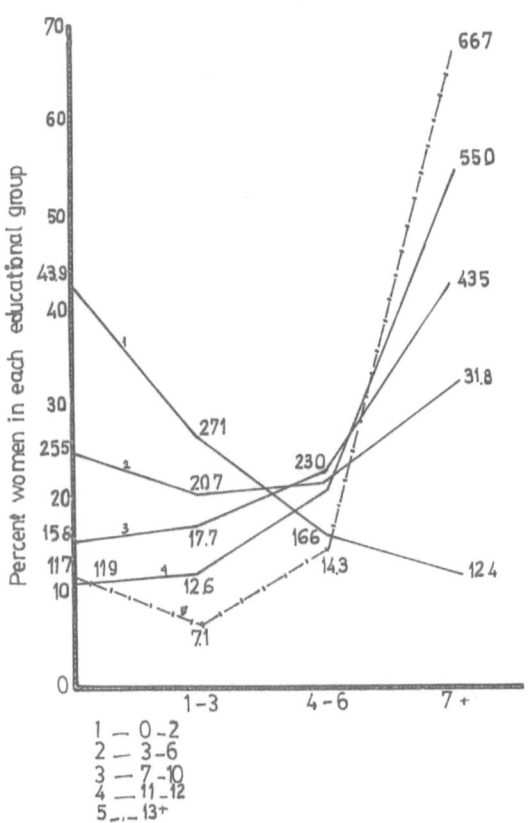

Figure 11.   Education and prenatal visits: outside
            Bandung.

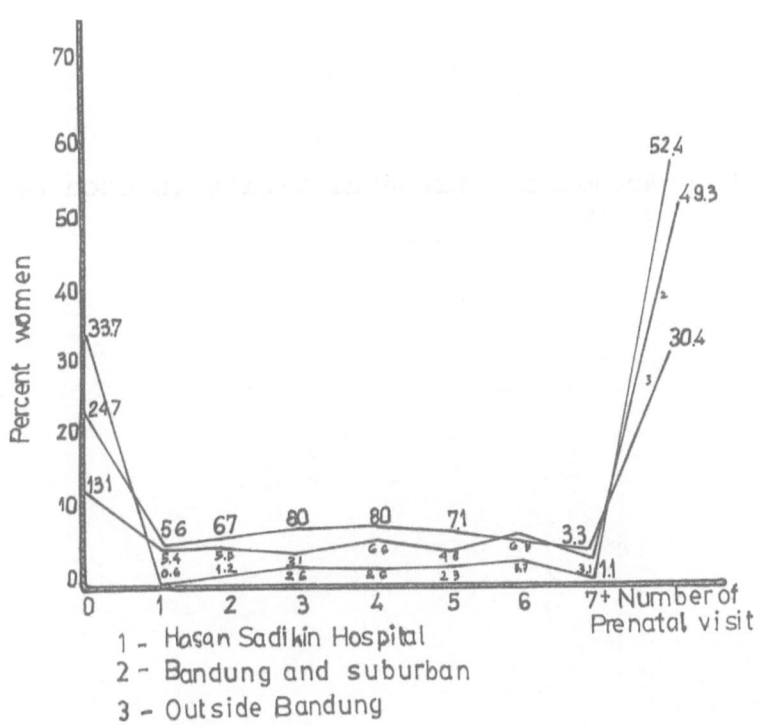

Figure 12.   Prenatal visits in each hospital group.

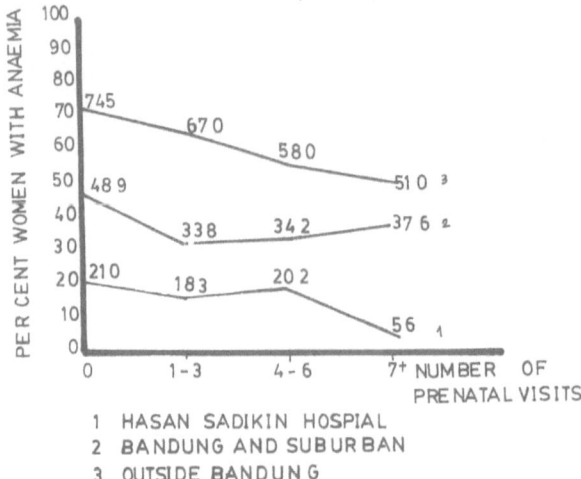

Figure 13.   Anemia and prenatal visits in each hospital
             group.

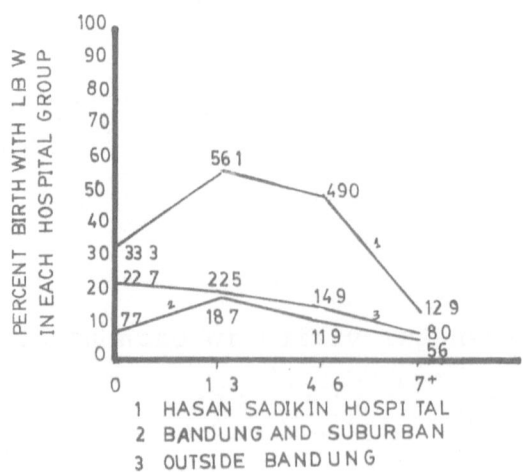

Figure 14.   Low birth weight and prenatal visits in each
             hospital group.

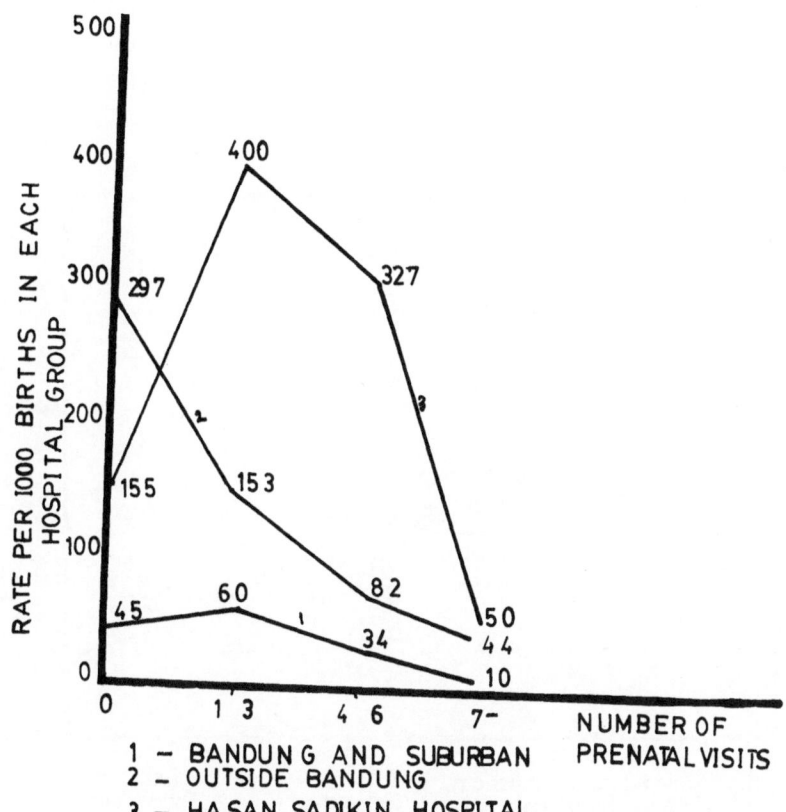

1 — BANDUNG AND SUBURBAN
2 — OUTSIDE BANDUNG
3 — HASAN SADIKIN HOSPITAL

Figure 15. Incidence of perinatal death by perinatal
visits.

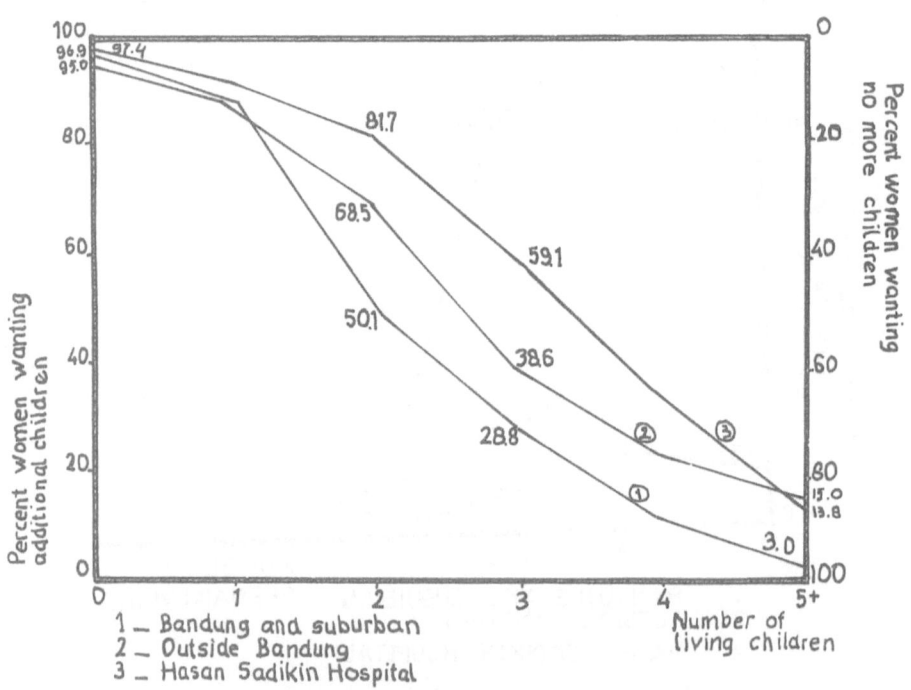

Figure 16. Incidence of women wanting additional
            children grouped according to number of
            surviving children.

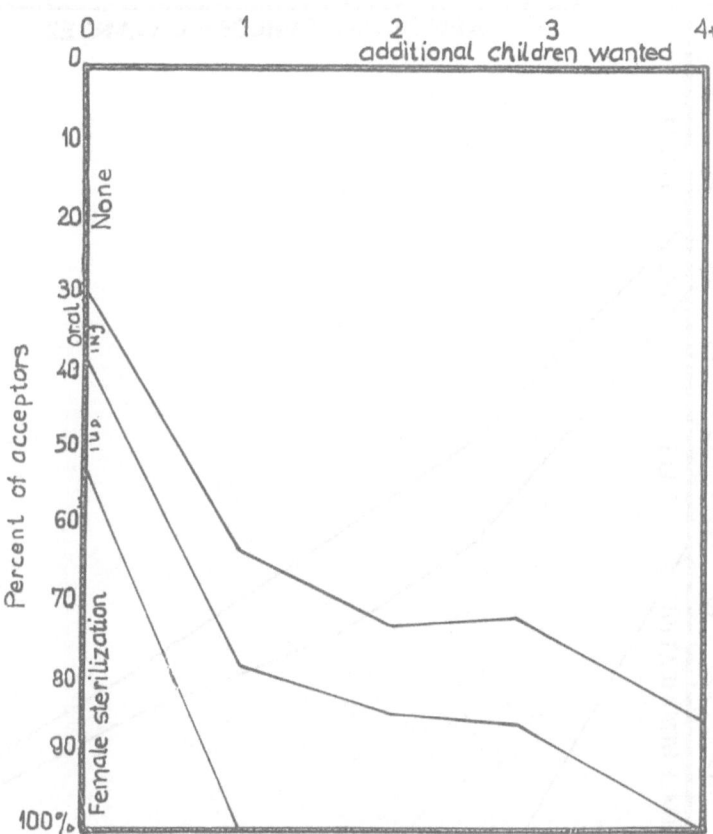

Figure 17. Contraceptive behavior by additional child-
           ren wanted: Hasan Sadikin.

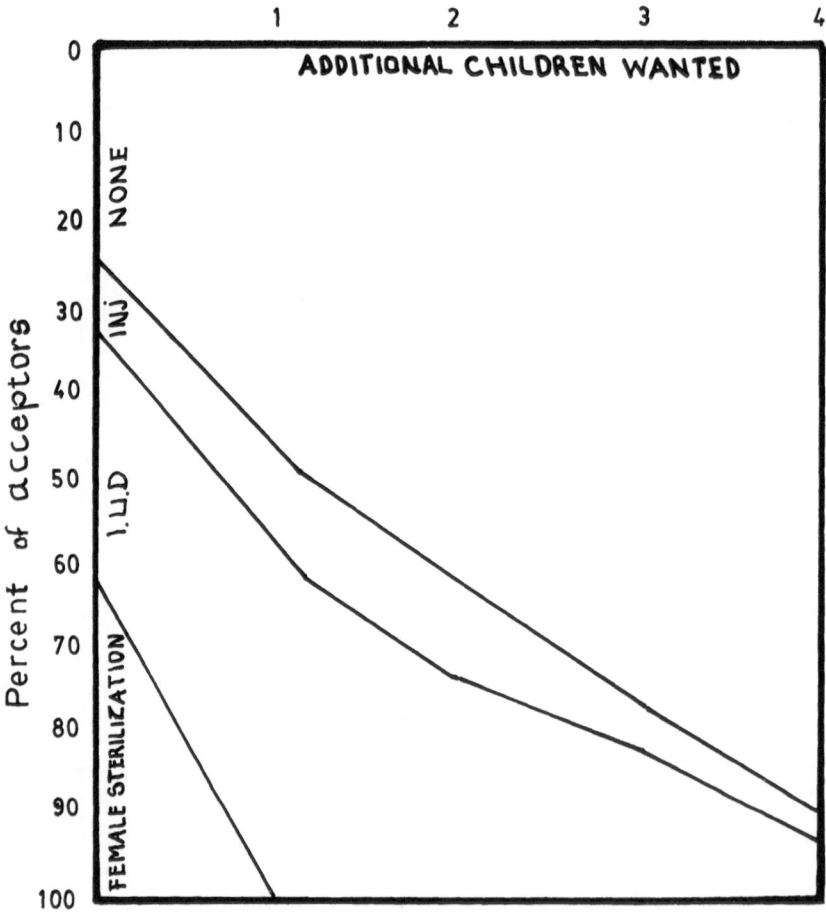

Figure 18.   Contraceptive behavior by additional child-
             ren wanted: Bandung.

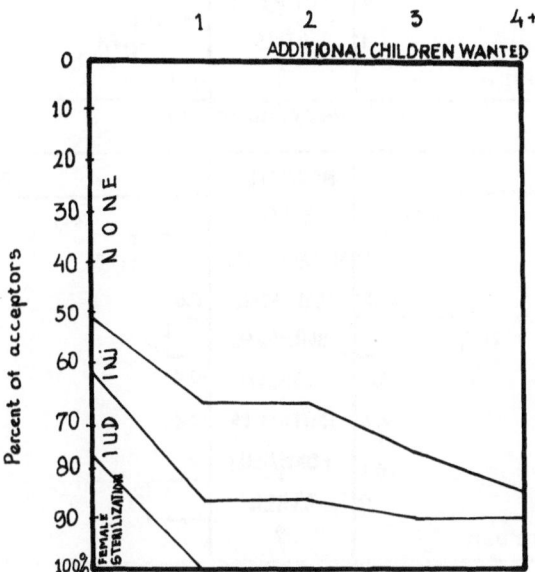

Figure 19. Contraceptive behaviour by additional
children wanted: outside Bandung.

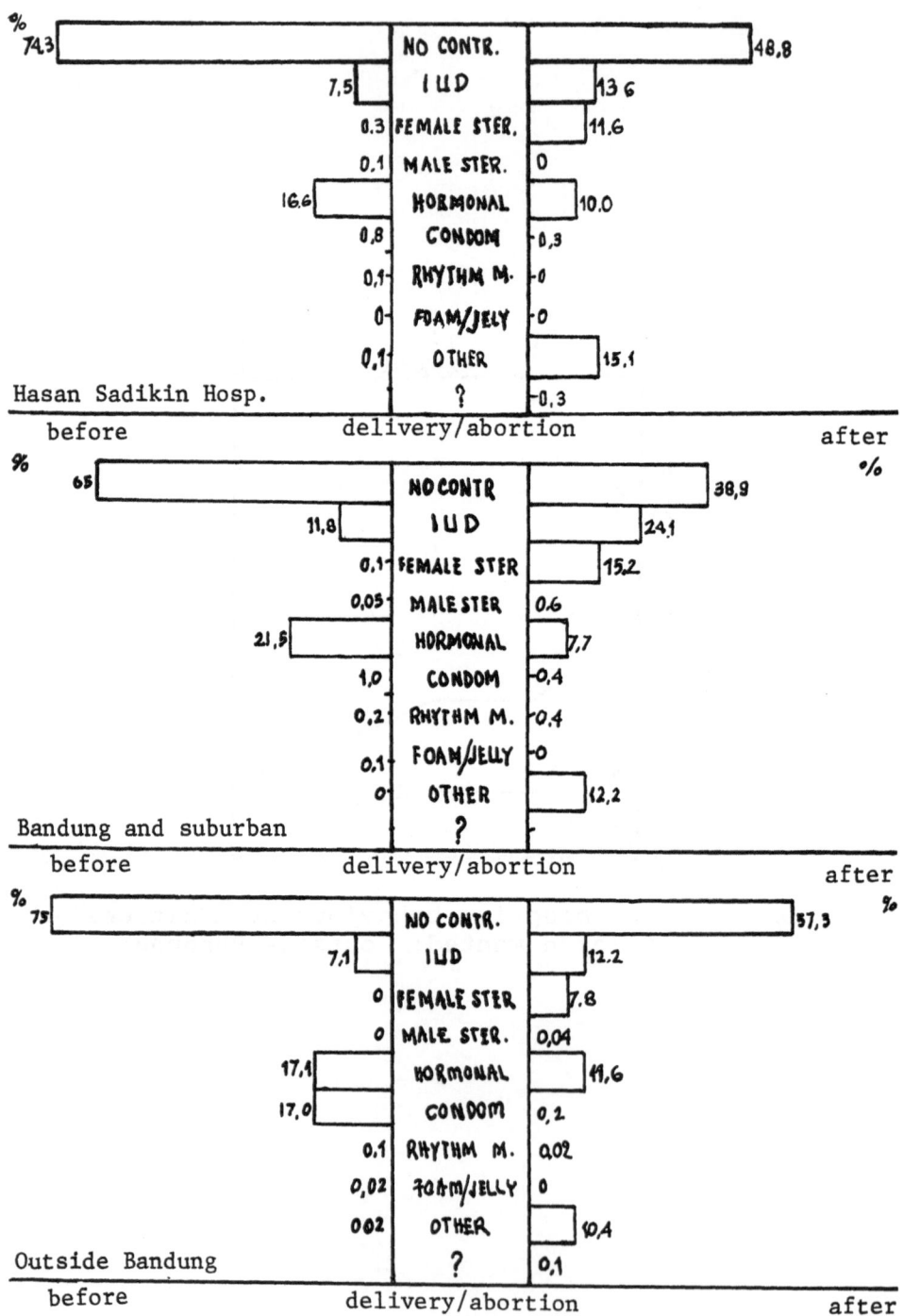

Figure 20.   Contraceptive performance.

the mean parity in the 25 to 29 age group had already
reached number of 1.9 to 2.5. Most of the patients have
had 5 to 6 years education.

Patient Characteristics and Prenatal Visits

Figures 3 to 8 show that grandmutiparous women and
elderly patients are the most neglected groups with
respect to prenatal care. Figures 9 to 11 reveal that
education has a positive effect on prenatal care. Figure
12 indicates that generally, the patients can be divided
into two groups: those who do not have any prenatal care,
and those who regularly visit prenatal clinics.

Relationship Between Prenatal Visits and Maternal and Child Health

The prevalence of anemia is very high (61 percent)
in the hospitals outside Bandung (Fig. 13). There appears
to be a correlation between anemia and prenatal care; in
those who had prenatal care, the prevalence of anemia is
lower. The same correlation is seen with birth weight
except for two groups who had no prenatal care. An acceptable explanation has not yet been apparent (Fig. 14).
A sharp decline in prenatal mortality is also associated
with prenatal care; again two groups with no prenatal
care have a relatively low perinatal mortality (Fig. 15).

Additional Children Desired

Figure 16 shows that a significant portion (28.8 to
59.1 percent) of mothers having three children still
wanted additional children.

Effects of Child Desire on Family Planning Acceptance

Figures 17 to 19 show that many patients including
those expressing no desire for additional children remain
without contraceptive protection even after contact with
the hospital. Only 8 to 15 percent wanting four or more
additional children choose to adapt family planning.

Postpartum Contraceptive Performance

Figure 20 compares contraceptive acceptance before
and after delivery or abortion, by the women in the three
groups. Contact with the hospital shows a gain of 18 to
25 percent in acceptance. Hospitals in Bandung and
surroundings provide 25 to 40 percent of the patients with
sterilization or IUDs while hospitals outside Bandung

provide these methods to only 20 percent.   Male
sterilization has a very low acceptance.

DISCUSSION

        The pregnancy wastage in 22 hospitals in West Java
is 20 percent.   This figure is not extraordinary, but the
termination of pregnancy by hydatidiform mole plays a much
more important role than in other countries and is
comparable with the prevalence of ectopic pregnancy.

        The age parity structure is still unfavorable, in-
fluencing the use of prenatal services and maternal and
child mortality and morbidity.   It seems that the small
family concept has not yet been fully appreciated.   Prenatal care, an important method of intervention to improve
maternal and child health, is still influenced by patient
characteristics, and less by center intervention.   The
importance of prenatal care for improving maternal and
child health is evident in Figures 13 to 15.   Anemia is an
important complication of pregnant mothers and one of the
factors affecting pregnancy outcome which should receive
serious attention.   The contact with hospitals gives only
an 18 to 25 percent gain in family planning acceptance.
The hospitals should try to increase acceptance for the
more stable methods of contraception, like sterilization
and IUDs.

CONCLUSION

        The high prevalence of grandmultiparity and the
great desire of having additional children reflects that
the small family concept is not yet appreciated.   Therefore health education should be intensified to prepare
future parents for their responsibilities.

        The postpartum contraceptive services should in-
crease their efforts especially to women not desiring
additional children.   As target, a 50 percent protection
rate should be achieved.   Sterilization and IUD should
cover 40 percent of the acceptors and male sterilization
should be encouraged.

        Prenatal care proves to be the most important method
of intervention to decrease perinatal mortality.   The
prenatal care services should implement the risk approach
giving special attention to grandmultiparous and elderly
women and those with low educational level.   The health

passport idea could be tested to improve the use of prenatal services.

Anemia is still a significant complication of pregnant women demanding our attention. Treatment of this complication should lead towards improvement of both mother and child health.

REFERENCE

1. Bernard RP, Sulaiman S, Agoestina T,Kendall EM (1980):
        Maternity Care Monitoring (MCM) in Indonesia -
        Early Findings and Implications for the 1980's.
        Majalah Obstetri dan Ginekologi Indonesia, 6:191.

CONCISE SCREENING SCALES FOR

HIGH-RISK MOTHERS AND NEWBORNS

A. B. Esguerra, A. N. Diamante, M. M. Ramos Jr.,
V. S. Doctor, C. B. Valdes, R. R. Pagorogon,
P. D. Macalino, M. S. Bautista, L. Pine-Tanseco

Department of Obstetrics and Gynecology
University of the East, College of Medicine
Quezon City, Phlippines

INTRODUCTION

The never-ending search for better ways of safe-
guarding the birth process goes on. Healthy mothers and
healthy neonates are aimed for by all childbirth
attendants. Lower maternal and perinatal morbidity and
mortality rates are major concerns of many agencies involved in total health care delivery. In response to this
need, medical science has developed advanced and expensive
technology designed to identify and rectify life-threaten-
ing conditions endangering the mother and her child, born
or unborn.

At present however, the supply of advanced technological services is much too limited in relation to the
demand for such services. Prosperous nations have limited
the availability of these modalities to regional centers
distributed throughout their territory. As for developing
nations, the number and quality of these services may be
constrained by inadequate economic resources. The strategy of limiting these sophisticated measures to those most
in need, with the view of optimizing their availability to
the greatest number of the population while diminishing
the cost of medical services has attained great relevance
and importance. Thus we have health care delivery
stratified into primary, secondary and tertiary levels.

In support of this move, instruments to identify

segments of the population in great need of specialized services from those who need only routine primary health care have been developed. In the area of maternal and newborn care, a number of high risk screening devices have evolved in recent years. This paper presents a concise screening scale system designed to identify high risk mothers and newborns, applicable in hospital settings; and with simplification, the system may eventually be applied in primary care settings, as a positive contribution to the ongoing search for better ways of safeguardng man's childbirth process.

Objectives

(a)   To develop a relatively simple and concise screening instrument to identify high risk mothers and newborns; and
(b)   To demonstrate that this instrument can be valid and reliable, stable yet flexible and ultimately useful in many levels of maternal and child health care.

Background

With the emergence of perinatology as a specialized area of concern with its own tools and perspectives, sole reliance on the old "clinical eye" of combined intuition and experience is fast becoming untenable. Although each practitioner has his own way of assessing maternal, fetal and neonatal well-being, a need for a standardized method of identifying high risk mothers and newborns that is common for all practitioners has become apparent.

Nesbitt and Aubrey (1) were among the first to present an antepartum risk scoring system related to maternal and neonatal outcome. This scoring system has enjoyed wide popularity. Modified scoring systems based on their work have been tried locally with varying degrees of success. The present authors have not been successful in the use of scoring systems of similar nature. Hobet el at (3, 4) have demonstrated that the inclusion of an intrapartum risk scoring produces better results. A number of authors (2, 5, 6, 7) have proposed a check-list format of a varying number of common risk factors as a simpler and less complicated screening method.

The present authors have found some of these scoring systems to be statistically unwieldy, with loose construction and non-comparable categories of risk factors, with subjective bias and lack of precision in some items, which may explain some of their unsatisfactory results.

They also believe that any scoring instrument to be acceptable and useful must first be precise, concise and statistically sound.

Expectations and Limitations

The screening scales for high-risk mothers and newborns presented in this paper attempt to fulfill the above criteria. These scales are constructed to be stable in format, concise in contents, comparable in categories, more precise and less subjective in application, clearly understandable, flexible and capable of further improvement, and able to stand statistical scrutiny.

Identified limitations are:

(a) Arbitary assignment of individual risk factors to some of the categories; these factors need further studies for confirmation or reassignment.
(b) Non-inclusion of other risk-factors;
(c) High degree of training required to administer the scales, and
(d) Applicability limited to hospital settings only, but with some modification, the system can be made applicable to rural settings where a greater need for screening and referral exists.

MATERIALS AND METHOD

Materials in the Construction of Instrument

(a) Known maternal and neonatal risk factors utilized in risk assessments (1-7, 10, 11).
(b) Common parameters of assessing postpartum and neonatal well being such as vital signs, length of hospital stay, elimination, etc.
(c) Sociological criteria used in classifying families into low, low-middle, high-middle and high income groups (8).
(d) Psychological factors deemed to have contributory relationship to increased risk in childbearing (9).

Method in the Construction of Instrument

Choice of format. After examination of the available risk screening devices, the rating scale format was decided upon as the most suitable and convenient form. A rating scale, with 4 columns representing increasing levels of added risk, labeled 0-3, arrayed against a 10

group classification of risk factors, giving a 40 category
framework, was constructed.

Assignment of risk factors. Only the more common
and representative risk factors were considered for
inclusion and then classified into 10 groups. Based on
their known or assumed relation with increased maternal or
neonatal morbidity, the individual risk factors were
assigned their corresponding places under the 4 columns of
increasing risk. In cases where the correlation coefficient was not established or was doubtful, the individual
risk factor was assigned a slot arbitrarily, based on a
consensus and recommendation of members of the hospital
perinatology committee.

Construction of screening scales. Three screening scales were devised. These are: the Antepartum Risk
Score (App. A) designed to identify high risk mothers in
the antepartum period; the Intrapartum Risk Score (App.
B) designed to identify high risk mothers intrapartum;
and the Neonatal Risk Score (App. C) designed to identify
high-risk neonates in the first 24 hours after birth.

Scoring. The individual risk factors were given
points according to the particular column representing
levels of added risk. Such that, those under the first
column (labeled "0") get a zero point; those under the
2nd column (labeled "1") gets a point and so on. These
points are tallied under the 5th and last column, then
added with the sum total of points representing the score
for that sheet. In the Antepartum Risk Score, where an
individual risk factor may be identified in the past and
also in the present, the past factor is given half a point
credited to that column. The present factor is given full
credit.

Cut-off point. A score of "6" points was selected
as a cut-off point in the Antepartum Risk Score and in the
Intrapartum Risk Score. A preliminary series of a small
number of cases using higher cut-off points in the score
failed to identify a significant number of mothers who
later on developed morbidity. Using a similar preliminary
screening, the score of "3" points was adopted as the cut-
off point in the Neonatal Risk Score. In these three
rating scales, scores below the cut-off point are rated as
"low-risk" scores, while those at or above the cut-off
point are labeled as "high-risk" scores.

Performance evaluation scales. For use in checking
on the risk screening scores as valid predictors of mater-

nal and neonatal morbidity, two rating scales designed to
evaluate postpartum and neonatal performance were constructed. These are: the Postpartum Performance Rating
Scales (App. D), and the Neonatal Performance Rating
Scales (App. E).

     For convenience and comparability, a rating scale
format, similar to that of the risk scores, was adopted.
Common parameters of assessing postpartum and neonatal
well-being, like vital signs, length of hospital stay,
feeding, elimination, were identified, weighed and distributed according to their presumed levels of increased
severity of complication. A cut-off point of "6" points
was adopted to distinguish between the "good performer"
and the "poor performer" in the Postpartum Performance
Rating Scale, to be administered on discharge. A cut-off
point of "3" points was taken to separate the "good
performer" or "non-morbid" from the "poor performer" or
"morbid" among the neonates in the Neonatal Performance
Rating Scale which is to be administered on discharge at
72 hours after birth. As designed, these scales are
simple and objective enough to reliably produce similar
results when administered by different evaluators.

Application and Validation

     The patient population used in this study were 145
mothers who delivered in the charity service of the Department of Obstetrics and Gynecology of the University of
the East Ramon Magsaysay Memorial Medical Center from
March 1 to August 31, 1981, and the 148 neonates including
3 set of twins born to these mothers and cared for in the
charity nursery of the Department of Pediatrics of the
same institution.

     In the method of risk assessment, all of the 145
mothers were assigned to an obstetric resident for assessment, using the Antepartum Risk Score and the Intrapartum
Risk Score. The mothers were classified into low-risk or
high-risk intrapartum groups. Another classification was
made, combining the antepartum risk with the intrapartum
risk group, obtaining a combined 4 group classification
which are: Group A (low-low group), low-risk antepartum
and low-risk intrapartum group; Group B (high- low
group), high-risk antepartum and low-risk intrapartum
group; Group C (low-high group), low-risk antepartum and
high-risk intrapartum group; and Group D (high-high
group), high-risk antepartum and high-risk intrapartum
group.

All of the 148 neonates were assessed during the
first 24 hours after birth by an assigned pediatric
resident, using the Neonatal Risk Score. These neonates
were classified into low-risk or high-risk groups.

Relation of Antepartum Risk and Intrapartum Performance

To determine whether a more complicated intrapartum
course could be predicted by an antepartum risk assessment, the intrapartum performance as measured by the
Intrapartum Risk Score (good <6, poor >6), of the two
antepartum risk groups (low-risk and high-risk) were
compared.

Relation of Maternal Risk Assessment and Postpartum Outcome

Postpartum morbidity rates. A comparison of the
postpartum morbidity rates of the low-risk antepartum
group with the high-risk antepartum group of mothers was
made. A similar comparison of postpartum morbidity rates
among the intrapartum risk groups was likewise undertaken.
The occurrence of postpartum complications among the 4
groups of combined antepartum-intrapartum risk groups of
mothers was also compared.

Postpartum performance rating. The postpartum
performance of the 145 mothers included in this study were
rated according to the Postpartum Performance Rating Scale
administered by other obstetric residence on discharge.
Using a 6 point cut-off score, the mothers were divided
into the "good performer" group (<6 points) and the "poor
performer" group (>6 points). The distribution of good
performers among the low-risk antepartum group and the
high-risk antepartum group of mothers was noted and compared. A similar comparison was made among the low-risk
intrapartum and high-risk intrapartum groups of mothers.
The distribution of "poor performers" and "good performers" among the 4 groups of combined antepartum-intrapartum
risk groups was also studied.

Relation of Maternal Risk and Condition of Newborn at Birth.

The distribution of low-risk neonates and high-risk
neonates among the maternal risk groups assessed in the
antepartum and intrapartum period, including the 4
combined risks was studied, compared and analyzed.

Table 1a. Distribution of Mothers According to
Antepartum Risk

Antepartum Risk	Number	Percent
High Risk	100	68.96
Low Risk	45	31.04
Total	145	100.00

Table 1b. Distribution of Mothers According to
Intrapartum Risk

Intrapartum Risk	Number	Percent
High Risk	58	40.00
Low Risk	87	60.00
Total	145	100.00

Table 1c. Distribution of Mothers According to
Antepartum-Intrapartum Risk

Antepartum-Intrapartum Risk	Number	Percent
A. Low-low	31	21.38
B. High-low	56	38.62
C. Low-high	14	9.66
D. High-high	44	30.34
Total	145	100.00

Relation of Neonatal Risk Assessment and Neonatal

Performance

To determine the value of neonatal risk screening in predicting neonatal morbidity and performance, all of the 148 newborns were evaluated using the Neonatal Performance Rating Scale administered by other pediatric residents on discharge at least 72 hours after birth. Those newborn scoring less than the cut-off score of 3 points were classified as non-morbid or good performers, while those scoring 3 points or more were classified as morbid or poor performers. A comparison was made of the distribution of non-morbid and morbid neonates into the two groups of new-

Table 1d. Distribution of Neonates According to
            Neonatal High-Risk Score

Neonatal Risk	Number	Percent
High	30	20.17
Low	118	79.73
Total	148	100.00

borns identified at birth as low-risk neonates or high-
risk neonates through the use of the Neonatal Risk Score
Sheet.

Relation of Maternal Risk Assessment and Neonatal Morbidity

To determine the relationship between maternal risk
assessment and neonatal outcome at 72 hours after birth
until discharge, the neonatal performance ratings, i.e.,
morbid or non-morbid, of the newborns of the different
groups of low-risk and high-risk mothers as gauged by
the Antepartum Risk Score, the Intrapartum Risk Score and
the 4 combined antepartum-intrapartum risk groupings were
compared.

RESULTS

Applying the Antepartum Risk Score on the 145 mothers
in the sample, 45 (31.04 %) were classified as low-risk
and 100 (68.96 %) as high-risk (Table 1a). The greater
preponderance of high-risk patients is a reflection of the
type of patients served by the authors' institution, which
is mainly a tertiary care university teaching hospital.

In the same sample, using the Intrapartum Risk Score,
87 (60 %) were in the low-risk group while 58 (40 %) were
classified as high-risk (Table 1b). The reversal in distribution of the low-risk and high-risk groups intrapartum
compared with the antepartum risk groupings may be a
result of the interventions instituted before and during
labor by those rendering care to the mothers.

Combining the antepartum and intrapartum risk assessment into a combined 4 group classification as suggested
by Hobel et al (2, 3), 31 (21.38 %) were found in the low-
low group, 56 (38.62 %) in the high-low group, 14 (9.66 %)
in the low-high group, and 44 (30.34 %) in the high-high
group (Table 1c).

Table 2. Relation of Antepartum Risk to Intrapartum
          Complications

Antepartum Assessment	No.	Intrapartum Risk			
		Good Score <6		Poor Score >6	
		No.	%	No.	%
High	100	56	56.0	44	44
Low	45	31	68.8	14	31.11
Total	145	87	60.0	58	40

p=>0.10

Table 3a. Postpartum Maternal Morbidity Rates by
           Antepartum Risk

Antepartum Assessment	No. of Cases	No.of Morbid Cases	Rates in Percent
High Risk	100	10	10.00
Low Risk	45	2	4.44
Total	145	12	8.27

Table 3b. Postpartum Maternal Morbidity Rates by
           Intrapartum Risk

Intrapartum Assessment	No. of Cases	No. of Morbid Cases	Rates in Percent
High Risk	58	10	17.24
Low Risk	87	2	2.29
Total	145	12	8.28

Table 3c. Postpartum Maternal Morbidity Rates by
           Antepartum-Intrapartum Risk

Antepartum-Intrapartum Risk	No. of Cases	No. of Morbid Cases	Rates in Percent
A. Low-low	31	0	0
B. High-low	56	2	3.57
C. Low-high	14	2	14.28
D. High-high	44	8	18.18
Total	145	12	8.27

Of the 148 neonates born to these 145 mothers, including the three sets of twins, 118 (79.73 %) were classified as low-risk and 30 (20.17 %) as high risk, using the Neonatal Risk Score (Table 1d). It is interesting to note that while similar to the intrapartum risk group in having greater numbers in the low-risk neonate group, the neonatal risk grouping also shows a reversal in distribution of low and high risk found in the antepartum risk groups.

Relation of Antepartum Risk and Postpartum Performance

A comparison of the intrapartum performance of the two antepartum risk groups in the study sample, using the Intrapartum Risk Score as an index of intrapartum complications shows that there were 56 (56 %) good performers among 100 high-risk antepartum mothers against 31 (68.81%) among 45 low-risk antepartum mothers (Table 2). It would seem that the Antepartum Risk Score exhibits a trend in predicting intrapartum morbidity but the relationship is not statistically significant ($p => 0.10$).

Relation of Maternal Risk Assessment and Postpartum Outcome

There were 12 mothers in the sample who developed morbidity in the postpartum period, giving a rate of 12/145 or 88.27 percent. All had urinary tract infection and one had drug fever. Table 3a shows postpartum maternal morbidity by antepartum risk. There were 10 morbid cases in the high-risk group, giving a 10 percent rate, which is 2 percent higher than the mean rate for the entire group. Of the low risk group, only 2 (4.44 %) developed complications which is about half of the morbidity rate for the group. It is apparent from the data that the occurrence of post-partum morbidity is positively correlated in a moderate degree with a high-risk score in the antepartum period ($p = <0.05$).

Table 3b shows postpartum maternal morbidity relative to intrapartum risk. There were 10 morbid cases in the high-risk group giving a rate of 17.24 percent which is 8.96 percent higher than the mean rate. Of the low-risk group, only 1 (2.29 %) developed complications which is 5.99 percent lower than the group morbidity rate. These figures indicate that the occurrence of postpartum morbidity is correlated to a significant degree with a high risk score in the intrapartum period ($p = <0.05$).

Table 3c shows postpartum morbidity related to the

Table 4a.   Relation of Antepartum Risk to Postpartum
            Performance

Antepartum Assessment	Postpartum Performance Rating			
	Good Score (<6)		Poor Score ($\geq$6)	
	Number	Percent	Number	Percent
High Risk	65	61.32	41	38.68
Low Risk	33	84.62	6	15.38
Total	98	67.59	47	32.41

p = <0.05

Table 4b.   Relation of Intrapartum Risk to Postpartum
            Performance

Intrapartum Assessment	Postpartum Performance Rating			
	Good Score (<6)		Poor Score ($\geq$6)	
	Number	Percent	Number	Percent
High Risk	22	37.93	36	32.07
Low Risk	76	87.36	11	12.64
Total	98	67.59	47	32.41

p = <0.05

Table 4c.   Relation of Antepartum-Intrapartum Risk
            to Postpartum Performance.

Antepartum-Intrapartum Risk	Postpartum Peformance Rating			
	Good Score (<6)		Poor Score ($\geq$6)	
	Number	Percent	Number	Percent
A. Low-low	30	96.77	1	3.22
B. High-low	46	82.14	10	17.85
C. Low-high	8	61.54	5	38.46
D. High-high	14	31.11	31	68.89
Total	98	67.58	47	32.41

p = <0.05

combined antepartum-intrapartum risk assessment. It also
reflects the influence of the combination of a weak predictor (antepartum risk) and a strong predictor (intrapartum risk) on the occurrence of postpartum morbidity. It
is interesting to note that there were no morbid cases in
Group A (low-low group). It can be said that in this

population of 145 mothers, a perfect inverse correlation
exists between the occurrence of postpartum morbidity and
low risk antepartum-intrapartum score. There were two
cases equivalent to 3.57 percent rate in the high-low
group, which is lower by 4.70 percent than the mean rate.
This merely indicates that despite the high-risk assessment in the antepartum period, the low intrapartum risk
determined the lower morbidity rate during the postpartum
period.

The low-high group showed a 14.28 percent rate (2/56)
which is 6.01 percent higher than the mean, while the
high-high group registered the highest morbidity rate of
18.18 percent (8/44) which is 9.91 percent higher than
(more than double) the mean rate. It appears that it is
the high-risk intrapartum score that determines the degree
of positive correlation that exists between maternal risk
assessment and the occurrence of postpartum morbidity.
However, the addition of the added factor of high antepartum risk has a slight contributory role in this relationship. This observation supports the view that the
inclusion of intrapartum risk screening enhances the value
of antepartal risk assessment in predicting postpartum
morbidity.

Relation of Maternal Risk to Postpartum Performance

Table 4a shows the postpartum performance rating of
the two antepartum risk groups of mothers. Good performance of the low-risk (84.62 %) and of the high-risk
(61.32 %) groups during the postpartum recovery period was
exhibited. Poor performance was shown by the high-risk
(38.68 %) as compared to the low-risk group (15.38 %).
Mean rate for poor performance is 32.41 percent. These
figures indicate that postpartum performance is
significantly correlated to antepartum risk (p = <0.05).

Table 4b shows the relation of intrapartum risk to
postpartum performance. Good postpartum performance was
rendered by 87.36 percent of the low-risk group as against
37.93 percent of the high-risk group. The mean rate was
67.59 percent. On the other hand, 62.07 percent of the
high-risk group were rated poor performers compared to
12.64 percent of the low-risk group. The mean rate was
32.42 percent. These figures indicate that postpartum
performance is related to intrapartum risk in a
statistically significant degree (p = <0.05).

Table 4c shows the relation of combined antepartum-
intrapartum risk to postpartum performance. Good

Table 5a. Conditions of Newborns in Relation to
           Antepartum Risk

| Mothers | | Neonates | | | |
| Antepartum | | Low Risk | | High Risk | |
Assessment	No.	No.	%	No.	%
High Risk	100*	83	81.37	19	18.63
Low Risk	45**	35	76.08	11	23.92
Total	145	118	79.73	30	20.17

p = >0.10
* = twin pregnancy

Table 5b. Condition of Newborn in Relation to
           Intrapartum Risk

| Mothers | | Neonates | | | |
| Intrapartum | | Low Risk | | High Risk | |
Assessment	No.	No.	%	No.	%
High Risk	58**	43	69.35	19	30.65
Low Risk	87*	75	87.21	11	12.79
Total	145	118	79.73	30	20.27

p = <0.05
* = twin pregnancy

Table 5c. Condition of Newborns in Relation to
           Antepartum-Intrapartum Risk

| Mothers | | Neonates | | | |
| Antepartum- | | Low Risk | | High Risk | |
Intrapartum Risk	No.	No.	%	No.	%
A. Low-low	32	25	78.12	7	21.88
B. High-low	56	50	89.29	6	10.71
C. Low-high	14	10	71.43	4	28.57
D. High-high	44	33	71.44	13	28.26
Total	145	118	79.73	30	20.27

p = 0.10

performance was rendered by 96.77 percent and only 3.22
percent of the same group had a poor performance; 82.14
percent of the high-low group were good performers with
only 17.85 percent of their group rated poor. The rate of

good performers was drastically reduced to 61.54 percent
among the low-high group while poor performers rose to
38.46 per- cent. In the high-high group, 68.89 percent
were tagged as poor performers against 31.11 percent of
good perform- ers. It would seem that the higher the
antepartum- intrapartum risks, the greater would be the
possibility of a poor performance in the postpartum
recovery period. This relationship is statistically
significant (p = <0.05).

Condition of Newborn and Maternal Risk Assessment

Table 5a shows the condition of newborns in relation
to antepartum risk; 83 neonates, including a set of
twins, born to 100 high-risk antepartum mothers were rated
low-risk neonates, giving a rate of 81.37 percent, while
19 or 18.63 percent of the same group were rated high-
risk; 35 neonates, including two sets of twins, born to
45 low-risk antepartum mothers were classified as low-risk
neonates, giving a rate of 76.08 percent. In the same
group, eleven or 23.92 percent were classified as
high-risk.

The rate of occurrence of low-risk neonates was almost similar among the high-risk and low-risk antepartum
group of mothers; 81.37 percent to 76.08 percent. The
difference is not statistically significant (p = >0.10).
Thus, this study is unable to show any correlation between
condition of newborns at birth and antepartum risk.

Table 5b shows the condition of newborns at birth in
relation to intrapartum risk. There was an observable
difference in the rate of occurrence of low-risk neonates
among the high-risk and low-risk intrapartum group of
mothers, 69.35 percent and 87.21 percent respectively.
The high-risk neonate rate was higher among the high-risk
intrapartum mothers than among the low-risk intrapartum
mothers, 30.65 percent and 12.79 percent. It can be
statted that the condition of the newborn at birth is
correlated with intrapartum risk (p = <0.05).

Table 5c shows the condition of newborns in relation
to antepartum-intrapartum risk. There was no demonstrable
difference in the occurrence of high-risk or low-risk
neonates among the 4 groups of combined anepartum-
intrapartum risk mothers. The difference was not statistically significant (p = >0.10). The addition of one
variable which has no relation to newborn condition
(antepartum risk) to one which is positively correlated
(intrapartum risk) does not result in increased predictive

Table 6. Neonatal Morbidity (Number and Rate) by
          Neonatal Risk

Neonatal Assessment	Total Number	Morbidity Number	Percent
Low-risk	118	14	11.86
High-risk	30	20	66.66
Total	148	34	22.97

Table 7a. Neonatal Morbidity (Number and Rate)
           By Antepartum Risk

Mothers Antepartum Risk	Number	Morbid Neonates Number	Percent
High Risk	100	22	22.00
Low Risk	45	12	26.66
Total	145	34	23.45

Table 7b. Neonatal Morbidity (Number and Rate)
           By Intrapartum Risk

Mothers Intrapartum Risk	Number	Morbid Neonates Number	Percent
High Risk	58	23	38.65
Low Risk	87	11	11.49
Total	145	34	23.45

Table 7c. Neonatal Morbidity (Number and Rate)
           By Antepartum-Intrapartum Risk

Mothers Antepartum-Intrapartum Risk	Number	Morbid Neonates Number	Percent
A. Low-low	31	6	19.35
B. High-low	56	5	8.92
C. Low-high	14	6	42.86
D. High-high	44	17	38.64
Total	145	34	23.45

capacity of the risk screening device but may even reduce
the effect achieved by use of the correlated variable
alone.

Relation of Neonatal Risk and Neonatal Morbidity

Table 6 shows neonatal morbidity grouped according to
neonatal risk. The figures show that the high-risk group
of neonates have a greater tendency to develop complications than the neonates low-risk at birth, 66.66 percent
and 11.86 percent respectively. This is statistically
significant (p = 0.05). It can be stated that the neonatal risk score is useful in predicting a greater
likelihood of developing diseases later on during the
neonatal period.

Relation of Maternal Risk and Neonatal Morbidity

Table 7a shows neonatal morbidity based on antepartum risk. Comparing the neonatal morbidity rate of the
149 newborns with the antepartum risk scoring of their
mothers, no significant difference in rates was found
among the low-risk and the high-risk groups, 26.66 percent
and 22 percent respectively. Thus, antepartum risk was
not shown to be correlated with neonatal morbidity (p =
>0.10).

Table 7b shows neonatal morbidity associated with
intrapartum risk. There was no observed difference in the
neonatal morbidity rates associated with the two
intrapartum risk groups of mothers. A 39.65 percent
morbidity rate was found among newborns of mothers rated
as high-risk intrapartum as against an 11.49 percent rate
among newborns of low-risk intrapartum mothers (0 = 0.05).
It can be stated that neonatal morbidity is correlated
with high intrapartum risk and that the Intrapartum Risk
Score can be useful in predicting the likelihood of
developing neonatal diseases.

Table 7c shows neonatal morbidity by antepartum-
intrapartum risk. A comparison of neonatal morbidity with
the combined antepartum-intrapartum risk groups shows that
higher morbidity rates are associated with low-high and
high-high groups (which includes high intrapartum risk
groups) as compared to the low-low and high-low groups
(which in cludes low-risk intrapartum groups). It would
seem that in predicting neonatal morbidity, the decisive
factor is intrapartum risk rather than antepartum risk.

CONCLUSION

In a group of 145 mothers delivered in the charity service unit of our hospital, including 148 neonates born to these mothers, had risk assessment by the Antepartum Risk Score, the Intrapartum Risk Score and the Neonatal Risk Score, and were later evaluated by the Postparum Performance Rating Scale and the Neonatal Performance Rating Scale. From this study conducted March 1 to August 31, 1981, the following conclusions can be made:

(a) Risk assessment of mothers and newborns can be made relatively simple, precise and statistically comparable by the use of the Antepartum, Intrapartum and Neonatal Risk Score systems developed in the study.

(b) Antepartum risk tends to be correlated to intrapartum morbidity and poor postpartum performance.

(c) Antepartum risk tends to be related to intrapartum morbidity but the relationship is not statistically significant.

(d) There is no relation between antepartum risk and condition of newborn at birth and neonatal morbidity.

(e) Intrapartum risk is positively correlated to postpartum maternal morbidity, poor postpartum performance, condition of newborn at birth and neonatal morbidity.

(f) The combination of antepartum-intrapartum risk is correlated to postpartum maternal morbidity and performance.

(e) Neonatal risk is correlated with neonatal morbidity.

The three risk screening scores in their present form may be useful in identifying high-risk mothers and new-borns in many health care settings with the following limitations:

(a) There is room for re-evaluation and modification of individual risk factors contained in the 40 categories of the risk score sheets.

(b) There is a need for improvement of the antepartum risk score in order to increase its predictive value in relation to neonatal outcome.

(c) Extensive follow-up of morbidity and mortality studies for each individual risk factor is in order.

(d) For eventual utilization as a useful screening instrument of maternal and newborn risk at a primary health care level, further simplification of content and form of the risk scoring system presented in this study is desirable.

REFERENCES

1. Aubry RH, Nesbitt RFL Jr (1969): High-risk obstet-
    rics. I. Prenatal outcome in relation to a
    broadened approach to obstetric care for patients at
    special risk. Am J Obstet Gynecol, 105:241.
2. Dela Paz JT, Micozzi MS (1977): Evaluation of
    maternal and child health care indices in the
    identification of high risk pregnancy. Phil J
    Obstet Gynecol, 1:315.
3. Hobel CJ, Hyvarinen MA et al (1973): Perinatal and
    intrapartum high risk screening. Am J Obstet
    Gynecol, 117:1.
4. Hobel CJ, Youkeles L (1979): Prenatal and intrapartum
    high risk screening. Am J Obstet Gynecol,
    135:1051.
5. Goodwin JW, Dunne JT, Thomas BW (1969): Antepartum
    identification of the fetus at risk. Can Med Assoc
    J, 101:57.
6. Morrison I, Olsen J (1979): Perinatal mortality and
    antepartum risk scoring. Obstet Gynecol, 53:362.
7. Sokol RJ, Rosen MG et al (1977): Clinical
    applications of high-risk scoring on an obstetric
    service. Am J Obstet Gynecol, 128:652.
8. Espiritu SC, Holensteiner MR, Huat CL, Lacar LQ,
    Quisumbing LR (1977): Sociology n the new
    Philippine setting. The Alemar-Phoenix Publishing
    House, Quezon City, Philippines, 105.
9. Brown WA (1979): Psychological care during pregnancy
    and the postpartum period. Raven Press, New York.
10. Aubry RH, Pennington JC (1973): Identification and
    evaluation of high risk pregnancy. The Perinatal
    Concept. Clin Obstet Gynecol, 16:3.
11. Babson SG, Pernoll ML, Benda GI (1980): Diagnosis
    and management of the fetus and neonate at risk, a
    guide for team care. The C.V. Mosby Co., Missouri.

[Appendices are available by direct correspondence with
    the senior author]

Appendix A

RISK FACTOR	LEVEL OF RISK				SCORE POINTS
	0	1	2	3	
1 AGE, YEARS	20–29	30–34	16–19	< 15 ≥ 35	
2 STATUS	married	live — in	separated/div.	Single	
3. PARITY	1–3	4–7	0	8+	
4 OBSTETRICAL HX	• Ps Pr	Ps Pr	Ps Pr	Ps Pr	
A. Toxemia	normotensive	mild	severe	eclamptic	
B Hemorrhage	usual blood loss	slightly increased blood loss	mod blood loss transfused 1 unit	severe blood loss transfused 2 + units.	
C Sepsis	none	PROM	transient fever or chills	persistent fever or chills	
D Labor	spontaneous	induced	precipitate	prolonged	
5 GYN/SURGICAL					
A Infertility	< 1 year	1-2 years	> 2-5 years	5 + years	
B Uterus/cervix	normal	malposition	incomp cervix	malformation	
– myoma	none	subserous	intramural	submucus	
– malignancy	paps I	paps II	suspicious	definite	
C Pelvis	normal	borderline	contracted	contracted	
D Operation	none	gen abdom	D & C Adnexal	CS/uterine	
6 MEDICAL/ENDOCRINE					
A. Systemic Illness	none	acute mild	acute serious	chr. debilitating	
B. Heart Disease	none	mild, class I	mod class II	severe, Class III-IV	
C Diabetes	none	family Hx	gestational	overt	
D STD	none	treated	untreated	at term	
7 NUTRITIONAL	90-150- lbs	151-180 lbs	70-89 lbs	<70 lbs/ > 180 lbs	
A Weight < non-preg total gain	20-30 lbs.	15-19 lbs	10-14 lbs.	<10 lbs/ >30 lbs	
B Anemia/Gms Hgb.	none/12.0	mild/10.1-11 9	mod/9-10	severe / <9	
C Smoking	non-smoker	<2 packs/day	2-5 packs/day	<5 packs/day	
D Alcohol/Drugs	negative	<2 years	2-5 years	<5 years	
8 FETAL FACTOR				stillbirth/	
A. Fetal wastage	none	abortion 1-2x	abortion 3 x +	neonatal death	
B Development	normal	malformation	large baby >9 lbs	preterm/post term multiple preg	
C. Delivery	all spont.	elective forcep	indic forcep/CS	breech Extr./dfc. forcep	
9 SOCIOECONOMIC	High Income	High-Middle	Low-Middle	Low Income	
A Land owned	Large farm	medium farm	small farm <2 ha.	farmtenant/worker	
B Business	Big businessman	aver. businessman	small proprietor store clerk	ambulant vendor household servant	
C Profession	Top professional	aver. professional	skilled laborer office worker/teacher	unskilled laborer	
D Govt service	High govt official	Minor govt official	govt. clerk	unemployed/handicapped	
10.PSYCHOLOGICAL		once	twice	3 x +	
A Nervous break/ number duration	none	<1 wk	1-2 wks	> 2 wks	
B Attitude to baby	wanted	accepted	tolerated	unwanted	
C Pregnancy fantasies	none	pleasant	unpleasant	terrifying	
D. Intellectual function	competent	low normal	mod retarded	incompetent	
E. Emotional tone	calm/confident	excited/dependent	sad/complaining	fearful/irritable	
F Support/husband	dependable	erratic	indifferent	absent	
G. Somatic S/S	good sleep/appetite	occas nauses/pica	occas vomiting perst. anorexia	perst. vomiting/insomnia	

*Ps = past history
Pr = present

EVALUATED BY: _____   TOTAL SCORE _____

Designation: _____   Risk Assessment: Low ☐ Moderate ☐ High ☐

Recommendation: routine ☐ special ☐ Intensive ☐

Figure 1.   Antepartum risk score sheet.

Appendix B

RISK FACTOR	LEVEL OF RISK				SCORE POINTS
	0	1	2	3	
A. MATERNAL					
1. Toxemia	normotensive	mild	severe	eclamptic	
2. Hemorrhage	usual blood loss < 250 cc.	sL. increased blood loss 200-500 cc.	− moderate blood loss − tachycardia	− excessive blood loss > 1000 cc. − transfusion	
3. Infection a. Membranes b. Temperature	intact normal	PROM 6-12 hrs. 37.5−37.9°C	PROM > 12 hrs. 38−39.9°C	amnionitis 40.0 + °C	
4. Course of Labor	normal 4−10 hrs.	− prolonged latent stage − dysfunctional Labor	− precipitous labor, < 3 hrs. − prolonged 2nd stage	Prolonged 18 + hrs.	
5. Intervention	none N S D	− elective induction − oxytocin augmentation − elective forceps − Spont. breech	− indicated Induction − elective CS. − indic. forceps − partial breech − man. removal of placenta	− CS hysterectomy − Emergency CS − difficult forceps − total breech extraction	
6. Anesthesia	none/ psychological	local infiltration pudendal block	saddle block spinal	general epidural	
B. PLACENTAL 7. Placenta	normal	− low implant. − marginal separation	− partial previa − abruption < 50%	− total previa − abruption > 50%	
8. Amniotic fluid	clear watery	cloudy thick	light meconium stained	dark meconium stained	
C. FETAL 9. Maturity a. Weight b. AOG	> 2,500 Gms. 38−40 wks.	2000-2500 Gms. 36−37 wks. 41−42 wks.	1,500-1,999 Gms. 32−35 wks. > 42 wks.	< 1,500 Gms. < 32 wks.	
10. Fetal welfare a. Heart rate in utero	normal 140-160/min	− transient tachycardia > 180/mm − transient bradycardia < 100/min	− tachycardia < 30 min. − bradycardia < 30 min	− tachycardia > 30 min. − bradycardia > 30 min.	

EVALUATED BY:

_____

TOTAL SCORE: _____

INTERPRETATION: ☐ Low Risk   ☐ Medium Risk   ☐ High Risk
RECOMMENDATION.   MOTHER   ☐ routine   ☐ special care
                  NEWBORN   ☐ routine   ☐ special care

Figure 2.   Intrapartum risk score sheet.

Appendix C

(Immediate - 1st 24 Hrs)

RISK FACTOR	LEVEL OF RISK				SCORE POINTS
	0	1	2	3	
1 BIRTH CONDITION					
a APGAR SCORE 5m	8 - 10	6 - 7	3 - 5	<3	
b Resuscitation	none/brief O_2 inhalation	prolonged O_2 inhalation	O_2 thru IPPB/ or ambu bag	Endotracheal intubation	
c Skin-Color	normal	mottled	pale	cyanotic	
-Jaundice	none	face	face, chest, abd.	generalized	
d Temperature		37.6-38.0	38.1-38.5	>38.5	
^{o}C Rectal	36.5-37.5	36.1-36.4	35 5-36 0	<35.5	
2. MATURITY AOG	38-40 wks.	36-37/41-42 wks.	32-35/$>$42 wks.	<32 wks	
. Weight, Gms	$>2500/<4500$	2000-2500	1500-1999	$<1500/>4500$	
3 ACTIVITY Motor	normal	weak tone/↑ active	Limp/hyperactive	flaccid/restless	
. cry	strong sustained	strong unsust./ weak sustained	weak unsustained	none	
4 RESPIRATION	normal	transient tachypnea	prolonged tachypnea	prolonged tachypnea w/persist cyanosis	
a Rate/min.	40-60	>60 1st 24 Hrs.	w/occ. cyanosis		
b Rhythm	regular	cyclic apnea	intermittent apnea w/occ. cyanosis	prolonged apnea w/cyanosis	
c Retractions	none	slight	moderate	severe	
5. CARDIAC· Rate/m.	140-160	161-180/110-119	181-200/100-109	$>200/<100$	
Murmur	none	present w/cyanosis	pres. w/occ cyanosis	pres. w/ persist cyanosis	
6 CNS: sensorium	normal	somnolent	Lethargic/ Irritable	stuporous/ comatose	
7. GIT STATUS . Feeding	1-1½ oz/5-15 m. every 3 Hrs	½-1 oz/$>$ 15m. every 3 Hrs.	½-1 oz/$>$15m. w/occ. regrgtn	½-1 oz/ $>$15m w/ frg regrgtn/abd. distn.	
8. HEMATOLOGIC a. Color/Gm. Hgb	pinkish/16-20	mild pallor/14-15 sl. flush/20-22	mod pallor/12-13 mod flush/22.1-24	severe pallor/<12 severe flush/>24	
b. Bleeding disorder	none	mild	moderate	severe	
9 METABOLIC STATUS a. clinical signs	none	tremors	convlsn/cyanosis <15 sec.	convlsn/cyanosis >15 sec.	
b. Laboratory - Bld glucose mg%	61-80	50-60	30-49	<30	
- Bld calcium mg%	9-11	8-8.9	7-7.9	<7	
10. GENETIC FACTOR a. multiple birth	single	twin	triplet	>3	
b congenital anomaly	none	external only	internal also/ vital organs free	vital organs involved	

EVALUATED BY _____   TOTAL SCORE _____

Designation _____

Risk Assessment   Low ☐ Moderate ☐ High ☐

Recommendation. routine ☐ special ☐ intensive ☐
       other_____

Figure 3. Neonatal risk score sheet.

Appendix D

EVALUATION FACTOR	LEVEL OF COMPLICATION				SCORE POINTS
	0	1	2	3	
DURATION OF CONFINEMENT (no. of days)	1 – 4	5 – 7	8 – 14	15+	
AMBULATION STARTED (days postpartum)	1 – 2	3 – 4	5 – 6	7+	
PEAK TEMPERATURE ≥ 38.0° C (no. of days)	none	1	2	3	
PEAK PULSE RATE ≥ 100/min (no. of days)	none	1	2	3+	
PEAK RESP. RATE ≥ 100/min. (no. of days)	none	1	2	3+	
URINATION	normal voiding	Frequency and/or dysuria	Catheterized	hematuria oliguria	
FLATUS/BM (day postpartum)	1st 2nd	3rd	4th	5th +	
ANEMIA/Gm. Hgb	none/12+	MILD / 10.1-11.9	Moderate 9–10	transfused or in shock < 9	
No. of DRUGS	none	1–2	3–4	5+	
OVERALL RESPONSE to CHILDBIRTH	satisfied	neutral/ tolerated	dissatisfied	regretful/ maladjusted	

EVALUATED BY: TOTAL SCORE: _____

_____

INTERPRETATION: ☐ low risk   ☐ Medium Risk   ☐ High Risk

RECOMMENDATION: ☐ routine care   ☐ special care

☐ other; specify_____

Figure 4.   Postpartum evaluation score sheet.

Appendix E

EVALUATION FACTOR	LEVEL OF COMPLICATION				SCORE POINTS
	0	1	2	3	
1 DURATION OF CONFINEMENT (no of days)	1 - 3	4 - 7	8 - 14	15+	
2 TEMPERATURE >37 5°C/<36.5°C (rectal-no. of days)	none	1 - 2	3 - 4	5+	
3. CARDIAC RATE >160/m or <120/m (no of days)	none	1 - 2	3 - 4	5+	
4. RESPIRATION RATE >60/m (no. of days)	none	1 - 2	3 - 4	5+	
5 WEIGHT LOSS % Birth Weight Day 3	3 - 5 %	6 - 7 %	8 - 10 %	> 10%	
6. G.I. TRACT a. feeding, Day 3	1-2 oz/5-15 m. every 3 hrs.	1/2 - 1 oz/5—15m every 3 hrs.	1/2 - 1 oz. fract.. feeding	<1/2 oz w/rgrgtn. or abd. dstn.	
b. meconium passage	normal amt <24 hrs	minimal amt < 24 hrs.	none < 24-48 hrs .	none < 48 hrs	
7. SKIN a. Color/Gms Hgb.	pinkish/16-20	Sl.⁴ flush/20-22 mild pallor/14-15	mod. flush/22 1-24 mod. pallor/12-13	Severe flush/>24 Severe pallor/<12	
b. Jaundice/ Bilirubin mg% (peak level)	none to mild (face, chest, abd)	Generalized slight	Generalized moderate	Generalized intense	
	Full Term 0 5-10 Pre Term 0.5-12	FT 10.1-12 0 PT 12 1-15	FT 12.1-15 PT 15.1-18	FT>15 PT>18	
8. ACTIVITY Day 3	normal	Sl. Sl.' increased/ weak tonus	hyperactive / limp	restless/ flaccid	
9. SENSORIUM Day 3	normal	somnolent	Lethargic/ irritable	stuporous/ comatose	
10. ACCEPTABILITY of CHILD	welcome	wanted but unprepared	unexpected/ indifferent	unwanted	

TOTAL SCORE

EVALUATED BY _____

Designation: _____

Complication Level Low ☐ Moderate ☐ High ☐
Recommendation . Further Care ☐ Discharge ☐
Routine ☐ Special ☐ Intensive ☐
Other _____

Figure 5. Discharge evaluation score sheet.

TEN TO FIFTEEN YEAR FOLLOW-UP OF CASES OF NEONATAL HYPERBILIRUBINEMIA TREATED WITH EXCHANGE TRANSFUSION

A. Genuino and E. N. Oteyza

Department of Pediatrics, University of the
Philippines College of   Medicine -
Philippine General Hospital
Manila, Philippines

INTRODUCTION

Hyperbilirubinemia remains as one of the most common problems in any neonatal unit. Its causal relationship with kernicterus and subsequent death has been well established. For those who survive kernicterus, the most commonly reported sequelae are choreoathetosis, asymetrical spasticity, sensorineural hearing impairment and mental and/or motor retardation.

There is a spectrum of tissue damage resulting from bilirubin toxicity and this may range from fatal kernicterus to subtle developmental and neurological abnormalities. The spectrum is so broad that toxicity of bilirubin to the brain, particularly the basal ganglia, hippocampus and cranial nerve nuclei, might not be detectable until later life. This is the reason why children who have survived kernicterus through exchange transfusion and phototherapy have been followed up for months or even up to five years.

The purpose of this study is to find out the long term effects of neonatal hyperbilirubinemia treated with exchange transfusion on the child's neurologic, psychologic, motor and psychiatric development. We have to stress at this point however, that there were significant number of babies who died within this study period because of severe jaundice and who did not undergo any exchange transfusion. It is a known fact that indirect hyperbili-

Table 1.   Profile of Children in the Study.

Variables	Number = 13 Exchange Transfusion	Number = 7 No Exchange Transfusion	Significance	
Mean age (years)	10	9.28	none	
Sex	3 males	2 males		
	10 females	5 females		
Age of gestation:				
Term	12	6	none	
Preterm	1	1		
Mean Birth Weight	6.4 lbs.	5.8 lbs.	none	
Mean age of mothers				
at delivery	31.3	31.8	none	
Condition at Birth:				
APGAR 10	11	4	none	
9	1	2		
8	1	1		
Mean: highest indi-				
rect bilirubin	24.4	17.1	.05	.1
Manner of delivery:				
vaginal	4	2	none	
forceps	5	2		
cesarian section	4	2		
breech	0	1		
Cause of jaundice:				
ABO	11	4	none	
EPJ	1	2		
Prematurity	1	1		

rubinemia if uncontrolled will lead to kernicterus and subsequent death. The focus of this research is not to prove that indirect hyperbilirubinemia causes brain damage because this has already been proven but to determine the long term effects of varying degrees of hyperbilirubinemia on the brains of children who survived and the role of exchange transfusion in altering the course of these long term effects.

MATERIALS AND METHOD

     The hospital records of two private medical centers in Manila, from 1963 to 1973, were reviewed and all babies born during this period with non-physiologic jaundice were listed. Those whom we were able to trace to their residences were notified and asked to come for examination.

Only 20 of those notified came for examination. Table 1 shows the profile of children with hyperbilirubinemia who were followed up for this study. Thirteen underwent at least one exchange transfusion and seven did not. The matched variables listed are those which can affect the bilirubin levels such as age of gestation (AOG), birth weight, condition at birth, manner of delivery, cause of the jaundice and maternal age at birth. The mean age of the children at the time this research was initiated was matched because it could also affect the IQ results. The T-test for significance was applied on each of the matched variables. It was found that there were no significant differences, meaning that the exchanged and the non-exchanged population groups are comparable for the purposes of this research. The only significant differ-ence between the exchanged and non-exchanged groups are the means of the highest bilirubin values attained during infancy. This suggests that the exchanged population represents the group of neonates subjected to higher bilirubin levels after birth. The non-exchanged group represents the children whose jaundice was not as severe such that exchange transfusion was not indicated at that time.

After a thorough physical examination and interview by a pediatrician, the children underwent a battery of psychological tests which included the Wechsler Intelli-gence Scale for Children - Revised (WISC-R), the Bender-Gestalt Visual Motor Test (BGVM) and the Draw-a-Person Test (DAP).

The WISC-R provides a measure of the general intel-ligence of a child in relation to his age group. It consists of 12 tests, 6 on verbal scale and 6 on perfor-mance scale. To determine the classification of an IQ obtained in the WISC-R, the following intelligence classification is presented:

Intelligence Quotient	Classification
130 and above	Very superior
120 - 129	Superior
110 - 119	High average (bright)
90 - 109	Average
80 - 89	Low average (dull)
70 - 79	Borderline
69 and below	Mentally deficient

The Draw-a-Person test was administered as an added measure of the intellectual status of these children, some

Table 2. Mean IQ Scores

IQ Scale	Exchanged	Non-Exchanged	Significance
VIQ	93	85	None
PIQ	107	101	None
FIQ	100	92	.05 (p) 0.1

Table 3. Mean DAP and BGVM Scores

	Exchanged	Non-Exchanged	Significance
DAP	11.3	11.4	None
BGVM	3	3	None

of whom may be discriminated against by the more culture-bound verbal tests. It may be used to get an initial impression of a young child's general ability and as an index of mental development of children for whom no standardized tests are available. The child's drawing reflects his concepts which mature with his mental level, experience and knowledge. A high DAP score is determined by the richness of details in the human figure drawings.

The BGVM was administered to assess the children's perceptual-motor functioning and culture. A high BGVM score means more errors in the reproduction of Gestalt figures printed in 9 standard sized cards, and indicates organicity.

The children also underwent psychiatric evaluation and the parents were asked to fill out a questionaire on behavior and neuorotic traits and asks the responder to select one of the 5 responses: No, or rarely; No, used to but not anymore; Yes, a little bit; Yes, a fair amount; Yes, very much. The questionnaire was scored by assigning a value of zero to the "Rarely" response and a two to the "Yes, very much" response. Values of 0.5, 1 and 1.5 were assigned to the in-between items.

An ear, nose and throat consultant did a thorough examination of the ears and performed an audiometry to detect any hearing loss and discriminate between conductive and sensory neural hearing loss, the latter of which is usually found in children who had high bilirubin levels in

Table 4. FIQ and Mean BGVM Scores

	Exchanged	Non-Exchanged
FIQ Range	78-125	69-108
Mean BGVM	0-8	0-13
Significance	None	None

Table 5. Scoring in the PIQ Subjects

	Mean Scores		
	Exchanged	Non-Exchanged	Significance
Picture Completion	10.1	9.7	None
Picture Arrangement	11.8	10.7	None
Block Design	11.6	9.7	None
Object Assembly	11	10.4	None
Coding	11.2	10.1	None
Mazes	8.5	8	None

Table 6. PQ Scores & Mean IQ Scores (Combined Population)

	Lower PQ (.047-.362)	Higher PQ (.38-.676)	Correlation
VIQ	97	81.3	.005
PIQ	111.9	97.2	.005
FIQ	104.2	89	.005

infancy. A neurologist performed a complete neurologic
examination and interpreted the EEG findings. An ophthal-
mologist conducted a thorough examination of the eyes to
determine visual impairments. A statistician was consult-
ed in the analysis of the results using tests of
significance.

RESULTS

     Table 2 shows the mean IQ scores of the exchanged
and non-exchanged groups. The mean IQ (FIQ) of the exchanged group is significantly higher than the mean IQ of
the non-exchanged group. This suggests that the mentation
of children subjected to high bilirubin levels are not so

Table 7. PQ Scores and Mean IQ Scores

	Exchanged		Non-Exchanged	
	Lower PQ	Higher PQ	Lower PQ	Higher PQ
VIQ	98.8	82	92.6	80
PIQ	113	99	109	94
FIQ	106.7	91	100	85.8

Table 8. Highest Peterson-Quay Traits

	Exchanged	Non-Exchanged
Skin allergy	8	
Self consciousness	9	8
Shyness, bashfulness	9	
Prefers play and younger children	8.5	
Temper tantrums	9.5	
Feelings easily hurt	9	7
Anxiety, fearfulness	8	
Irritable, hot-tempered	9	
Stomach aches	8.5	
Specific fears	9.5	
Difficulty with arithmetic	9.5	
Cries over minor annoyance		7.51

much affected as long as prompt management is instituted. Although the mean IQ of the verbal (VIQ) and performance (PIQ) of the exchanged group are higher than the non-exchanged group, the differences were found to be not significant statistically. Probably some children scored higher in the verbal or performance scale and lower in the other.

The performance IQ is a better gauge of organic brain damage than the verbal IQ because the latter is more affected by the child's cultural background level of education and environment. In Table 2, it is therefore the PIQ which should indicate more the presence of damage to the brain by high bilirubin levels.

Table 3 shows the mean Draw-a-Person and Bender-Gestalt Visual Motor scores among the exchanged and non-exchaged groups. Normal children should score lower in the BGVM test and higher in the DAP test. There is no statistical difference between the scores of the exchanged

Table 9. Typical Peterson-Quay Traits
in Minimal Brain Damage

Hyperactivity
Short attention span
Distractibility
Overreaction to emotional stimuli
Impulsiveness
Inconsistency/unpredictability
Difficulty getting through or reaching
Muscular incoordination
Speech defects
Lack appropriate fear
Lack learning from experience
Lack response to punishment
Perceptual deficits
Temper tantrums

Source: Gross & Wilson (1974): Minimal Brain Dysfunction

Table 10. BGVM and PQ Scores (Exchanged Population)

BGVM	PQ	Significance
0 - 2	0.301	
4 - 8	0.314	None

and non-exchanged groups. These indicate that there are probably no evidences of organic brain damage in both population groups.

Table 4 is meant to show correlation between the mean IQ (FIQ) and the BGVM scores in such a way that if a child has a high FIQ, the BGVM score should be low (less error). By using the coefficient of correlation (r), the result was negative. Children in either the exchanged or non- exchanged groups with higher IQ did not necessarily make less errors in the BGVM, and vice versa. This suggests that the lower mean IQ score in the non-exchanged group is not due to an organic brain problem but to some other factors like schooling and environmental stimulation.

Since there was no significant difference between the mean PIQ scores of the exchanged and non-exchanged groups, the performance IQ is a better gauge of previous

organic brain damage than the verbal or full scale IQ. We
looked into each subtest of the PIQ to find out if any of
the population groups scored higher in a particular
subtest. As seen in Table 5, the mean scores were almost
similar and we found no significant differences. All of
the subjects scored almost the same in all subtests.

The mean Peterson-Quay (PQ) scores which are suppose
to indicate any behavioral disturbances in any of
our population groups were also tabulated. Children with
behavioral problems usually have higher PQ scores. The
mean PQ scores of 0.3146 for the exchanged group and
0.3721 for the non-exchanged group were not found to be
significantly different.

Table 6 attempts to determine if those children with
higher IQ scored lower in the PQ questionnaire, not discriminating whether a child was exchanged or not. The PQ
scores were arranged from highest to lowest and the mean
IQ scores were taken for the higher PQ group and the lower
PQ group. We found that children with higher IQ scored
lower in the PQ questionnaire. This was significant at
alpha .005.

Table 7 differentiates between the exchanged and
non-exchanged groups. The exchanged group had higher mean
IQ scores regardless of whether the PQ score was high or
low. However, when these figures were statistically
tested, we found no significant difference. This probably
means that having higher biliburin values at birth or
undergoing an exchange transfusion does not determine
subsequent performance in the IQ scoring. The two preceding tables suggests that those children with lower IQ
are more vulnerable and can cope less, therefore
manifesting more behavioral problems.

Table 8 gives an enumeration of the most frequently
observed behaviors among children who scored high in the
PQ questionnaire and compared these with a table prepared
by Gross and Wilson (Table 9) on the typical PQ trait in
minimal brain-damaged children. It seems that the brain-
damaged traits were not found in any of our population
groups except for temper tantrums which we occasionally
observe in any normal child. We also tried to find out if
those children who committed errors in the BGVM test
(higher BGVM scores) had more behavioral problems resulting in higher PQ scores. As seen in Table 10, we found no
significant differences. This reinforces the fact that
none of the children in any of the population groups had
evidences of brain damage.

Table 11. Results of Audiometry Testing.

	Exchanged	Non-Exchanged	Total
w SHNL	5	4	9
w/o SNHL	3	1	4
Total	8	5	13

Table 12. Audiometry and Mean IQ Scores of Children with Sensory Neural Hearing Loss and of Children With Normal Audiograms.

	VIQ	PIQ	FIQ
SNHL	86.9	99.8	92
Normal	104	120	113
Significance	.01 .025	.005	.005

Table 13. Audiometry and Mean IQ Scores of Exchange and Non-Exchanged Populations.

	SNHL			Normal	
	Non-Exch.	Exchanged	Significance	Non-Exch	Exchanged
VIQ	81.8	91	None	96	107.3
PIQ	98	101.2	None	121	119.7
FIQ	88.5	95.8	None	108	114.7

Seventeen of our study population of 20 were examined by an audiologist to test for sensory neural hearing loss which is a common accompaniment of indirect hyperbilirubinemia. Three from both groups were not tested. Four in the exchanged group showed findings consistent with conductive hearing loss and was evaluated by the audiologist as probably due to upper respiratory tract infection. Five children in the exchange group (Table 11) and four of the non-exchanged group had sensory neural hearing loss (SNHL) but mostly at high frequency levels of 6000 Hz, which is not used in our normal listening range. These findings are very similar to the report of Koaster et al who found high frequency SNHL in his follow-up of

jaundiced babies. The frequency of SNHL in the exchanged
group which also represents the group with higher indirect
bilirubin values, is not significantly different from the
frequency of SNHL in the non-exchanged group. The Z-test
between two proportions was used.

The IQ scores of those children with SNHL were compared with those with normal audiograms. As seen in Table
12, the mean IQ scores of children without SNHL were
higher than those who had SNHL. When these were separated
into an exchanged and non-exchanged population groups
(Table 13), the mean IQ scores of the children without
SNHL were still higher than those with SNHL. Although the
mean scores of the exchanged population were still higher
than the non-exchanged population in children with or
without SNHL, these probably were found to be insignificant statistically. This means that the factor of being
exchanged or not or having higher or lower bilirubin
values does not alter the subsequent IQ of children who
survive an episode of hyperbilirubinemia without frank
evidences of organic brain damage. The two preceding
tables suggest that although the hearing losses were at
the high frequency levels not usually used in a normal
listening range, these may affect the child's performance
later on.

The ophthalmologic examinations of the children did
not reveal any abnormalities with visual perception nor
strabismus. These visual problems were reported by Human
et al in their four-year follow-up of babies with hyperbilirubinemia. The neurologic examination and EEG
tracings showed no abnormalities.

CONCLUSION

This study reinforces the fact that prompt management of hyperbilirubinemia from whatever cause can still
result in well-adapted children with even high IQ.
Children who undergo an exchange transfusion for severe
jaundice are not necessarily the same group who would
perform poorly later in life. As pointed out by Odell et
al, the maximum bilirubin concentration does not reflect
the subsequent occurrence of brain damage. A better gauge
probably would be the maturation of the serum proteins
with bilirubin during infancy.

Our other long-term parameters of organic brain
damage such as BGVM and DAP test, PQ scoring, EEG, audiometry and ophthalmologic examinations failed to

demonstrate any harmful effects of hyperbilirubinemia in both our exchanged and non-exchanged population groups. This does not suggest however that there was not an even slight damage previously. This could have happened, but with education and environmental stimulation, these children from a relatively upper socio-economic status could have overcome their handicaps and turned out to have an even higher IQ in our present examination. It was also demonstrated that SNHL, although in the high frequency level, may still affect the performance of seemingly normal children.

This study does not imply that the severity of jaundice does not matter in the subsequent performance of children who survive; nor that an exchange transfusion does not alter in any way the infant's subsequent development. On the contrary, exchange transfusions are a major reason for the increased survival of severely jaundiced babies. This paper suggests that the bilirubin concentration is not an absolute gauge in determining the severity of jaundice. We have to use better parameters like the protein saturation by bilirubin. This paper also suggests that children with a history of severe jaundice who turn out well should still be evaluated on a long-term basis for the finer aspects of brain damage such as sensory neural hearing loss of the high frequency type, slight behavioral disturbances and poorer performance in IQ testing. Lastly, it is also suggested that slight developemntal lags due to severe jaundice in infancy may be overcome years later by proper education and environmental stimulation.

REFERENCES

Odell BB et al (1970): Studies in kernicterus. The saturation of serum proteins with bilirubin during neonatal life and its relationship to brain damage at five years. J Pediat, 76:12.

Valaes T, Hyte M (1977): Effect of exchange transfusion of bilirubin binding. Pediatrics, 59:881.

Upadhyay Y (1971): A longtitudinal study of full-term neonates with hyperbilirubinemia to four years of age. Johns Hopkins Med J, 128:273.

Hardy JB, Peeples MO (1977): Serum bilirubin levels in newborn infants. Distributions and associations with neurological abnormalities during the first year of life. Johns Hopkins Med J, 128:265.

Genuino AS (1968): Preliminary follow-up of 25 cases of hyperbilirubinemia in the newborn treated by

exchange transfusion for the past four years.
Phil J Pediat, 17:176.

Weiner B (1970): The relationship of birth weight and
length of gestation to intellectual development at
age 8 to 10 years. J Pediat, 76:694.

Hyman S et al (1969): CNS abnormalities after
neonatal hemolytic disease or hyperbilirubinemia.
A prospective study of 405 cases. Am J Dis
Child, 117:406.

Keaster N et al (1969): Hearing problems subsequent
to neonatal hemolytic disease or hyperbilirubinemia. Am J Dis Child, 117:406.

Gross MB, Wilson WC (1974): Minimal brain dysfunction. A clinical study of incidence, diagnosis
and treatment in over 1000 children. Brunner/Mazel,
New York.

Oski FA, Stockman JA (1981): Yearbook of
Pediatrics. Year Book Medical Publishers,
Chicago.

Koppitz EM (1964): The Binder-Gestalt test for young
children. Grune ·and Stratton, New York.

Harris DB (1963): Children's drawings as measures of
intellectual maturity. A revision and extension
of the Gooerough Draw-A-Man test. Hardcourt, Brace
and World, New York.

Glasser AJ, Zimmerman IL (1967): Clinical interpretation of Wechsler Intelligence Scale for children
(WISC). Grune and Stratton, New York.

PRESENT PERSPECTIVE OF MATERNAL AND NEONATAL HEALTH IN PAKISTAN AND AN APPROACH TO THE PROBLEM THROUGH PRIMARY HEALTH CARE

A. K. Awan

Chairman, Maternal and Child Welfare
Association of Pakistan
Lahore, Pakistan

INTRODUCTION

Pakistan, a land of 84 million people, like most other developing countries, exhibits poverty-culture, and has a poor health status (1, 2, 3, [Table 1]).

EVOLUTION OF HEALTH SYSTEM IN PAKISTAN

Heavy mortality of troops in India led to the appointment of a "Sanitary Commissioner" in 1869 (4). The British administrators concerned themselves, not with a health policy for the people as a whole, but only with health services for their countrymen. The exceptions were the fortunate individuals admitted into their ruling heirarchy who were allowed to benefit from official medical services. A few private citizens were also permitted to use these facilities, either as charity or on payment.

In Pakistan our health policy has basically remained the same. It is mainly the state employees that get medical care as a matter of right, while ordinary citizens get it only as a matter of grace (5).

Because of high maternal and child mortality, the Lady Chelmsford All-India League for Maternity and Child Welfare (a voluntary organization) was established in 1920 (6). It helped to develop institutions for training maternity supervisors.

Table 1.   Health Status as Depicted by Some
            Basic Indicators.

No.	Type of Indicator	Measurements	Year Recorded or Estimated
1	Crude birth rate	42.6 per 1000	1979
2	Crude death rate	13.0 per 1000	1979
3	Infant mortality rate	105 per 1000	1978
4	Population served with potable water supply	26.9%	1978
5	Population served with sewerage system	9.7%	1978

Source: Statistical Profile of Children in Pakistan (1).

In 1961, the Maternity and Child Welfare Association
of Pakistan was established (7). This voluntary organization succeeded in influencing governmental policy related
to maternal and child health (8). Thus, the evolution of
maternal and child health (MCH) services has been through
voluntary efforts initially. The governmental support
came later.

Maternal and Neonatal Health

Life-expectancy of females, at birth, is not only
markedly lower as compared to developed countries, but
also lower than that of males within Pakistan (9). Age
specific mortality rates are higher in females during the
age-period 15 to 39 years, as compared to males, and this
situation has remained unchanged during the last 45 years
(10, 11).

A committee, constituted in 1938, came to the conclusion that maternal mortality rate in the Indo-Pakistan
sub-continent was 20 per 1000 live births as compared with
4.9 (per 1000 live births) in England and Wales (12). In
1960, maternal mortality rate was estimated to be 15 to 20
(per 1000 live births) in Pakistan (13). At present, the
rate is 6 to 8 (per 1000 live births (14). By comparison,
in 1975, the rate in the U.S.A. was only 0.13 (15). High
maternal mortality is accompanied by excessive morbidity.
The annual number of deaths among women in Pakistan associated with pregnancy and child bearing, was 200,000,

Table 2.   Spontaneous Pregnancy Wastage Rates Calculated
           by Life Table Method, Saddar Pregnancy Study,
           Lahore, 1963-1965.

No.	Type of Pregnancy Wastage Rate	Rate/1000 Fetuses At Risk
1	Total pregnancy wastage rate	200.81
2	Total fetal loss rate	176.21
3	Late fetal loss rate	32.08
4	Early neonatal loss rate	29.86
5	Perinatal loss rate	60.98

Source: Awan (18), 1974.

while the number of women who have to undergo varying degrees of disability and suffering from the same causes
every year was likely to be about 4 million (16).

Our extensive population control program has as yet
produced little impact on the rate of population growth,
which has remained 3 per cent per annum during the last
two decades (17).

Pregnancy wastage rates are high as shown in Table 2
and perinatal loss rate is 4 times higher than in the
U.S.A. or Singapore(19).

Type of Health System

There exist in the world today three basic systems of
medical care: public assistance, health insurance, and
national health service. These in turn are associated
with and correspond to three basic economic systems extant
in the world today: precapitalist, capitalist, and
socialist" (20).

The public assistance system is dominant in 108 countries, having 1962 million people, or 49 percent of the
world's population. These countries mainly have agricultural economies and feudal or semi-feudal land- holding
systems; and in them, whatever available medical care is
provided through a public assistance system primarily for
the poor. Pakistan belongs to this category. President
General Mohammad Zia-ul-Haq said it was his earnest desire
that medical assistance be provided to all those who were
sick, particularly the poor (21).

The system and its facilities have limited coverage,

are underfinanced, overcrowded, and have insufficient
personnel. The quality of service that is offered does
not compare favorably with what is generally available in
developed countries. There is little involvement or
participation of people in the formulating policy or
enactment of decisions. The culture of poverty suppresses
desire for participation of expression of needs due to
fatalism, low self-esteem, ignorance or past experiences,
and acceptance of one's lot in life as immutable. Modern
allopathic health services seem remote in place, time and
cost, and hence unavailable. Whatever is available may be
cherished as charity or a blessing, and however inadequate, is considered as a lucky chance at magical cure.
One's health is part of one's fate determined by God, and
so not to be questioned by any mortal, as God is surely
not accountable.

It is difficult to visualize how most of the
countries with a public assistance system can develop
either toward national health service or national health
insurance under the prevailing socio-economic and
political situation (22).

Conceptual Basis of Our Efforts

Political culture or orientation of the social system
has "input" and "output" functions. The "input functions"
are interest articulation, interest aggregation, political
socialization and communication (23). Interest articulation takes place through various groups and organizations,
and this in turn aggregates into demand for programs which
are expressed through manifestos by various political parties. The "input functions" of the system are possible
in cultures where individuals can freely express their
views, and form groups which can organize their activities
and articulate their demands. Once a group is in power, it
seeks to translate its program into public policy, and
then endeavours that the policy be implemented. The
implementation of the policy occurs through "output functions" which are carried out by the executive machinery.

In the Indo-Pakistan sub-continent during the four
hundred years of Mughal rule, the public policy was by
large, a consequence of the "output functions" of the
social system, and the welfare of people was the
responsibility of the crown.

During the succeeding 100 years of British rule, the
public policy was the benevolent act of the alien government, and the people by large expected that the government

would take measures on their behalf. Thus our people
remained attuned to the "output functions", and developed
a "subject political culture".

Pakistan at its inception, inherited a running tradition of a "subject political culture" of over 500 years
(24). Since the time of independence, events have been
such that political process has hardly created the climate
wherein the "input functions" of the political system
could occur. Consequently the "output functions" of the
state are conducted on the basis of assesments made by
bureaucrats and power groups.

Health Facilities in Pakistan

At the time of independence, health conditions in Pakistan were very unsatsfactory. Only about three million
people in towns had the luxury of protected water supply.
We have come a long way since 1947 (25) but are yet far
from our destination (26). For example, 16,800 MCH stations are needed, whereas we have only 858 such units
offering primary health care to mothers and children.

We have 15,500 registered doctors and dentists (1:
5400 persons), and 51,600 hospital beds (1:1628 persons).
A tiny network of social security services was developed
in 1965, but a major portion of the medical care services
is provided by private clinics, on a fee-for- service
basis. A small stratum of landowners, businessmen, officials, and professionals use specialists and private
hospitals for personal medical care.

Besides qualfied doctors, a large number of healers
of "indigenous system" practise medicine in Pakistan.
There are 43,000 hakims and ayurveds, and 13,000 homeo-
paths. Furthermore, a very large sector of the population, especially in rural areas, go to quacks, faith
healers and priests for medical care (27).

Health insurance is not in existence in Pakistan
except for those covered by the tiny network of social
security services. Our public sector expenditure on
health (including medical education) is 1 percent of the
GNP; semi-public sector spends 0.3 percent of the GNP,
and private sector financing is roughly estimated to be
1.8 percent of the GNP. The total expenditure of health
care (excluding environmental protection) is estimated to
be 400 million U.S.$ or 3 percent of the GNP (28).

In Pakistan, about 99 percent of deliveries take

place at home. In cities, better social-class women, or
those who have complications, may seek hospital admission.
Home confinements are generally attended by dais, i.e.,
TBA's. Mishaps are attributed to the "will of God", and
"bad fortune", and not to the dai.

Inspite of being undesirable, it is impossible to
banish dais, because they are what rural women and most of
urban mothers are able to get or afford. People pay a
small compensation for their services. It is estimated
that more than 25,000 to 30,000 indigenous dais are at
present practising in Pakistan. Almost all villages have
them. Only about 3000 of them have been formally trained.

The most economical and rewarding approach for improving maternal and neonatal health is through the
mother. Antenatal care should enable the attendant (even
when a dai) to put a mother in low or high risk category.
It is the high risk mother carrying a high risk fetus
whose health is in jeopardy who would be in need of
special arrangements for care from a better qualified
professional person.

The success of the dai's work and the quality of
maternal and neonatal care rendered by her depends on her
training and supportive supervision. She must have within
reach a referral individual or static MCH unit so that
when in doubt or dealing with a high risk case, she is
able to solicit consultation and help (31). This is the
basis which we are now developing in our MCH services as
an integral part of our health care program.

Motivated by the Alma Ata Conference, our experts
have proposed the provision of minimal acceptable health
facilities for all people by the year 2000 shown in Table
3 (32) through the agency of a national health service.

An expenditure of 7,630 million US dollars would be
needed for trying to convert our dreams into a realty.
Our present ambitions are laudable but are not easy to
fulfill in the light of our past achievements (33), economic constraints, multiple competing priorities, subject
political culture and lack of relevant political will
among those who make decisions.

SOCIAL MECHANISMS FOR ATTAINING OBJECTIVE

Primary health care requires a drastic reordering of
priorities and a change of attitudes at all levels of

Table 3. Health Facilities: Existing and Projected

Facility	Year 1980 (Existing)	Year 2000 (Projected)
Hospital beds	51,610	130,000
Doctors/dentists	15,500	65,000
Nurses	5,100	43,000
Population per doctor	5,334	2,000
Paramedics	35,000	100,000
Basic Health Units and Rural Health Centers	7,000	26,000
Community Health Workers	2,000	130,000

Source: S.H. Mahmood and M.F. Zaidi (16) 1981.

government and legislature, beginning at the very top.
Primary health care is in fact, a complete system. Even
if we succeed in selling primary health care concept to
the political elite or those who rule, the chances of success will lie on how strong that determination is. Wah
Wong (34) from the UNICEF remarked: "Will it be strong
enough to resist demands from other sectors who claim for
priority attention and funding? Will it withstand the
pressure to cut back first on social services, when bud-
getary reductions have to be made? Will it be recognized
that health programs are an investment for a stronger future? Will there be, in short, the political will to stay
with the program?" (34) Strong leadership and political
will are essential to achieve goals (35).

Primary health care is essential health care made universally accessible to all members of a community by means
acceptable to them, through their full participation and
effort, and at a cost that the community can afford (36).
But community self-reliance and participation in the determination of direction and goals are not feasible in
developing countries where political process is not functional. An excerpt from a report of a mission to study
needs assessment for population assistance (37) states
that "... people in their own development in Pakistan have
faced some fundamental problems in the structure of the
society, in the diverse characteristics of ... communities
throughout Pakistan, and in the economic and social
conditions of the people."

Mechanisms that are found suitable in alien political
system may not fit our political and economic situation.

The Third World are at different levels of social, technological and economic development. Our capability profile
has relationship with the level of our cultural evolution.
We have tried community health-care methods generated in
other cultures long enough without great success. We need
to develop our own strategy based on our own philosophies.

     After unsuccessful attempts at offering universal
coverage through successive national health service plans,
our planners have responded to realities. Attempts at
primary health care in Pakistan is likely to be in the
framework of a public assistance type of a health system,
with support from the private medical sector, social security agencies, limited compulsory health insurance (38),
efforts of voluntary and philanthrophic agencies, and
funds raised through "Zakat and Ushar" taxation. We will
have to rely on a composite approach, using all possible
mechanisms to improve health coverage through pooling of
resources. With government backing and support and with
integrated planning, coordination and good organization,
more resources will become available and better outputs
would result, increasingly meeting the deficiencies of a
public assistance type of health system. The Federal
Minister has urged the private sector to invest in the
development and expansion of medicare. He thinks that
"... large scale induction of the private sector will go a
long way in reducing the acute shortage of medical aid
facilities" (39). It is important that "... the
government should make a serious effort to increase its
spending on health so that a real expansion of health
facilities can take place" (40).

     Governor Jilani (41) announced a donation of five lac
rupees (US $50,000) and made an emotional and touching
appeal urging people to conceive and implement plans for
the treatment and rehabilitation of ill persons and thus
render service to the suffering humanity (41).

     "Zakat and Ushar" taxation, a charitable but reli-
giously ordained assessment and taxation on certain types
of wealth, is a new source which is being increasingly
mobilized for financing the health care of the poor,
indigent, widows and orphans (42).

CONCLUSION

     What is needed is the development of an integrated
health plan permitting maximum exploitation of every
mechanism and available resource for attaining primary

health care goals in developing countries. More than that, a substitute for the missing political will for successful policy formulation and implementation is needed. If the ruling group and lawmakers who influence decision making can be motivated, the missing input function of the political process in a subject culture may be substituted or short-circuited and the country may be considerably helped to develop in a direction for taking appropriate decisions. The World Health Organization, the International Association for Maternal and Neonatal Health and other international agencies, in collaboration with national voluntary health organizations, may possibly be mobilized so that, besides educating, inspiring and motivating professionals, these agencies may also perform similar functions for the concerned key persons who play important roles in the decision-making process. Carefully planned conferences, seminars or workshops involving vital leaders of the developed and developing world, and a few specially selected health professionals and social scientists, may be able to help develop determination or commitment essentially required for practising primary health care philosophy in the developing countries. The involvement of leaders of the developed countries will be beneficial because of the catalytic role which they are likely to play.

REFERENCES

1. Government of Pakistan (1980): Statistical Profile of Children of Pakistan, Islamabad. Planning and Development Division, Health, Demography and Social Welfare Section, Pakistan Basic Country Data.
2. Awan, AH (1978): Conceptual basis of planning for rural health. In: Proceedings of 14th National Health Conference, Planning Rural Health Services, Lahore. Public Health Association of Pakistan, p. 6.
3. Robinson WC (1967): Recent mortality trends in Pakistan, Part 1. In: Studies in the demography of Pakistan, Pakistan Institute of Development Economics, Karachi, p. 5.
4. Niaz-ud-Din (1960): In: A manual of hygiene and preventive medicine, Ripon Book Depot, Lahore, 413-419.
5. Report by the Health Study Group, Lahore (1970): Government of West Pakistan, Suptd. Govt. Printing Press, 1-2.

6.   Young R (1923): The health school, Delhi.
     Maternity and Child Welfare Journal, 211.
7.   Government of Pakistan (1960): Annual Report of
     the Director of General Health, 1966-67. Health
     Division, Biostatistics Section, Islamabad,
     181-182.
8.   Hasan CK (1980): "Presidential Address". Proceed-
     ings of the 21st National MCH Conference,
     Lahore, MCWAP.
9.   Ghosh BN (1966): In: A treatise on hygiene and
     public health , 15th Edition, Scientific
     Publishing Co., Calcutta, 703.
10. Awan AK (1979): Maternal and child health.
     Muzaffar Medical Publications, Lahore, 16.
11. Govt. of Pakistan (1980): Statistical Profile of
     Females in Pakistan. Planning and Development
     Division, Health and Social Welfare Section,
     Islamabad, 20.
12. Central Advisory Board of Health(1938): Report on
     maternity and child welfare work in India by
     Special Committee. Simla, Manager, Govt. of
     India Press, 25.
13. Niaz-ud-Din: op. cit., 346.
14. Planning Commission of Pakistan (1978): Health and
     health related statistics of Pakistan, 2nd
     edition, Islamabad.
15. Ministry of Health and Welfare (1979): Statistics
     relating to maternal and child health in Japan.
     Children and Families Bureau (Maternal and Child
     Health Division), Tokyo, 46.
16. Mahmood SH, Zaidi MT (1981): Health system. Past
     performance and present capability profile. In:
     Proceedings of the 15th National Health
     Conference, Lahore. Public Health Association
     of Pakistan.
17. Report (1979): Mission of needs assessment for
     population assistance: Pakistan. United Nations
     Fund for Population Activities, 115.
18. Awan AK (1974): Some biologic correlates of
     pregnancy wastage. Am J Obs Gyn, 119:527.
19. World Health Organization (1980): World health
     statistics. WHO, Geneva.
20. Terris M (1980): The three world systems of medical
     care, Trends and Prospects. World Health
     Forum, 1:78.
21. Pakistan Times: Poor must have medical aid - Zia.
     Pakistan Times 35:178.
22. Terris M: op. cit. 85.
23. Cabriel GA, Vergas (1963): The Civic Culture.
     Little, Brown & Co., Boston, p. 17.

24. Naseer S (1978): Our political heritage and public policy. Rural Health as a case study. In: Proceedings of the 14th National Health Conference, Planning Rural Health Service. Public Health Association of Pakistan, Lahore, 25-28.
25. Govt. of Pakistan (1977): Primary health care in Pakistan. Planning Commission, Health Section, 2-3.
26. Mahmood SH, Zaidi MF: op. cit.
27. Awan AH (1969): The system of local health services in rural Pakistan and planned administrative and technical support. Public Health Association of Pakistan, Lahore, 85.
28. Siraj-ul-Haw M (1978): In: International conference on primary health care, Alma Ata, USSR. Primary Health Care, Islamabad. Government of Pakistan, Planning Commission, 3.
29. Awan AK (1979): Maternity and child welfare. Muzaffar Medical Publications, Lahore, 31, 36.
30. Report: Mission on needs assessment for population assistance, Pakistan, op. cit, 49.
31. Ibid., 49-50.
32. Mahmood SH, Zaidi MF, op. cit.
33. Government of Pakistan (1976): Health services in Pakistan. Planning Commission, Health Section, Islamabad, 1-35.
34. Wong W (1979): Problems of children in Asia. In: Symposium on child welfare in commenration of the International Year of the Child. Ministry of Health, Tokyo, 11-21.
35. World Federation of Public Health Associations (1978): Conference Bulletin No. 4, 2.
36. Ibid, 3.
37. Report: Mission on needs assessment for population assistance. Pakistan, op. cit., 97.
38. Report: Health study group recommendations, op. cit., 60.
39. Dawn (1981): Health care for all, Editorial, Aug. 27, Column I.
40. Ibid, Column II.
41. Jilani (1981): Realize duty towards sick brethren. Pakistani Times, Lahore, 35:213.
42. Report: Mission on needs assessment for population assistance. op. cit. 100.

CAUSES OF MATERNAL DEATHS AND

STRATEGIES FOR THEIR PREVENTION

V. C. W. Wong

Senior Lecturer and Consultant
Department of Obstetrics and Gynaecology
University of Hong Kong, Hong Kong

INTRODUCTION

There has been no paucity of publications on maternal mortality from various parts of the world. Most of them showed definite improvement in the mortality rates since the Second World War. Over the past decade, the reported maternal mortality rate ranged from <10 to 600/100,000 maternities, depending on the standard of obstetric care in that locality(1). Many factors can affect the incidence either directly or indirectly. Before discussing the actual causes of maternal death, one must consider the pitfalls in data collection, and the limitations in comparison of figures as a result of the differences in the definitions of maternal deaths and their causes as presented in published reports.

DATA COLLECTION

The maternal mortality rate and the causes of such deaths in a particular country or locality depend on the accuracy of the data collected, which in turn depends on the method of collection of information.

Among published figures, some are derived from maternity services directly, some from family health service and some from the death registry. Deaths as a result of ectopic pregnancy or abortion may not be included in the statistics of a maternity service because these women may not have presented themselves to an

antenatal clinic yet, and if an abortion is performed
illegally the cause of death may not be linked to the
abortion, unless a proper necropsy is performed. If the
death register is used, maternal deaths associated with
other diseases may be missed because it is the main cause
of death that is entered; besides the fact that the deceased is pregnant may not have been recorded in the death
certificate. Therefore a more comprehensive approach is
needed in order to obtain information from all sources.

According to the Report on Confidential Enquiries
into Maternal Deaths in England and Wales, (2) a maternal
death is defined as "one occuring during pregnancy, or
during labour, or as a consequence of pregnancy within one
year of delivery or abortion." By taking the duration of
one year after delivery or abortion, one may include
deaths entirely unrelated to the pregnancies. The definition by the Internation Federation of Gynaecology and
Obstetrics (FIGO) is more practical, because it only
includes deaths within the first 42 days after delivery or
termination of pregnancy.

In some published reports on causes of maternal
deaths, data derived before the 28th week of pregnancy
were not included; therefore a large number of deaths
from abortion and ectopic pregnancy had been excluded with
possible distortion of the figures showing the prevalence
of the principal causes of death.

In order to facilitate future comparison of vital
statistics in relation to medical care, a standardization
of the definition of maternal mortality and the
classification of causes is needed.

CAUSES OF MATERNAL DEATHS

The main causes of maternal deaths are the same all
over the world, namely: hemorrhage, infection, complication of preeclampsia, and in some countries, pulmonary
embolism. Despite the availability of safe blood transfusion techniques and the widespread use of antibiotics,
most mothers still die of hemorrhage and/or infection.
Other less frequent causes include complications of
anesthesia, cardiac disease, renal disease, diabetes
mellitus, malignancies, amniotic fluid embolism, suicide,
etc.

"Hemorrhage" is a very broad term. It may include
bleeding as a result of abortion and ectopic pregnancy in

the first and second trimester. In the third trimester,
bleeding may occur antepartum or postpartum resulting from
placenta previa, accidental hemorrhage, disseminated in-
travascular coagulation, uterine atony, retained placenta
and genital tract trauma. In some analysis, bleeding
associated with special events such as rupture of the
uterus, or caesarean section are separately classified and
discussed.

On the other hand, there may be several factors
contributing to the death of a single individual, e.g.,
infection and hemorrhage can occur as a result of an
abortion, and the cause of death may be classified under
only one of the above three categories. That is why it is
difficult to compare data from different countries concerning the causes of maternal mortality, unless specific
definitions are adopted by all countries concerned.

CLASSIFICATION OF MATERNAL DEATHS

For the purpose of analysis and audit, causes of
maternal mortality have been classified as:

(a)   true and associated;
(b)   direct, indirect and unrelated; and
(c)   avoidable and unavoidable.

In the "Confidential Enquiries into Maternal Deaths
from England and Wales"(2), the deaths are classified
under a single main cause coded according to the International Classification of Diseases (3) of the World Health
Organization. Those that fall under the chapter "Complications of Pregnancy, Childbirth and the Puerperium" are
labelled as true maternal deaths; deaths with a main
cause coded elsewhere are called associated maternal
deaths.

Under this system of classification, ambiguity may
arise because the pregnant mother may die from an
associated disease, e.g., cardiac disease, but the
pregnancy may have aggravated the disease thus contributing directly or indirectly towards the death. Hence it is
more explicit if the causes are separated into the three
classes: direct, indirect, and unrelated.

Another approach is to review all the cases and to
determine whether the deaths were avoidable or not. By
the term "avoidable" is meant that the risk of death could
have been lowered if some part of the management did not

fall short of an accepted standard of practice. The term
may define deficiencies in the system, or errors from an
individual due to either ignorance or negligence, with a
view to induce changes to promote future improvements in
medical care.

After a review of published reports on avoidable
causes of maternal deaths, one may classify them under
three levels of failure of care:

(a)   failure of the mother;
(b)   failure of the medical staff; and
(c)   failure of the health administrator.

The mother may fail to consult regularly at the antenatal clinic to heed the doctor's advice for admission
into hospital for observation or treatment, or to seek
medical advice at the earliest suggestion of a problem.
In countries with high mortality rates, it is recognized
that "delay" is a very important killing factor.

The medical staff or traditional birth attendant may
fail to take advantage of services available, thus treatment is delayed if they cannot select the high risk
patients for hospital delivery before problems arise.
Complications must be detected early so that proper
management can be instituted in time, e.g. calling in a
flying squad or consulting a senior person (obstetrician).
The management can still be unsatisfactory if the consultant fails to respond and act promptly, or the therapy is
inappropriate or outdated.

On the other hand, the health administrators may have
failed to provide an effective flying squad service with
efficient transportation for patients and attendants to a
hospital adequately staffed and equipped to deal with such
emergencies.

PREVENTION STRATEGIES

Within the scope of primary health care, much can be
done to decrease maternal mortality from the three main
causes: hemorrhage, infection, and hypertensive diseases
in pregnancy. Strategies for their prevention can be
undertaken according to the three levels of care as stated
above.

Education of Mothers.

     Health education programs should be directed special-
ly towards the high-risk population, i.e., teenagers,
those with advancing age and parity, those of low social
class and those at risk of having illegitimate pregnancies. In order to reach these target groups, education
should be conducted in schools, youth groups, maternal and
child health clinics, community centers, social service
distribution centers, and social hygiene clinics.

     This type of program is difficult to organize in
countries that need them most. In many developing countries, because of cultural inhibitions, social attitude
and economic constraints, women are poorly educated and
ill-informed and do not appreciate the value of structured
education program such as antenatal classes.

     In a recent report from South Iran where the maternal
mortality rate is 250/100,000, none of the women had any
antenatal care (4). In another report from Colombia with
a similar mortality rate, only 11 percent of the mothers
had antenatal care; 84 percent of the deaths were avoidable, 64 percent of which were attributed to the failure
on the mother's part (5, 6). These figures serve to
illustrate the importance of educating the public concerning the basic principles in health care. In villages
where people do not attend clinics and classes, different
media have to be chosen, e.g., the use of television in
some rural areas where villagers share a communal television set and in the evenings it is an important form of
entertainment with a captive audience. For stubborn
villagers, it would be useful to solicit the help of
village elders and traditional birth attendants, to spread
the "gospel" because they command trust and respect from
the villagers. Where necessary, home visits to pregnant
women may be the only answer. For those who can be contacted, they should be taught the importance of early and
regular antenatal visits.

     The most important signals of danger such as pain,
hemorrhage and fever should be emphasized, and the mother
should be instructed to attend the nearest health care
center or call for medical help as soon as those symptoms
arise.

     From available reports, between 20 to 40 percent of
the total maternal deaths are due to abortion and its
associated complications. Therefore, the dangers of

illegal abortion has to be underscored to both the young and the old. This has to be coupled with strong support in the advice for a reliable method of contraception for spacing of children. Sterilization should be encouraged as a simple and effective method of contraception when the family is completed.

The dangers facing a grand multigravida should be spelled out, especially the problems of obstructed labor, rupture of the uterus, and antepartum or postpartum hemorrhage. To those with medical diseases such as hypertension and cardiac abnormalities, the risk is even higher. From "Confidential Enquiries", about half of those who died from cardiac disease were in their fourth or subsequent pregnancy.

In countries where the abortion law is very strict, more emphasis should be placed on the promotion of contraception. This is made more difficult by restrictions from the Catholic Church. In places where this faith is prevalent, the physician and primary health care personnel must recognize the limitations of the sympto-thermal method in the detection of ovulation and the women should be advised accordingly.

Infection plays an important part in maternal deaths, amounting to 40 percent in some reports. Illegal abortion with sepsis is an important contributing factor, and as emphasized earlier this should be stamped out either by education, appropriate legislation (perhaps as the legalization of abortion in Bangladesh), or an effective sterlization program to decrease unwanted pregnancies in the multiparae. For the prevention of puerperal sepsis, both mothers and birth attendants should be taught the basics of hygiene in looking after the perineum after delivery. The use of herbs and other poultices should be discouraged; proper antiseptics should be made available.

Education of Medical and Paramedical Staff

The problem of training traditional birth attendants need to be tackled with more vigor. Perhaps lessons can be learned from China where such programs are successfully organized. These potential birth attendants, be they mothers, teachers, or students, should be taught specific tasks such as basic antenatal care, aseptic delivery procedures in the home environment, and advice on contraception. Refresher courses and discussions of problems should be conducted under the supervision of experienced midwives or doctors, so that they can improve and attain higher standards of practice.

In places where mothers attend antenatal clinics, it is essential that midwives and family doctors are aware of the high-risk group of patients such as grand multiparae, those with medical diseases, previous caesarean section, second and third stage abnormalities, etc., and they should be selected for closer antenatal monitoring and proper hospital confinement.

The medical and paramedical staff should be well-trained to recognize the early signs of complications such as mildly increased blood pressure and proteinuria, vaginnal spotting, premature leaking of amniotic fluid, and pyrexia; these may need immediate hospitalization.

With deliveries conducted at home, or clinics in remote areas, the birth attendants must be trained to deal with acute emergencies such as postpartum hemorrhage or retained placenta. They should ask for help as early as possible, and a "flying squad" service would be invaluable. This squad must be staffed by experienced obstetricians, with necessary equipment and drugs for resuscitation, including blood and blood products. Efficient transporta-tion is essential since this may be the crucial factor between life and death. In places where road transporta-tion is either congested or poor, and for those on isolated islands, the use of a helicopter service may be the only solution.

Improvement of Facilities and Practice

The provision of flying squad service with proper transportation facilities has been discussed. The health administrator must ensure a simple and effective referral system so that patients can be referred from the home or the local health center to a base hospital.

As for the base maternity hospital, it must be served by competent residents, anesthetists and perinatal consultants 24 hours a day, with adequate supporting equipment and staff, including the service of a blood bank. The service of experts should be available e.g., a haematologist in case of D.I.C or a microbiologist in case of uncontrolled infection.

The hospital consultants must shoulder the responsi-bility to ensure an acceptable standard of practice. For example, methods to minimize intrapartum infection may include stringent aseptic technique in vaginal examina-tion, shortening the interval between rupture of membranes and delivery of the baby, the use of prophylactic anti-biotics in selected cases and taking appropriate specimens for bacteriological examination when the need arises.

In cases of ectopic pregnancy, an immediate laparotomy must be performed while blood replacement is instituted. Delay in stopping the bleeding may push the patient into irreversible shock, which may result in another avoidable death.

Finally, when deaths do occur, the cause and the circumstances surrounding the death must be elucidated. Postmortem examination should be done, and it would be helpful if a standard protocol is established for necropsy of this nature. The health authority should exercise control over the details included in the death certificate. A panel of consultants can act as assessors to examine the reports and help in the analysis of the cause of death. The purpose of this exercise is not to attribute blame on a particular party, but to find out the level of failure or inadequate attention, and whether improvements can be made so that the risk of death can be materially lessened in the future. Unbiased discussion can be encouraged if the medical staff is assured of full confidentiality regarding information presented for the audit, and that they need not worry about the problems of litigation.

This type of audit is practiced to a certain extent in most developed countries, but this is beneficial only if adequate feedback is conveyed to the units concerned so that proper measures can be taken to correct any breakdown in exisiting practice.

CONCLUSION

Maternal deaths can be prevented through appropriate health education for the masses, adequate obstetric training for the birth attendants, supported by standard facilities and a reliable surveillance program, under the supervision of the health authorities.

Looking at the problem from a global point of view, more than 50 percent of the deaths can be prevented or we can save more than 200,000 lives every year if all women in Asia, Africa and South America are taught: to have their children between the age of 20 and 24; to attend prenatal clincs; and to`have sterilization after the second or at most the fourth pregnancy.

REFERENCES

1. World Health Statistics Annual (1979).
2. Tomkinson J, et al: Report on confidential enquiries
       into maternal death in England and Wales, 1973 –
       75, Her Majesty's Stationery Office, London.
3. World Health Organization (1967): International
       Classification of Diseases, 8th Edition, World
       Health Organization, Geneva.
4. Borazjani G, Javey H, Sadjadi HE, Daneshbod K (1978):
       Maternal mortality in South Iran – A seven-year
       survey. Int J Gynaecol Obstet, 16:65-69.
5. Hasbun AJ, Sanchez MC (1978): Maternal deaths at a
       University Hospital. Rev. Colomb Obstet Ginecol.
6. Sanchez Torres F (1977): Maternal mortality (Analysis
       of 30 consecutive deaths). Rev Colomb Obstet
       Ginecol, 28:217-229.

SYSTEMATIC MATERNAL HEALTH CARE IN SHANGHAI

X. Puqiu

Head, Department of Maternal and Child Care
Shanghai First Hospitalof Maternal and Child
Care
Shanghai, People's Republic of China

INTRODUCTION

Our government pays much attention to the protection
of mother's and children's health and considers it to be
an important part of the people's health services. Right
after the liberation, we started to train primary health
workers, established the three-grade maternity health
network and popularized modern midwifery and scientific
methods of bringing-up children, so as to decrease the
incidence of major diseases (such as puerperal fever, neonatal tetanus, etc.) which threaten the life of the mother
and child. As a result of these efforts, the mortality
rates of both mother and child were reduced. In recent
years, following the practice of family planning to reach
the objective of decrease in birth rate, maternal health
care has been enriched and perinatal health care has
gradually evolved.

SYSTEMATIC HEALTH CARE MODEL

Shanghai is a city with a population of 11 million.
There are 9 maternity hospitals, 3 children's hospitals
and a number of Obstetrics and Gynecology, and Pediatrics
Departments in general hospitals at different levels led
by the MCH Division of the Shanghai Municipal Health
Bureau, with a total of 4794 obstetric and gynecologic
beds and 2587 pediatric beds (Fig. 1).

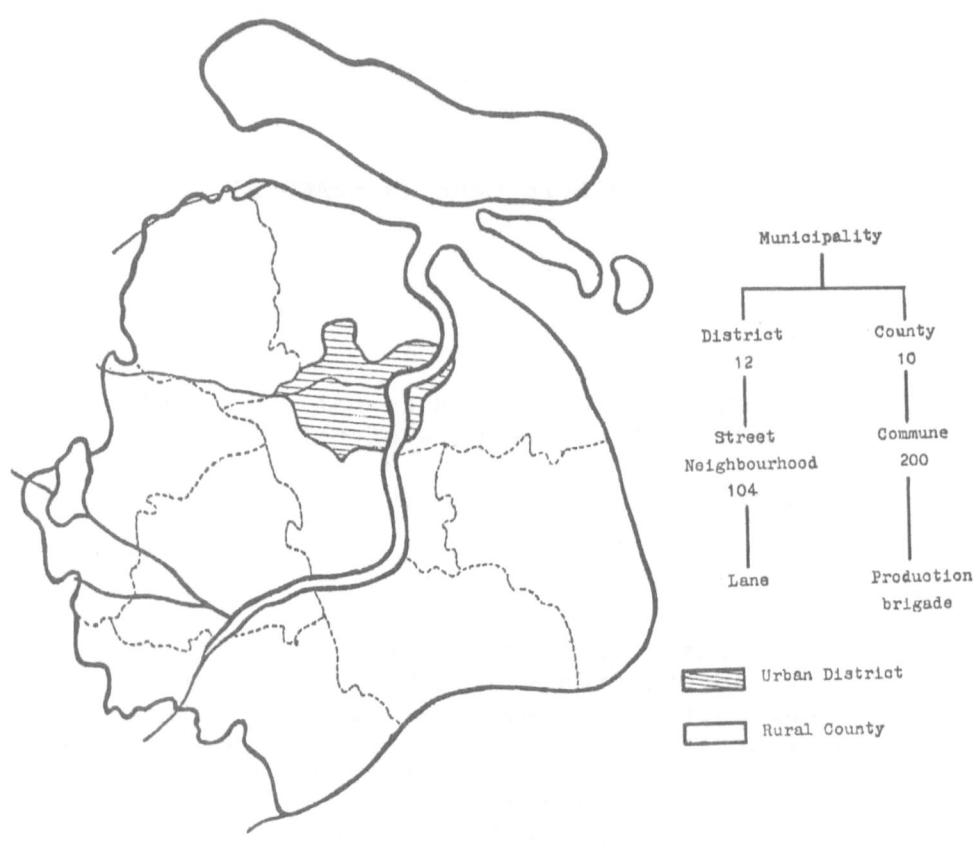

Figure 1.   Map of Shanghai

The Shanghai First Maternity and Infant Health
Institute and the Shanghai Children's Hospital are
responsible for technical supervision in the field of
maternal and child health care for the whole city. The
following changes were implemented for improvements in
this field.

Establishment and Consolidation of the Maternal and Child Health Network

Each district and county has its own MCH center in
close cooperation with the clinical departments of the
district or county hospitals. The center is responsible
for therapeutic and preventive procedures as well as medical training and research studies in that area (Fig. 2).

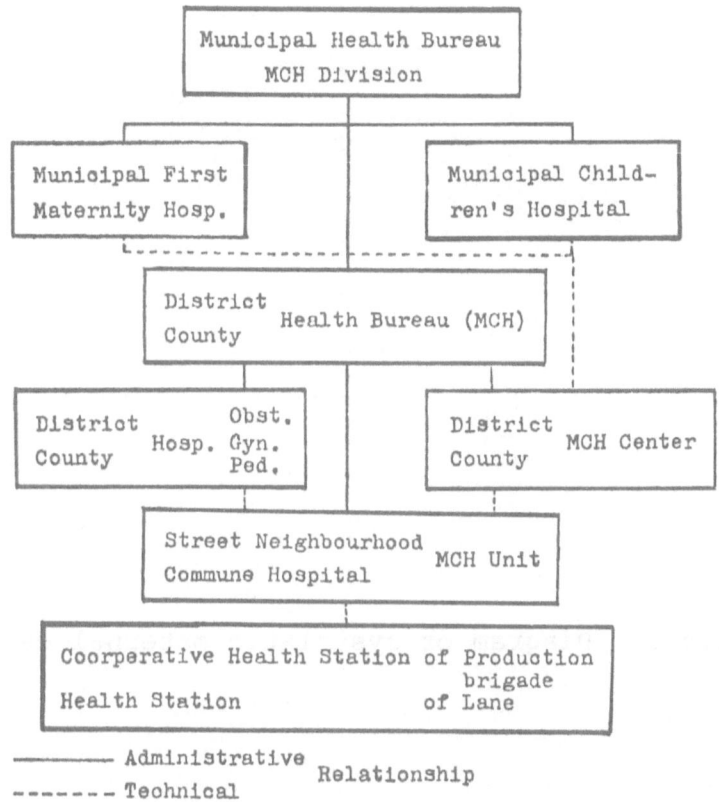

Figure 2.   Shanghai maternal and child health care network

At the primary level, there are 104 sub-district hospitals in urban districts and 200 commune hospitals in the rural counties, with a MCH group in each of them. Each MCH group has 3 to 5 members working as a team. All commune hospitals have obstetrical and gynecologic and pediatrics clinics and in addition, a hospital delivery service. The MCH groups of the sub-districts and commune hospitals are responsible for the training and technical supervision of the primary health workers. They are also responsible for systematic maternal health care, mass screening and treatment of gynecological diseases, systematic health care for children, regular check-up, physical examination and hygiene direction in the nurseries and kindergartens, regular prophylactic vaccinations, control of contagious diseases, accumulation of data and information and primary statistical work pertinent to MCH and family planning.

THE DIAGRAM OF SYSTEMATIC MATERNAL CARE

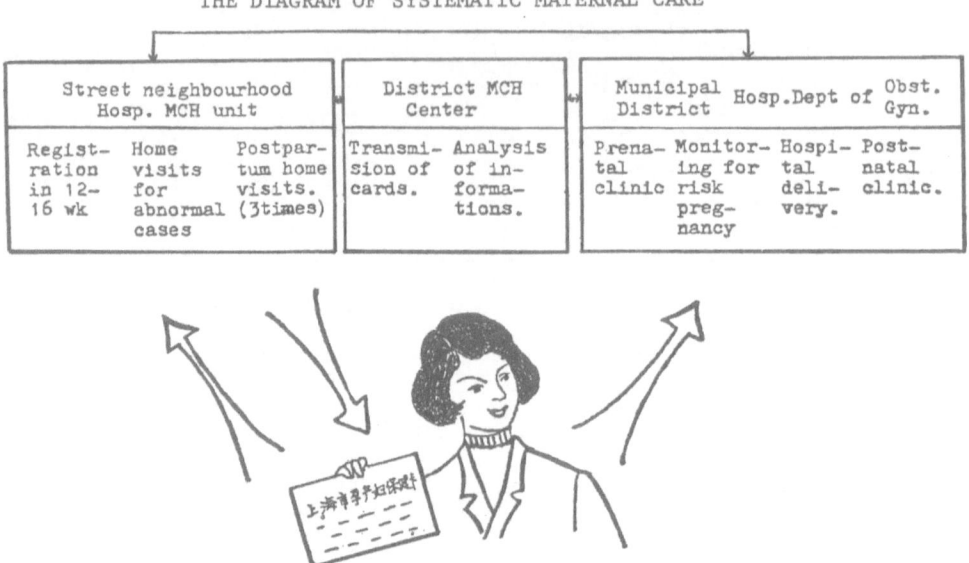

Figure 3.   Diagram of systematic maternal care.

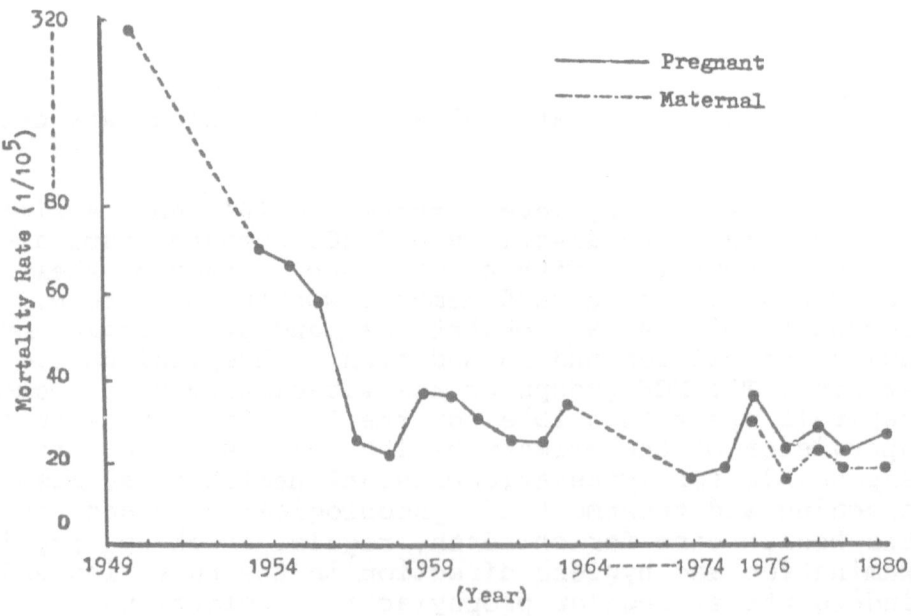

Figure 4.   The annual maternal mortality rate in Shanghai.

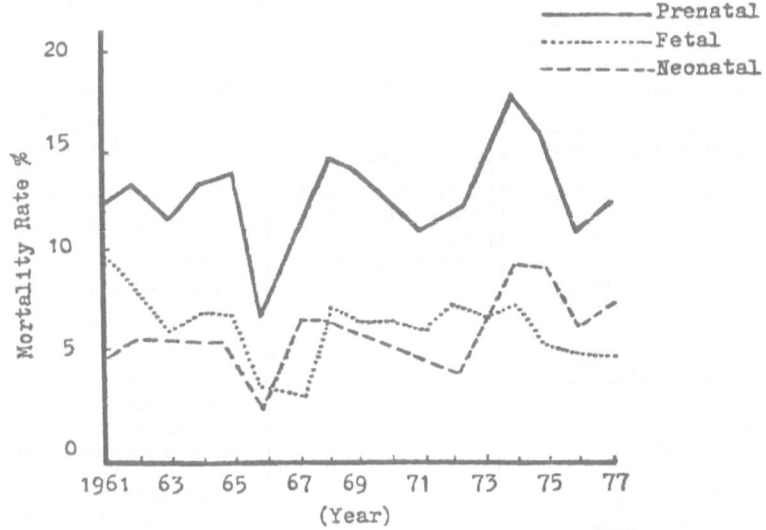

Figure 5.   Fetal, neonatal and prenatal mortality, 1961-77.

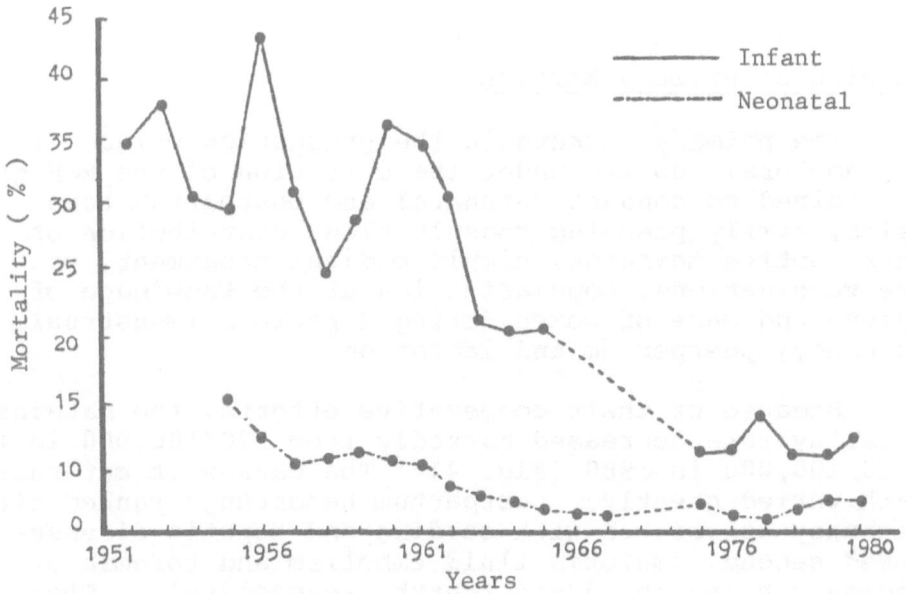

Figure 6.   Neonatal and infant mortality in Shanghai.

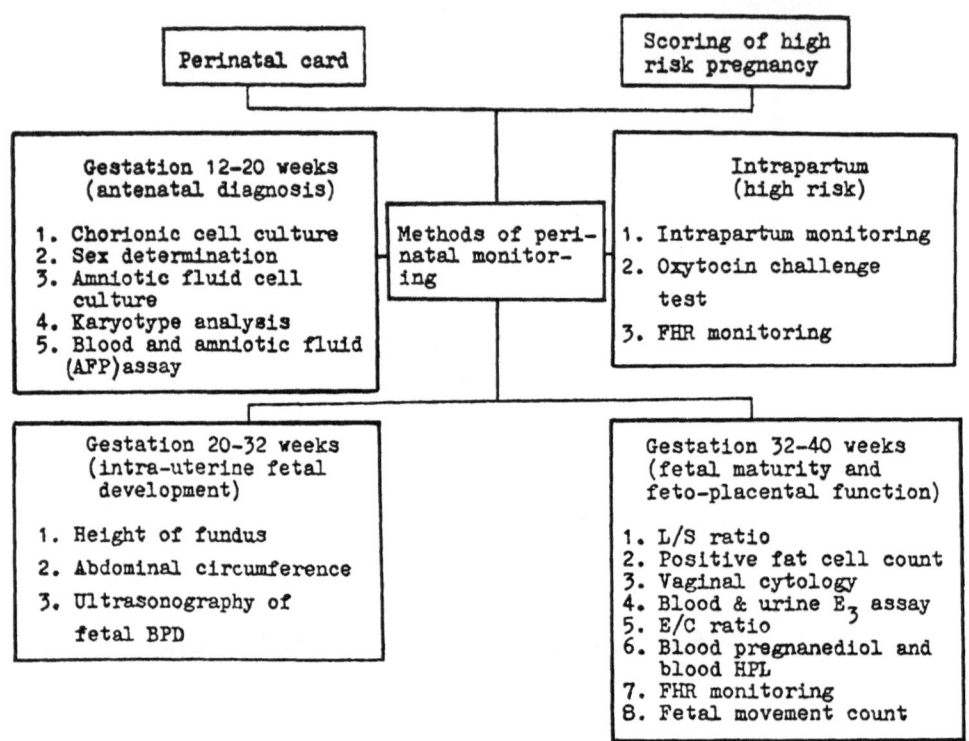

Figure 7.   Perinatal care

Training of Primary Workers

The primary workers in the production brigade (barefoot doctors) who are under the direction of the MCH group
are trained to conduct antenatal and postpartum home
visits, family planning consultation, distribution of
contraceptive measures, simple medical treatment, preventive vaccinations, popularization of the knowledge of
hygiene and care of women during 4 periods (menstrual,
pregnancy, puerperium and lactation).

Because of their cooperative efforts, the maternal
mortality rate decreased markedly from 320/100,000 in 1949
to 30/100,000 in 1980 (Fig. 4). The causes of maternal
death varied greatly; postpartum hemorrhage ranked first,
pregnancy associated with cardiac and hepatic diseases
ranked second, amniotic fluid embolism and toxemia of
pregnancy being third and fourth, respectively. The
neonatal mortality rate decreased from 68/1000 in 1949 to
13.8/1000 in 1980 (Fig. 5). The causes of fetal deaths
were prematurity, pneumonia, birth injury, anoxia and

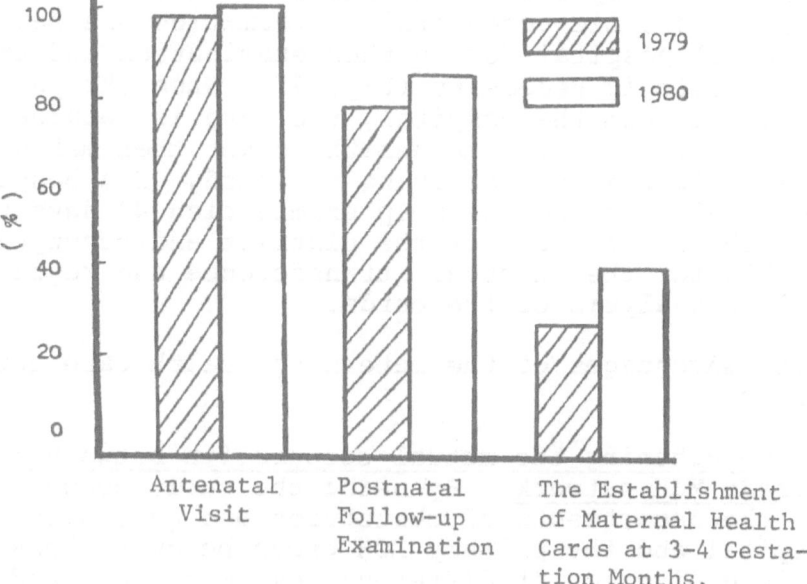

Figure 8. The perinatal care during 1979-80 in Shanghai.

congenital malformation in the decreasing frequency of
their occurrence.

        According to the retrospective statistics, the peri-
natal death rate in our hospital during 1961 to 1977 was
12.8/1000 (Fig. 6). The causes of deaths were anoxia,
malformation, dystocia, prematurity, postmaturity, antepartum fetal hemorrhage, macerated fetus, neonatal
diseases and death of unknown causes.

Adoption of a Maternity Health Card

        For further promotion of the quality of maternal
health work and maximization of the function of the
primary organization, the MCH personnel of our hospital
designed a maternity health card which was began to be
used in the urban districts in 1978. Every pregnant woman
is registered at the primary maternity health group where
the midwife takes the history, performs a preliminary examination and gives health directions for early pregnancy.
After the registration procedure, the card is given to the
mother. The normal pregnant woman is sent to the district
or county hospital for regular prenatal examination and
hospital delivery. The main findings and procedures done
in the hospital are recorded on the card (Appendix).

Those who have complicated medical diseases, hereditary
diseases or possible congenital malformation are sent to
the municipal hospital for further examination and prenatal diagnosis if necessary (Fig. 7). When the patient
is discharged from the hospital, the card is returned to
the primary MCH group. The health worker then makes a
home visit right after receiving the card. The hospital
is responsible for the check-up examination 42 days postpartum. The MCH centers of the district and county are
responsible for the punctual transference and regular
statistical analysis of the cards.

     The advantages of the maternity health care card are
as follows:

     Strengthening the mutual cooperation between the
three grade MCH network. By using the card, cooperation
between the departments of obstetrics and gynecology of
the hospital and the primary MCH group becomes closer.
The MCH organization of different levels support and help
each other in the management and prevention of complicating diseases. Under the guidance of the obstetricians and
gynecologists of the hospital, the quality of the primary
MCH network is much improved. On the other hand, the
hospital gets more information and suggestions from the
primary care level, which will further improve the obstetrical quality of their department. Thus, through the
card, the MCH work is consolidated, and the mothers and
newborns receive the benefits from the systematic health
care.

     Promoting the quality of the work of the primary
MCH group. By using the card, the mother can receive
systematic health care from early pregnancy up to 42 days
after delivery. Some district hospital teams conduct
home visits right after marriage. Once amenorrhea occurs,
the woman makes an early visit and is registered to obtain
a maternity health card. In 1980, 42.79 percent of the
cards were completed during the third month of pregnancy
(Fig. 8). On the average, prenatal examination was 100
percent averaging 10.5 visits; postpartum visit rate was
73.1 percent, averaging 2.6 times. Minor diseases such as
thrush, diaper rash of newborn, maternal breast disten-
sion, etc. can be managed at home. Many primary MCH
groups establish well-baby clinics and perform postpartum
follow-up 42 days after delivery.

Accumulation of data and information.

     By conducting systematic statistical analysis of the

cards, knowledge is gained as to how the MCH work is progressing, their quality levels and the results, so as to improve the work further. For example, from data gathered in 1980, the primipara rate is 89.3 percent, the incidence of hypertension syndrome of pregnancy is 29.3 percent (mild 16.8 percent, moderate 5.1 percent, and severe 7.4 percent), post-term birth (42 weeks) 5.0 percent, premature birth (37 weeks) 5.0 percent. These figures indicate the focal points of health care the Shanghai MCH service is doing at the present. In view of the high incidence of primipara, attention is directed on prevention and management of the complications specific for the primiparas.

In addition, by using the card, one can develop the direction of perinatal health care. For example, the card provides information on the scoring system of the high risk pregnancy, genetic consultative clinic, prenatal examination diagnosis and treatment of intrauterine growth retardation, laborgram and record of fetal movements.

Our hospital is the only municipal maternity facility affiliated with the Health Bureau of Shanghai. We have 200 beds for the mothers and 110 beds for the newborns. We take the responsibility of directing and supervising MCH work of 4 sub-districts and 70 factories and enterprises with which we had established contact, accept the referred high risk mothers and supervise the technical work of MCH of the whole municipality. We conduct training classes, write propaganda materials, carry out mass survey according to the plans, keep informed on MCH work and the quality of the obstetrical service in the entire municipality. We also conduct investigational studies on diseases and problems related to maternal and neonatal health in order to improve the situation.

CONCLUSION

In the past 32 years, maternal and child health care in Shanghai has improved. The adoption of this systematic health care model has played a great role. The maternity health card is now widely used throughout the city.

[Appendices are available by direct correspondence with the author]

SHANGHAI MATERNAL HEALTH CARD DISTRICT O.P.D. No ANTENATAL VISITS (Summary) SPECIAL VISITS

Name _____ No. _____

Working Unit

Kind of Work

Last menstrual period _____ Expected date of confinement _____

Basal blood pressure _____ Hemoglobune _____ Gm.

Address. No. _____ Lane, _____ Road, _____ Street, _____ District.

Confinement residence: as above No. _____ Lane, _____ Road, _____ Street

Early pregnancy: viral infection, Rubella medications _____ Yes _____ No

Drugs taken:

X-ray exposure. _____ Chemicals

Hereditary disease: Familial phycosis, _____ Hemophilia, _____ others( )

Abnormal obstetrical history _____ see* _____ Yes _____ No

Chronic illness _____ see** _____ Yes _____ No

Propaganda and education: A.N.Visits, _____ Care of nipples, _____ coitus,

physical exertion

Gestation Wk. _____ Clinic

Note:

Date:

*Abnormal Obstetrical History:

ANTENATAL VISITS (Summary) table — columns: No. of visits | Date | Gestation weeks | Blood pressure | Edema | Protein-urea | Abnormal condition | Appointment for next visits | Clinic of Examination

Rows numbered 1 through 14

SPECIAL VISITS — columns: Date | Condition

Last Antenatal Visits
Date

Propaganda and Education:
Coitus
Personal Hygien
Signs of labour
The preparation of baby clothes

Abortion(gestation week)
Spontaneous abortion   0
Artificial abortion   0
At early Pregnancy   0
At late Pregnancy   0

Gestation wk:
First sign of Toxemia of Pregnancy
24 — 0   28 — 0   32 — 0   36 — 0   38 — 0   40 — 0

Number of Antenatal Examinations
0 — 0   1 — 0   3 — 0   5 — 0   7 — 0   9 — 0   11 — 0   13 — 0   15 — 0
(0 — 0 marked)

Chronic illness
(   )   0
Hypertention   0
Hyperthyroidism   0
Diabetes mellitus 0
Anemia   0
Tuberculosis   0
Nephropathy   0
Hepatitis   0
Cardic disease   0

Anomaly   0
Neonatal Death   0
Stillbirth   0
Fetal Death   0
Obstetrical Hemorrhage 0
Eclampsia   0
Operative Delivery   0
Spontaneous Abortion   0
Artificial Abortion   0

AGE   GRAVIDITY   PARITY   BASAL B.P. gestation wk   The Gestation Week when card is made ( )
20—   1—   1—   0-12   0-12
25—   2—   2—   0-16   0-20
30—   3—   3—   0-20   0-28
35—   4—   4—   0-33
40—
0 0 0 0 0   0 0 0 0   0 0 0 0   0 0 0   0 0 0 0

Genetic Factors   0
History of Abnormality Family History Positive   0
Marriage of Close Relative   0
During 2nd Trimest of Pregnancy   0

APPENDIX A. Shanghai Maternal Health Card, Page 1.

Gestation Week at Delivery | Within 28 30 32 34 36 38 40 42

Ways of Delivery: Spontaneous Delivery, Vacuum extraction, Forceps Delivery, Breech Delivery, Breech Extraction, Caesarean section ( )

Condition of Mother: No laceration, III Perineal tear, Postpartum Hemorrhage, Infection, Prolonged labour ( )

Toxemia of Pregnancy: Mild, Moderate, Preeclampsia, Eclampsia

Postpartum Follow-up: 0 1 2 3 4 Within three days visits; Normal, Abnormal

Conditions during Labour

Name of Hospital for Delivery

Date of Delivery: day,   month,   year,   (gestation week   )

Way of Delivery: Spontaneous Delivery, Vacuum extraction, Forceps, Breech extraction, Caesarean section, Others

Laceration of perineum   0, I, II, III, Episiotomy   Suture   resumed   retained. Internal stitches   External stitches

Complications: Postpartum Hemorrhage, Toxemia of Pregnancy(mild, moderate, Pre-eclampsia, Eclampsia),
Infection(external genitalia, Endometritis, Parmmetritis, Septicemia), Prolonged labour

Miscellaneous

Newborn   male   female   Apgar score   Body wt.   gram   Special condition: Anomly, Trauma, Infection

Maternal Death   Date: Hour: Cause of Death: Fetal death, Still birth.

Note.   Date of Discharge: Signature:

Postpartum Follow-up(Mother)   Substitute   District

Date	Postpartum Day	Temperature	Breast Milk	Nipples	Uterine Retraction	Perineum	Lochia	Instruction	Signature

Special condition of infant: Cause;   Date:

Card Receiver: Remarks:

Condition of Newborn: Normal, Asphyxia, Anomaly, Injury of labour, Infection

Body Weight: <1000, 1000—, 1500—, 2000—, 2500—, 3000—, 3500—, 4000—

Unusual Condition: Abortion, Fetal Death, Stillbirth, Maternal Death

Day: Within one day, 1—7 days, 7—28 days

APPENDIX B. Shanghai Maternal Health Card, Page 2.

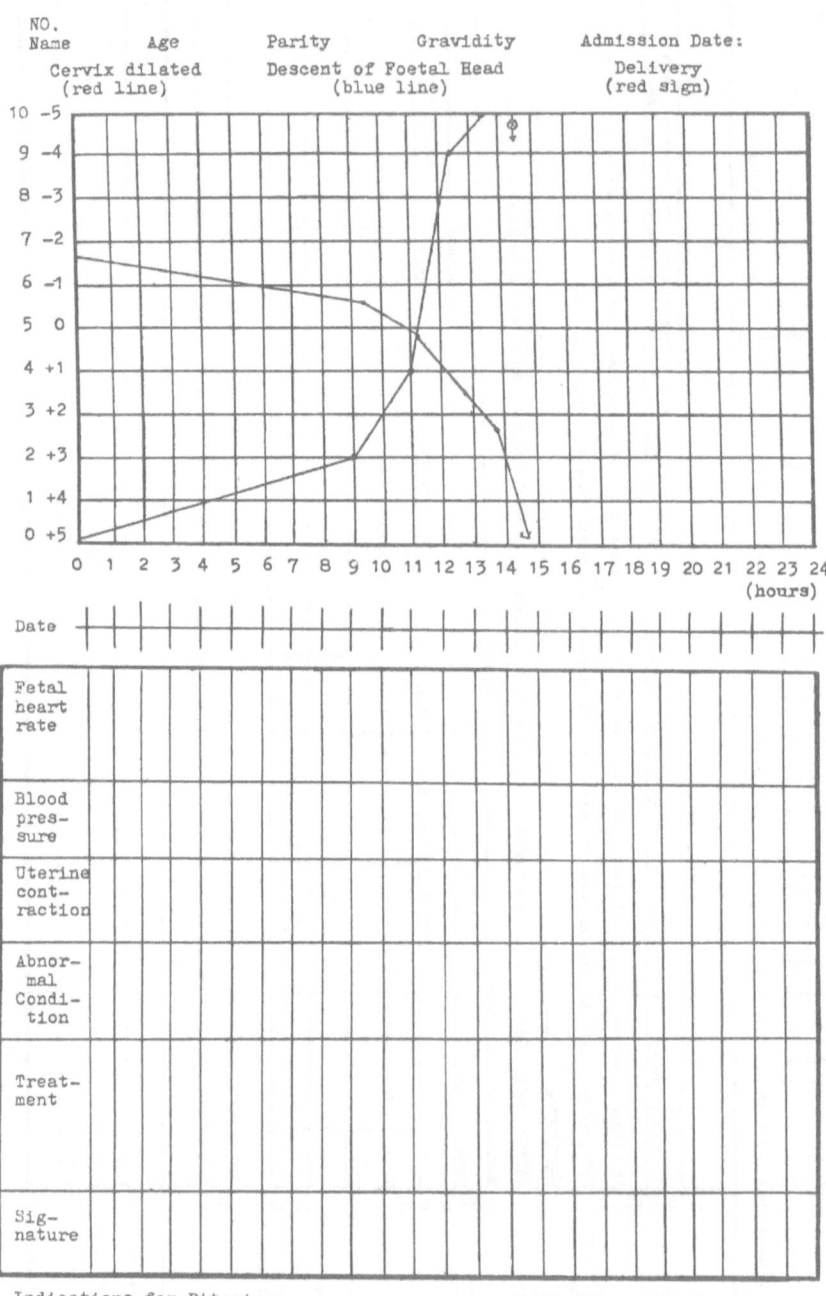

APPENDIX C.   Partogram.

I. FIXED FACTORS	5'	10'
	General conditions: 1. Age <20>35 yrs. old. 2. 3. Infertility for 3 yrs. or pregnant without treatment.	 >40 Body length <145 cms. Infertility for 3 yrs. or pregnant after treatment.
	Complications of Obs and Gyn origin: 1. Had delivered abnormal fetus or with hereditory disease. 2. Cesarian section 2 yrs. or more. 3. Abortion twice or 1-2 prematurity with no living fetus. 4. Intracranial hemorrhage, still-birth, neonatal death. 5. Induce labor at medium period, D&C, difficulty in labor through vagina. 6. Repair of uterus 2 yrs. or more. 7. Uterine myoma, ovarian cyst or history of operation. 8. Hemolysis ABO>1:128	 Fatal fetus with anomely. Cesarian section within 2 yrs. Abortion thrice or prematurity with no living fetus. Pregnant chest, spinal malformation, pelvic deformity. History of rupture of uterus. Repair of uterus within 2 yrs. Vagina, soft canal deformity. (Double uterus or vagina). RH hemolysis.
	Associated medical diseases: 1. Cardiac diseases: Heart function I-II. Sequalae of myocarditis (complete right or incomplete left bundle) (ventricular premature beat 5 times or more), (auricular premature beat 10-12 times). 2. Essential hypertension 130/90 (present). 3. Chronic persistant hepatitis or SGPT >80 units. 4. History of renal disease (over 12 yrs. of age). 5. Diabetes: control by intake. 6. Anemia, 6-8 grams. 7. Hyperthyroidism, no medication. 8. Psychosis. 9. History of lupus erythmatosus. 10. Fever of 39°C, less than 3 days.	Heart function III-IV or accompanying valvular lesions, cyanotic type, complete left bundle block, ventricular premature beat more than 10 times. Essential hypertension 160/100. Hepatitis proved. Renal function impaired. Control by drug. Hemoglobin beyond 6 grams, aplastic anemia. Controlled by drug. Attacks during pregnancy. No damage to the fetus. Fever for more than 4 days or influenza.
II. DYNAMIC FACTORS	1. Toxemia of pregnancy, mild, moderate. 2. Antepartum hemorrhage of unknown cause. 3. Premature rupture of the membrane. 4. Unmarried or no prenatal examination. 5. Fetal heart rate >160/m. 6. Foetus movement <30 times/12 hours or less than 50% of normal level. 7. Fetal growth retardation: Height of fundus and biapiculate diameter < the 10th perdentile.	Severe (BP 160/100. Albuminurea ++). Placenta previa, placenta abruptio. Double pregnancy; Excessive or less amnionic fluid. Transverse position after 32 weeks gestation, breech presentation. Fetal heart rate <120/m. Foetus movement absent. Height of fundus and biapiculate diameter below the 10th percentile-significant variance.

APPENDIX D. Perinatal Scoring

ACHIEVEMENTS IN PERINATAL AND MATERNAL HEALTH:

SURVIVAL IN JAPAN

T. Wagatsuma

Head and Chief Consultant
Department of Obstetrics and Gynecology
National Medical Center Hospital
Tokyo, Japan

INTRODUCTION

Probably one of the greatest tragedies for a family or a local community is the death of a child, a mother, or both during pregnancy, parturition, or after the child has been born. To some extent, the quality of obstetrical care of a region or a country can be evaluated by studying the area's perinatal and maternal mortality rates. It can be said that the lower these mortality rates, the better the obstetrical care available in that area.

FACTORS ASSOCIATED WITH PERINATAL AND MATERNAL MORTALITY

The following factors are considered to be closely associated with perinatal and maternal mortalities according to studies conducted in various countries.

Parity and Age

Perinatal and maternal mortalities tend to be high in population grous in which the mother is younger than 20 or older than 35 years of age. Perinatal mortality is minimum in cases of paragravida two and three, but increases thereafter. Maternal mortality rate tends to rise with increasing parity. In Japan, the increased risk of mother is significant after the third birth; in Great Britain it is after the fifth. In Japan, majority of women have their first child between 20 and 29 years of age and 83 percent of married women have only two children.

Socio-economic status

Perinatal and maternal mortality rates tend to be
high among mothers from the socio-economic classes with
relatively low standards of living, limited education, and
with little concern for her health.

Birth Interval

The shorter the birth interval, the higher is the
perinatal mortality risk of the next child. The significance of a short birth interval extends beyond an increase
of perinatal mortality, for if the child survives, it
tends to replace its immediately older sibling on the
breast, which may lead to the death of that sibling from
infection enhanced by malnutrition. The short birth
interval can also increase the frequency of low birth
weight infants. Proper instruction of contraception for
child spacing is essential in this respect.

Antenatal Care

The factor most closely associated with the incidence
of perinatal and maternal mortalities is the availability
of high quality antenatal care. Unfortunately, the group
which has the highest mortality rate tends to be the group
least likely to receive antenatal care. If the mother
receives antenatal care at appropriate interval from the
early stage of pregnancy, it would be possible to detect
and treat or even prevent complications that may arise.

Medical Facilities and Environmental Factors

A study of perinatal and maternal deaths in order to
determine whether they were avoidable or not, indicates
that in many cases, death could have been avoided if
medical facilities and the social environment had been
different. Social factors leading to death can be said to
arise from the mother herself, her family, and the doctor,
midwife or nurse participating in the delivery.

Medical Causes of Perinatal and Maternal Deaths

Most of the conditions which can cause maternal death
would, at the same time, threaten the life of the fetus or
the newborn. Antepartum hemorrhage, toxemia of pregnancy,
cardiovascular and renal disease, and infections are the
most frequent causes of deaths.

STRATEGIES TO REDUCE PERINATAL AND MATERNAL MORTALITIES

The reduction of perinatal and maternal mortalities in Japan was achieved by the implementation of the following strategies.

Education

As stated previously, perinatal and maternal deaths tend to occur in cases in which the mother is not concerned with her health, and/or in cases in which the mother does not receive appropriate antenatal care. Therefore, multidisciplinary health education should be provided starting at the school level and extending to the communities. In this course, which should be taken by both sexes, the physiology of human reproduction, human sexuality, family planning and the health impact of nutrition and hygiene should be stressed. Those providing primary health care must participate directly in educating the public and must also offer appropriate advice. In order to reduce perinatal and maternal deaths, it is necessary to inform women of the desirability of having children at an appropriate age, of limiting the number of children, and the importance of family planning in general. Education of nurses, midwives, traditional birth attendants, medical students, primary physicians, and other providers of health care, is also cruicial.

Fortunately in Japan, literacy rate is as high as 99 percent and the term of compulsory education is 9 years of elementary and junior high schools. In April 1979, 94 percent of junior high school graduates entered senior high schools or technical colleges. At present, a certain level of health education is available at these schools, although there are many difficulties in particular areas, such as sexuality and family planning education for the teenagers.

The Provision of Primary Health Care

It is said that primary health care is the forefront of medical care since it must not only provide appropriate care to local residents, but must also contribute to promoting their health condition through education and disease prevention. The person who plays that important role in the provision of primary health care differs according to the circumstances of various countries. Regardless of who is important in providing primary health care services, the measures which must be taken in order to reduce perinatal and maternal mortality is the same.

There are some 6000 obstetricians/gynecologists in Japan
who provide obstetric services required in primary health
care. Majority of these obstetrician/gynecologists
practice in private clinics which are equipped with beds
and facilities for surgery and delivery. Forty-three
point seven percent of the total deliveries in Japan are
performed in these clinics, 50.6 percent in hospitals,
5.1 percent in maternity homes, while 0.5 percent of the
births occur in private homes.

Proper Antenatal Care and Indentification of Potential High Risk Mothers

Mothers who are under 20 or over 35 years of age,
unmarried, overweight or underweight, of low socio-economic standing, having poor obstetrical history or who
suffer from preeclamptic toxemia, diabetes, cardiovascular, renal or hypertensive disease, or grandmultiparae,
tend to be high risk cases. It is necessary through the
provision of antenatal care from the early stages of pregnancy to identify the potential high risk mothers and to
prevent or detect at the early stages the occurrence of
such complications as toxemia of pregnancy. Screening for
anemia and/or treating anemia by providing iron supplements can reduce the risk of postpartum hemorrhage. Cases
who suffer from significant vaginal bleeding during
pregnancy should be placed in, and treated at an appropriately equipped medical institution. Recently, the
ultrasonic scanning equipment significantly improved the
diagnostic technique of placenta previa, which is one of
the major causes of perinatal and maternal mortality.

As to the historical background of maternal and
neonatal health activities in Japan, the institute (called
AIIKU Institute) was established in 1934, from funds do-
nated by the Emperor in commemoration of the birth of His
Majesty, the Crown Prince. AIIKU means "love and tender
care" in Japanese. The Institute and its affliated
organization became a center for Maternal and Child Health
(MCH) activities in Japan during the prewar period and has
been continuously contributing a great deal to the improvement of maternal and child health in this country. A
certain number of villages throughout Japan were chosen as
model villages for maternal and child health activities.
These so-called AIIKU villages, have a leader, and together with volunteer housewives, organize a team to
cooperate with local midwives, MCH workers, and public
health nurses, to promote community health activities.
They disseminate information on maternal and child hygiene
and family planning, encourage the expectant mothers to

attend the antenatal clinics or the mothers to take their
children to the well-baby clinics.

These systems of "women's club" were quite successful
in promoting the maternal and child health activities at
community level in Japan, until the industrialization and
urbanization started. Such AIIKU activity could sufficiently function only in an agricultural community, where
a close human relationship among farmers existed. At
present however, most Japanese are living in the highly
industrialized urban communities, where personal communication among neighbors are quite ineffective. Majority of
young couples are living in a row of apartments as nuclear
family groups. Young wives or expectant mothers suffer
from lack of sufficient knowledge of maternal and child
health, which their elder sisters had obtained personally
from their mothers or grandmothers when they lived together. Therefore new procedures for of approaching these
MCH targets in the industrialized urban communities are
now urgently required.

To promote early attendance to the antenatal clinic,
a woman is issued what could be called "a mother-child
passport" or "health booklet", when she reports her pregnancy to a regional health center. This booklet contains
not only necessary information for the pregnant woman, but
also a record of her physical findings, laboratory results
during her antenatal care, and a history of her labor and
delivery. It also contains records of the development and
immunization of the child during preschool period. According to the 1979 statistics, of all the reported cases
of pregnancy, 23.6 percent of the mothers reported her
pregnancy by the third month, while 90 percent reported
by the fifth month and received the booklets. Most local
authorities provide the expenses for one to three obstetrical visits for antenatal care. The average Japanese
woman tends to be concerned about her health and is
enthusiastic about receiving antenatal care. As stated
previously, antenatal care in Japan is provided by
obstetricians in private practice, at hospitals, and by a
few midwives in private practice.

The Provision of Emergency Health Services Through an Adequate Referral Network

Although maternal and fetal deaths can be prevented
to a certain extent through education and proper antenatal
care, there are also many deaths due to unpredictable
causes. Hypoxic condition of the fetus occurs most frequently during labor and delivery. Constant recording of

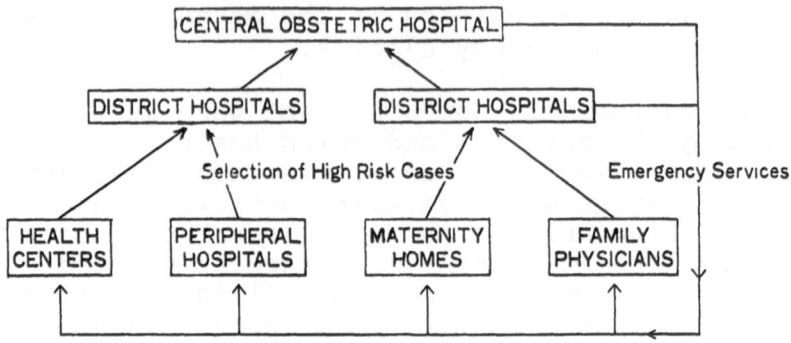

Figure 1. Referral network of obstetric care in Japan.

both the fetal heart rates and uterine contractions during labor makes it easier to detect the onset of fetal hypoxia due to placental dysfunction or cord compression. With the sudden onset of postpartum hemorrhage, there is little that a skilled and experienced obstetrician can do alone.

In bleeding cases, maternal death can often be prevented by two or more relatively less experienced physicians and an adequate supply of blood for transfusion. It is necessary to allocate the mothers accordingly. For example, low risk mothers are assigned for private or maternity home deliveries, while potentially high risk mothers are assigned to well-equipped and well-staffed hospitals. In addition, in cases when sudden complication such as fetal hypoxia or postpartum hemorrhage occur during a private or maternity home delivery, it is necessary to have an available mobile service such as the Flying Squad in Great Britain which can transport mothers with their babies to medical centers. In 1950, Japanese institutional deliveries comprised 4.6 percent of all births while they presently comprise 99.4 percent of all births. Domiciliary deliveries have fallen from 95.4 percent in 1950 to 0.5 percent in 1978. As previously stated, 43 percent of present institutional deliveries occur in private clinics. This poses no problem for low risk cases. However, in emergency situations which require cesarean section, neonatal intensive care, or transfusions of large quantities of blood, immediate referrals to larger hospitals become necessary. At present, the lack of official coordination between these private clinics and nearby large hospitals is considered a problem.

Table 1.   Maternal Mortality Rates in Selected Countries.
           (per 10,000 live births)

Country	1965	1970	1975	1977
Japan	8.8.	5.2	2.9	2.3
U.S.A.	3.2		1.3	
Federal Republic of Germany		5.2	4.0	3.4
Netherlands	2.7	1.3	1.1	1.3
England and Wales	1.8	1.9	1.3	1.3
Sweden	1.4	1.0	0.2	0.1
Switzerland	3.8	2.5	1.3	0.4
New Zealand	2.2	3.2	2.3	

Table 2.   Perinatal Mortality Rate in Selected Countries.
           (per 1000 live births)

Country	1965.	1970	1975	1978
Japan	30.1	21.7	16.0	13.0
U.S.A.	28.5	27.8	20.7	
Federal Republic of Germany	29.0	26.7	19.4	13.8
Netherlands	23.4	18.8	14.0	
England and Wales	27.3	23.8	19.9	
Sweden	19.9	16.5	11.1	9.6
Switzerland	23.1	18.3	13.5	10.7
New Zealand	22.5	19.8	16.5	

Statistical Survey

     Conducting a statistical survey on perinatal and
maternal mortalties as is done in the United States can
lead to a reduction in mortalities. Through such a survey, it is possible to raise the consciousness of laymen,
physicians, midwives, and health care workers to the
problems of perinatal and maternal deaths. Besides the
annual statistics of the entire country reported by the
Ministry of Health and Welfare, the Committee on Perinatal
Statistics (Japan Society of Obstetricians and Gynecologists) has compiled annual reports on the perinatal deaths
among selected registry hospitals in Japan since 1974.
Through this registry it became possible to analyze the
detailed causes of perinatal deaths, leading to a steady
decline of the perinatal mortality at these registry
hospitals.

     Compared to the decrease of perinatal deaths, the
rate of decline in maternal mortality in Japan has been

rather slow. The Japanese Association of Physicians for
Maternal Health organized a special committee in 1971 to
conduct a study of 455 cases of maternal deaths occurring
between 1968 and 1970 in a certain region. The Committee
reported that the major causes of maternal deaths correspond to those of the United States and Europe. A
significant number of deaths were found to be among cases
involving mothers younger than 20 or older than 30 years
of age and/or experiencing three or more pregnancies. The
largest number of deaths was due to hemorrhage. Although
the Ministry of Health and Welfare's study based on death
certificates gave toxemia of pregnancy as the cause of the
largest number of death, the Committee's Report showed
that the incidence of hemorrhage was 37.5 percent which
was twice that of the incidence of toxemia. At the time
the study was conducted, Japan still had a relatively high
rate of maternal mortality as a developed nation: 8.8 per
10,000 live births in 1968 and 5.2 per 10,000 in 1970.
However the incidence has gradually declined over the
years: 4.1 in 1972, 2.9 in 1975, 2.3 in 1979 and 2.0 per
10,000 live births in 1980. Although this rate is still
higher than that of the Netherlands, Great Britain or
Switzerland, it is lower than that of West Germany and is
said to be equal that of New Zealand (Table 1).

        Further efforts to reduce the tragedies of perinatal
and maternal deaths through the provision of adequate and
appropriate health care should be a major goal for us.
Table 2 represents the perinatal mortality in selected
countries.

CONCLUSION

        In the last twenty years, perinatal and maternal mor-
tality rate in Japan have significantly decreased with the
aid of various health strategies that include education,
provision of primary health care, proper antenatal care
with the identification of potentially high-risk mothers,
the provision of emergency health services through an
adequate referral network and statistical surveys.

REFERENCES

1.   Llewely-Jones D (1974): Human reproduction and
        society. Faber and Faber, London.
2.   Sakamoto S and Maeda K (1981): Perinatal statistics
        of registry hospitals of Japan in 1974 to 1978 by
        the Committee on Perinatal Statistics of the Japan

Society of Obstetrics and Gynecology.
<u>Asia-Oceania J Obstet Gynec</u>, 7:29-41.

3. Ministry of Health and Welfare (1981): <u>Statistics
    relating to Maternal and Child Health in Japan</u>.
    Maternal and Child Health Division, Children and
    Family's Bureau, Bosieisei Kenkyukai, Tokyo.

4. Wagatsuma T (1977): Advances in MCH and family
    planning. In: <u>Proceedings of 4th SEAMIC Seminar,
    Health Aspects of Community Development in
    Southeast Asia</u>. H Katsunuma and N Maruchi,
    Editors, Southeast Asian Medical Information
    Center, Tokyo.

5. Wagatsuma T (1979): Maternal mortality and primary
    health care. In: International Congress Series No.
    512, Gynecology and Obstetrics, <u>Proceedings of the
    IXth World Congress of Gynecology and Obstetrics</u>.
    Sakamoto, Tojo, Nakayama, Editors, Excerpta Medica,
    Amsterdam-Oxford-Princeton.

ACHIEVEMENTS IN MATERNAL AND NEONATAL HEALTH:

SURVIVAL IN SRI LANKA

K. P. Wickramasuriya

Medical Officer, Family Health Bureau
Colombo, Sri Lanka

INTRODUCTION

The Democratic Socialist Republic of Sri Lanka
(Ceylon) is an island situated in the Indian Ocean,
separated from the southern part of the Indian sub-
continent by a narrow strip of shallow waters. It has an
area of 65,640 sq. km. (25322 sq. miles) and a population
density of 232 per sq. km. (586 per sq. mile). Thirty
percent of the area is agricultural land of which tea,
rubber, coconut and paddy comprise the major crops. The
country is divided into wet and dry zones based on the
annual rainfall.

Sri Lanka has been under foreign domination since
the 16th century and became a politically independent
nation in 1948. In 1978 a new constitution was promulgat-
ed with the country becoming a Democratic Socialist
Republic, but continued to remain within the Commonwealth
of Nations.

POPULATION

The 1981 census revealed the population of Sri Lanka
as 14.86 million, of which 72 percent are distributed in
the rural areas. The urban and the plantation sectors
comprise 21.5 percent and 6.5 percent of the population
respectively.

The people are of different ethnicity, the major
ethnic group being the Sinhalese (74 percent). The Sri

Table 1. Percentage of Literary in Sri Lanka

Census Year	Both Sexes	Males	Females
1881	17.4	29.8	3.1
1891	21.7	36.1	5.1
1901	26.4	42.0	8.5
1911	31.0	47.2	12.5
1921	31.9	56.6	21.2
1946	57.8	70.1	43.8
1953	65.4	75.9	63.2
1963	71.6	79.3	63.2
1971	78.1	85.2	70.7

Source: Department of Census and Statistics

Lanka Tamils constitute 12.6 percent, the Indian Tamils 5.6 percent, Moors 6.1 percent and the balance being comprised of Burghers, Malays and other nationalities.

The population of Sri Lanka is young, with approximately 50 percent being less than 20 years of age. This contributes to the high dependency rate of 78 percent. The overall literacy is high for a developing country, with a rate of 85 percent for males and 71 percent for females as indicated in the census of 1971 (Table 1).

In the early part of the century, illiteracy was high among females. With the introduction of free education, the literacy rate and educational attainment of the population showed a significant improvement over the past four decades.

Population Growth and Fertility

Census enumerations have shown a rapid increase in the population during the last four decades. The population recorded at the first census in 1871 was 2.4 million. Since 1946 the population has shown an increase from 6.6 million to 14.85 million in 1981. The natural increase has been the main contributory factor for this rise.

Expansion of health care services together with social and economic development since the 1940s contributed to the dramatic decline in the crude death rates and appreciable increases in the life expectancy at birth. These levels are comparable with those in developed countries. It is conventional to generally attribute such

Table 2.   Pattern of Fertility in Sri Lanka

	1953	1963	1971	1977
General Fertility Rate	189.5	166.5	138.7	108.8
Marital Fertility Rate	256.2	239.4	215.0	187.3
Total Fertility Rate	5.3	5.04	4.22	3.8
Gross Reproduction Rate	2.6	2.5	2.1	1.9
Crude Birth Rate	38.7	34.1	30.1	28.4

Source: The Registrar General's Department

improvements to the impact of effective health sector
inputs. These achievements together with socio-economic
development have resulted in a change in the fertility
pattern in the country (Table 2).

The crude birth rate has decline from 39.7 per 1000
in 1950 to 27.6 per 1000 in 1980. The general fertility
rate has shown a decline of 42.6 percent during the period
1953 to 1977. The total fertility and the gross reproduction rates have decreased by 28.3 percent and 26.9 percent
respectively during the same period and the age specific
fertility rates in the highly fecund age groups have shown
a similar pattern.

Organization of Health Services

In Sri Lanka, health is a state concern and it is
the responsibility of the government to provide comprehensive health care to the people. Approximately 1.5
percent of the GNP was spent on health care during the
last few years. The health budget as a percentage of the
total budget has been 5.5, 3.4, 3.7 and 3.2 in 1977, 1978,
1979 and 1980 respectively. Seventy-five percent of the
health budget was directed to patient care services, while
only 20 percent was made available for the community
health services.

In the past, due to emphasis being placed mainly on
the curative services, the preventive health services did
not receive the priority attention it deserved. Lately,
however, there has been a shift of emphasis towards health
promotion and disease prevention, both in thought and in
action.

Table 3. Medical Institutions and Medical
Personnel in Relation to Population

Year	Number of Hospitals	Number of Dispensaries	Doctor/Population Ratio
1935	98	72	18000
1945	246	209	11000
1955	380	283	9100
1965	417	293	8200
1978	451	352	4000

Source: Ministry of Health

DEVELOPMENT OF MATERNAL AND CHILD HEALTH SERVICES

The origin of the organized program for maternal and child health dates back to 1906 with the establishment of a Maternal and Child Health Department in the Colombo Municipality. The first health unit was established in 1926 for field health activities, and by 1936 eight such health units were functioning in the country. With the outbreak of malaria epidemic in 1935, extension of maternal and child health services was channelled through the Malaria Control program to cover all districts in the country. Medical officers recruited under this scheme serviced a large number of health centers which proved to be very popular. Trained public health midwives were appointed to the health units and improved health care was provided for women, during the prenatal, natal and postnatal periods.

The health unit scheme was further expanded reaching a total of 91 health units by 1950. Presently there are 104 such units. This scheme provided the framework for the establishment of a large number of institutional and field clinic centers throughout the country (Table 5). Trained health personnel (both medical and paramedical) employed showed a significnt increase. The doctor/population ratio decreased from 1 per 18,000 in 1935 to 1 per 4000 in 1979. The specialist services also expanded rapidly, resulting in a remarkable improvement in the quality of health care provided within the country.

A separate section for maternal and child health was

established within the Ministry of Health in 1968 and this was subsequently redesignated the Family Health Bureau. The establishment of a separate Ministry for family health activities in 1977 was an expression of the commitment and concern of the government for maternal and child health activities in the total health program.

Health Administration System

Sri Lanka has a well developed health infrastructure to provide an efficient family health service within the country. Health care is available within a radius of 2.8 miles and access to a government medical institution is possible within a radius of six miles.

The country is divided into 19 divisions for the purpose of health administration. Each division is in the charge of a Superintendent of Health Services (SHS) who is responsible for the total health care within the division.

The SHS division is further subdivided into health areas with populations ranging from 40,000 to 200,000. These health areas are in the charge of Medical Officers of Health (MOH) who are responsible for all promotional and preventive health activities including maternal and child health. He is supported by a team of trained paramedical staff comprised of public health inspectors (PHI.I), public health nurses (PHN) and public health midwives (PHM.M).

The public health midwife is the "grass root worker" and provides routine domiciliary and clinic care in the community. Each PHM area is comprised of several villages and has a demarcated area, with a population ranging from 3000 to 8000. Some of her major functions would include:

(a) provision of prenatal, natal and postnatal care;
(b) health education;
(c) motivation for family planning and distribution of conventional contraceptives (pills and condoms); and
(d) assist at the maternal and child health clinics within the area.

Each health area is provided with a network of family health centers which function regularly. The clinics are conducted by medical officers assisted by area field staff (PHI, PHN and PHM.M) and provides antenatal, postnatal and child care services, including immunization and provision of food supplements to medically selected beneficiaries. Any abnormalities are refered to medical

institutions for specialized care. Family planning
facilities are available at most of these clinics. The
services afforded by trained personnel in the field of
maternal and child care are observed to be high in Sri
Lanka in comparison to that of most of the developing
countries.

Sources of Data Related to Maternal and Child Health

Prior to 1880, collection of data on births and
deaths was incomplete and disorganized. The Birth and
Death Act of 1887 provided legal sanction for the
registration of vital events. The collection and processing of statistics with respect to births and deaths is the
responsibility of the Registrar General's Department.
Thereafter, a remarkable improvement in the registration
has been observed. A survey conducted to assess the com-
pleteness of birth and death registration showed that 98.7
percent of births and 92.3 percent of deaths were registered in 1967 as compared to 88.1 and 88.5 percent
respectively, in 1951.

Information with respect to morbidity is limited to
hospital in-patient statistics. In view of this, only
little consideration has been given to morbidity in the
assessment of achievements in the field of maternal and
neonatal health.

ACHIEVEMENTS IN MATERNAL AND NEONATAL HEALTH

A significant improvement in the field of maternal
and neonatal health has been observed in Sri Lanka during
the post war period. Since 1945, the mortality rates have
demonstrated an appreciable decline from 16.5 per 1000
live births to 0.8 in 1978, showing a reduction of 95
percent.

Maternal Mortality

The high rate of maternal mortality that prevailed
during the early part of the century may be attributed to
the interactions of a multitude of pernicious factors.
Inadequate maternal care services, poor nutritional status, unhygienic environmental conditions and general state
of social poverty were among the major determinants for
these high rates of mortality. In addition to the above
risk factors, a high prevalence of malaria contributed to
this high mortality.

Table 4. Percentage of Maternal Deaths Due to the
          Three Major Causes

Year	Total Maternal Deaths	Maternal Deaths (3 major causes)	Percent of Total Maternal Deaths
1940	3423	2878	84.1
1950	1692	1189	70.37
1960	1094	705	64.4
1972	514	286	55.6
1975	385	210	54.5

In the past, the main causes of maternal mortality
were puerperal sepsis, toxemias, hemorrhage of pregnancy
and child birth. Statistics for the period 1940 to 1975
are given in Table 4. A 35 percent decline in the percentage of maternal deaths due to the three major causes
has been recorded over a period of 35 years.

Mortality due to the three major causes have demonstrated an interesting pattern during the past four decades
(Table 5). In the early forties, toxemia was the main
cause of maternal deaths with sepsis and hemorrhage taking
the second and third places, respectively. During the
1970s this pattern changed. Hemorrhage became the main
cause of maternal deaths, as deaths from sepsis showed a
dramatic decline.

The age specific maternal mortality rate have shown
a reduction in all age groups since 1954 (Table 6). The
decline was most marked in the under 20 age group where an
89 percent reduction has been observed.

Expansion of and improvement in the maternal and
child health services in the country resulted in the improvement of care to both mother and child. The quality
of maternal care provided improved considerably over the
last few decades. At present there are over 2100 fully
trained Public Health Midwives providing domiciliary care.
The proportion of mothers delivering in medical institutions increased from 25 percent in 1950 to about 76
percent in 1976.

Statistics for 1979 reveal that approximately 62
percent of pregnant women in the country received prenatal
care from the health centers and 55 percent had received
domiciliary care provided by the field midwives. It was
observed that each field midwife on the average had made

Table 5.   Maternal Mortality by Major Causes
Rate per 10,000 Live Births

Year	Toxemia	Sepsis	Hemorrhage
1935-44	80.86	56.72	13.25
1945	72.17	38.62	11.16
1950	15.96	11.20	10.71
1955	12.35	7.16	9.13
1960	7.50	3.30	8.71
1965	6.45	2.33	6.80
1972	2.63	1.70	3.13
1976	2.11	0.48	2.37

Source: Registrar General's Department.

Table 6.   Age Specific Maternal Mortality

Age Group	1954	1960	1966	1972
Under 20 years	4.7	2.5	1.1	0.5
20 and under 25	3.6	2.6	1.5	1.4
25 and under 30	3.7	2.4	1.9	1.3
30 and under 35	5.0	3.1	2.2	1.3
35 and under 40	7.7	4.7	3.8	2.1
40 and under 45	9.5	6.9	6.5	3.6
45 and over	14.2	15.1	12.5	5.8

Source: Registrar General's Department.

4.2 visits per pregnant mother during the prenatal period.

The National Sample Survey conducted by the Family
Health Bureau in 1977 revealed that 89.9 percent of
primagravida women in the sample had delivered in medical
institutions where satisfactory midwifery services were
available.   It was also revealed that the proportion of
deliveries conducted by untrained personnel was highest
among the high parity group: 31.7 as compared with 3.7
for primagravidas.   These observations would illustrate
the utilization and coverage of organized MCH services in
the country.   The reduction in the age specific mortality,
and mortality due to sepsis and toxemia was the result of
improved maternal care facilities provided during
prenatal, natal and postnatal periods.

Perinatal Mortality

In Sri Lanka, stillbirths are recorded only in
certain selected areas of which there are 82.   As a

Table 7. Infant and Neonatal Mortality

Year	Neonatal Mortality Rate	Infant Mortality Rate	Proportion to IMR
1940 – 44	76.1	133.0	57.1
1945 – 49	62.5	112.2	55.7
1950 – 54	45.4	77.0	58.9
1955 – 59	38.6	65.6	58.8
1960 – 64	33.2	55.0	60.4
1965 – 69	32.0	51.6	62.0
1970 – 74	29.7	47.2	62.9
1975 – 78	26.0	42.0	61.9

Source: Registrar General's Statistics.

result, available statistics do not reveal the complete picture. Stillbirths were high during the 1930s with a rate of about 83 per 1000 births. Thereafter the rate declined steadily reaching a level of 20 per 1000 births by 1978. Perinatal mortality showed a similar pattern, the rate declining from a level of 77 per 1000 births to 60 in 1966. It may be relevant to refer to a study conducted in one of the major maternity hospitals in the country where a similar pattern was observed: 2431 perinatal deaths were analyzed and the mortality observed was lowest in the under 30 age group, and was highest in the 40 and over age group. The study also revealed that the lowest mortality was among the primagravidas.

Neonatal mortality

Since 1940, a decrease of 66 percent was observed in neonatal mortality rates (Table 7). During the period 1940 to 1944, the mean neonatal mortality rate was 76.1 per 1000 live births. This showed an appreciable decline reaching the present rate of 26 per 1000 live births for the period 1975 to 1978.

Throughout the period 1940 to 1978, the neonatal mortality represented approximately 60 percent of the infant deaths. Furthermore it has been observed that 68 percent of all neonatal deaths occurred during the first week of life. The general pattern observed in other countries is reflected even in Sri Lanka where the decrease in infant mortality rate was mainly in the post neonatal period, while the proportion of early and late neonatal mortality remained consistently high.

The death rates from immaturity and debility, infec-

Table 8.   1966 Neonatal Mortality by Cause
(Deaths per 1000 Live Births)

Immaturity and congenital debility	18.69
Infections of newborn and convulsions	6.96
Tetanus, birth injuries, postnatal asphyxia	3.10
Congenital malformations	0.50
Other Causes	5.37
Total	34.62

Source: Registrar General's Department

tions of the newborn, convulsions and birth injuries were
high among the neonates in the early part of the century
(Table 8).   Deaths due to neonatal tetanus were reported
to be high during this period.

With improved aseptic techniques adopted by trained
health personnel at the time of delivery, together with
immunization of tetanus toxoid during pregnancy, the incidence of neonatal tetanus remarkably declined.   Mortality
rates due to infections of the newborn, birth trauma and
postnatal asphyxia have been reduced with improved maternal care facilities.   Inspite of better maternal care,
neonatal deaths due to immaturity still continues to be
high.

Breast feeding is encouraged and promoted.   Studies
undertaken have shown that 85 percent of the babies are
breast fed during the first six months and are thus
protected from exogenous infections.

The neonatal mortality in the plantation sector
increased during the period 1972 to 1975, and remains high
in comparison with the non-estate sector.   The factors
which contributed to this difference would probably be:
greater degree of malnutrition among mothers in the estate
sector;   lack of proper maternal care facilities in most
estates;   shortage of trained personnel (midwives);   and
low level of institutional births.

This unfavorable situation and disparities have been
taken into consideration in the launching of the estate
sector family health program.   A package of services is
ensured through the expansion of services to the
plantation sector.   It would not only reduce the
mortality, but would also help raise the general standard
of living enabling the under-served population to lead a
more socially and economically productive life.

Table 9.   Expectation of Life at Birth in Years.

Years	Male	Female	Female Excess Over Males
1920 - 22	32.7	30.7	-2.0
1945 - 47	46.8	44.7	-2.1
1952	57.6	55.5	-2.1
1962 - 64	63.3	63.7	+0.4
1967	64.8	66.9	+2.1
1971	64.2	67.1	+2.9

Source: Department of Census and Statistics.

Life Expectancy

Expectation of life at birth has shown a two-fold increase since 1920, reaching a level of 64.8 for males and 67.2 for females. It is of interest to note that during the early period (1920 to 1960), the life expectancy of males was higher than that of females, the difference narrowing gradually with the passage of time. The first time female life expectancy exceeded that of males was during the period 1962 to 1964. Thereafter the difference further increased up to 2.9 in 1971. These figures are comparable with those of developed countries.

CONCLUSION

The achievements in the field of maternal and neo-natal health are the results of a multitude of factors, such as expansion of health facilities; control of communicable diseases; improvement in literacy and educational attainments especially among females; introduction of food subsidies; and other socio-economic welfare measures adopted during the past five decades. These factors have contributed to the reduction of neo-natal and maternal mortality and fertility in Sri Lanka.

This brief presentation is a synoptic expression on the organization of family health services in the country along with some general achievements in the field of maternal and neonatal health recorded during the past few decades. While the attainment reached provides a certain degree of satisfaction, maternal and neonatal mortality still remains high when compared to that of developed contries.

The figures for infant and maternal mortality over

the past few years show apparent stagnation. It is
assumed that investments in neither medical nor health
care by themselves would bring about appreciable
improvement in maternal and neonatal mortality in the
near future. New strategies will have to be conceived and
new programs will have to be implemented. Multi-sectoral
and multi-disciplinary approaches may have to replace
conventional medical and curative interventions. Primary
health care with its major thrust on the family health
component would probably be the answer, not only to reduce
morbidity and mortality, but also to ensure a minimum and
a reasonable level of health for every individual enabling
him to optimize his potential for decent living.

REFERENCES

1. Department of Census and Statistics (1974): The
      Population of Sri Lanka (For the C.I.C.R.E.D).
2. Bulletin on Vital Statistics (1978).
3. Reports of the Registrar General, Sri Lanka.
4. E.S.C.A.P. Country Monograph Series 4: Population of
      Sri Lanka.
5. Director of Health Services: Reports. Sri Lanka.
6. Meegama SA (1980): Socio-economic determinants of
      infant and child mortality in Sri Lanka. An
      analysis of post-war experience. Scientific
      Report No. 8.
7. Rajanayagam S (1971): Perinatal mortality . Ceylon
      Medical Journal, December.
8. Perera PAD (1965): Maternal Health Science in Sri
      Lanka. Journal of Ceylon Public Health Association
      5, 1964-65.

CAUSES OF PERINATAL DEATHS AND PREVENTION

IN THE CONTEXT OF PRIMARY HEALTH CARE IN GHANA

S. Ofosu-Amaah

Professor of Pediatrics and Chairman of the
Department of Community Health
University of Ghana Medical School
Accra, Ghana

INTRODUCTION

In 1977, the World Health Assembly meeting in Geneva
decided upon a plan to achieve "Health for all by the Year
2000" through the strategy of Primary Health Care. The
international meeting in Alma Ata in 1978 (1) gave renewed
emphasis to the campaign for Primary Health Care (2, 3).

The concept of Primary Health Care envisioned a
countrywide system with a high degree of community
involvement to ensure social control of the health infrastructure. There should be mobilization of all possible
resources in the country - both material and personnel,
within and outside the health sector.

The strategy was to ensure that all members of
families, communities and their leaders as well as trained
health professionals have defined roles to play. There
has to be the selection and adaptation of technologies
appropriate for solving primary health care problems
within the given community (2, 3, 4).

In the preface to the FIGO publication "Maternity
Care in the World" (4), Dr. Mahler, the Director General
of the World Health Organization, noted that "in the
second half of the 20th century, ... some 80 percent of
women in certain countries in the Third World go through
pregnancy and delivery without receiving any form of care
from a health professional and most of these unfortunate

women rely almost exclusively on the services and goodwill of untrained traditional birth attendants (TBA) and village handywomen. ... If present trends in health services are allowed to continue, the future of some 80 percent of the world's children will be jeopardized, particularly in regard to physical and mental growth and development" (5). The majority of births take place outside institutions specially adapted for the purpose in developing countries. The immediate problems of the newborn are similarly handled.

Out of 110 million babies born alive each year in the developing world, 12 million do not survive the first year of life (6), 40 percent of whom die within 28 days of birth. Puffer and Serrano in their classic study in 10 South American countries reported that 36.1 percent of deaths in the first year of life happen within the neonatal period (7). In our own studies in Danfa (rural Ghana), the neonatal mortality rate was 55 per 1000 live births (8). This was about half of all the deaths in the first year of life. Such rates may be found in many developing countries. What make the data sobering indeed is the high fertility rates and high neonatal mortality rates in developing countries.

The major causes of neonatal mortality in the Third World are low birth weight, infections and birth injuries. Low birth weight is a serious and pervasive problem in the developing world. Of the estimated 21 million low birth weight infants born in 1975, 19 million were born in developing countries (9). The mortality rate of these infants may be as high as 20 times that of normal weight infants.

Neonatal infections are another important cause of death. In some parts of the world, neonatal tetanus may cause about 10 percent of neonatal deaths. The underlying factors for this are the poor techniques of untrained attendants, cultural factors, and the unavailability of the most simple services such as the immunization of pregnant women with tetanus toxoid. The combination of low birth weight and infection is obviously synergistic. Another problem related especially to low birth weight infants is poor temperature control, which can easily lead to hypothermia and death.

The advances made in the field of obstetrics and perinatal medicine during the past decade are enormous. The uses of oxygen, blood transfusion, antibiotics, fetal monitoring, fetocopy amniocentesis, ultrasound techniques,

etc., are yielding impressive results. There also is
better knowledge of the physiology of the newborn leading
to improved techniques of heat regulation, nutrition,
resuscitation and prevention of infection. Another area
of development has been in the field of epidemiology
relating to mothers and the children. The employment of
the "risk approach" as a managerial tool in this field is
a major advance.

IMPROVING NEONATAL CARE AT PRIMARY HEALTH CARE LEVEL

     To achieve the aim of the primary care movement with
respect to the problems of the newborn would demand the
application of technology that is appropriate for the
given community. So great are the variations between
countries and even within a country that there can be no
universal set of instructions. What we must not lose
sight of is the fact that advances, even the most basic in
character discovered many years ago and being used
routinely even within institutions in the developing
countries, have yet to reach millions of mothers and
infants in many developing countries. We are all so
mesmerized by the brillant technical innovation, that in
the race towards the use of futuristic equipment, we
forget the newborns in the villages who may never see a
trained health worker to prevent its perishing within a
few days after birth.

     For some countries within the developing world,
widespread primary health care services are within sight.
There may also be adequate numbers of trained health personnel. The issue here then is to determine how to raise
the level of care employing the Primary Health Care
strategy. For many countries on the other hand, the
situation is more intractable. Eighty percent of deliveries may be performed by the TBAs. The question is how
the recent knowledge and technology could reach all the
newborns in the least favored countries. This is where
the role of obstetricians and pediatricians will be
critical in achieving the aim of "health for all".

     Let me illustrate this point by an example from Ghana
of work of physicians in an Obstetrics and Child Health
center. In the Danfa rural area where we worked since
1970, we realized that our maternity unit, serving a population of 13,000, should be delivering from 600 to 700
babies per year. The midwives at the Health Center were
delivering only about 100 babies. We found that most of
the babies were being delivered by women and even men in

the villages. We decided to identify these birth attendants and learned about their practices. We identified 68
attendants of which only 5 were literate. We then
instituted a training program which was completed by 60 of
them. The aim was not to abandon their old knowledge and
supplant it with modern maternal care, but rather to
strengthen their areas of weakness and discourage harmful
practices. These included the identification of women at
risk, care of the cord, aseptic techniques, care of the
newborn, family planning and the encouragement of mothers
to have their babies immunized. Midwives provided the
training and supervision of TBAs which was not an easy
task. Eventually a manual of the process was produced and
it has been adopted by the Minister of Health. By 1972,
in a population of nearly 40,000, there were identified
263 TBAs and 26 assistants. Half of the TBAs were males
and only 6 percent were literate. A system of referral
from the TBAs to the Health Center and to the nearest
hospital was instituted. Records were kept with the help
of village school children or other literate villagers who
assisted the TBAs with the paper work.

The physician or medical expert has many roles to
play in the program of raising the level of neonatal care
in the developing countries. They can provide the inspiration, be the researcher, teacher, planner and evaluator
of the program. The first step is for the physician to
absorb the philosophy of the primary health care movement,
and be enthused by the vision of "health for all" by the
end of this century. The next step is for him to find out
about the state of neonatal care at the primary health
care level - in the home and in the community. This will
entail studies involving the use of epidemiological
methods, knowledge, attitude and practices of the existing
primary health care practitioners, TBAs, community health
aides, etc. He will, on identifying these practitioners,
understand their constraints and realize what technology
and new knowledge he might have to introduce. Nothing is
more chastening for the physician than to work at the
local level under the same limitations as the local practitioners. It is easy to theorize as to what improvement
should occur at that level. The final test is to
experience the system and be able to apply scientific
principles, and to make improvements that would be sus-
tainable by the local attendants when the expert
withdraws.

These studies may be elaborate or simple depending on
local circumstances but they should lead to several decisions. These would include a determination of which

workers in the field to cooperate with, what new knowledge and technology to adopt, what support systems to build up, what process of management to employ, what resources will be needed if the scheme is to be countrywide, and the plan of development of the total system.

Having determined which groups to train, the methods of training should be evolved. It might mean the production of manuals, audiovisual aids, etc., depending on local circumstances. The training would include the actual technical features of improved neonatal care as well as an understanding of important preventive measures such as the immunization of women with tetanus toxoid and the critical importance of antenatal care, birth spacing, and nutrition. It should include training in the very important areas of adequate data collection, evaluation of any program and feedback to the local practitioners. The support system, including communications, transportation, referral, and the movement of supplies should be carefully studied. The adoption of appropriate technology is not merely the introduction of new equipment and technical procedures but also the application of improved managerial arrangements. Nothing will stifle the development of the primary health care system quicker than the lack of a continuous contact to the higher levels of referral of cases and problems and an expectant and considerate attitude of health workers at the district hospital. There should be adequate and sustained arrangements for supporting the primary health care level, for feedback, and for visits of supervision and teaching.

Other groups that will need training or coordination in primary health care are medical students, residents in training, and all other health professionals during their formative training. It is indeed necessary that these groups spend part of their time working at the primary health care level.

The development of improved techniques for primary health care is continuous and requires that experiences be shared between different parts of the same country, and also among health workers from different countries. This will also involve publications such as the type produced presently by ARTAG for diarrheal diseases.

CONCLUSION

The task of improving the level of health care and ensuring that all newborns are reached is a daunting one but it can be done if the well-trained experts in maternal and child health would work with those at the primary health care level. These medical experts have to adapt new procedures and methods appropriate to care at that level, but they need to have a vision of a world where the unnecessary suffering of the poor and those distant from centers of excellence, can be largely alleviated. A century ago, Rudolf Virchow said that doctors are the natural advocates of the poor. This is still true today and the ferment that we can achieve is even more urgently needed.

REFERENCES

1. Alma Ata (1978): Primary Health Care.
2. World Health Organization (1981): WHO Chronicle, 35:4, Geneva.
3. World Health Organization (1981): Global strategy for health for all by the year 2000. WHO, Geneva.
4. FIGO (1976): Maternity care in the world. Second Edition, FIGO,ACM, England.
5. World Health Organization (1976): New trends and approaches in delivery of maternal and child care in health services. WHO Technical Report Series 600, Geneva.
6. Population Reference Bureau (1980): World Population Data Sheet, Washington, D.C.
7. Puffer RR, Serano CV (1973): Patterns of mortality in childhood. PAHO Scientific Publication No. 262, Washington, D.C.
8. Danfa Project Final Report (1979): Accra and Los Angeles.
9. Rooth G, Engstrom L (1977): Perinatal care in developing countries. Uppsala.

MATERNAL MORTALITY AT IFE UNIVERSITY

TEACHING HOSPITAL COMPLEX

C. O. Adeoye

Department of Obstetrics and Gynaecology,
Faculty of Health Sciences, University of Ife
Ile-Ife, Nigeria

INTRODUCTION

Although the past has seen a steady decline in
maternal mortality rate near the so-called "irreducible
minimum" in the developed countries (7), maternal mortality rate in Nigeria is still alarmingly high (8, 12).
Lagos had a rate of 1600/100,000 in 1977. Certain observations became immediately apparent. First, is the fact
that organized antenatal care is not yet universally
acceptable to all our communities. Second, even where
this is acceptable, adequate facilities are not often
accessible. As a result, hospitals tend to be looked upon
as a place of last resort, where sick patients from
distant points, after surmounting several logistical
problems, converge in a state of extremis. Finally, the
inadequate facilities do not meet the needs of such
patients.

The objective of this study is to examine the causes
of maternal deaths at the two obstetrical units of the Ife
University Teaching Hospital Complex, in order to identify
as well as suggest solutions for the key problems in the
antenatal health care delivery system of the Teaching
Hospitals Complex.

METHODS

All cases of maternal deaths (excluding deaths from
abortion) at Ife State Hospital (Ile-Ife), and Wesley

Guild Hospital (Ilesha), were reviewed over an 18-month
period from January 1979 to June 1980. Where the case
notes were not available, the causes of death were obtained from the ward register and diagnostic index from
the medical records department.

        Because of paucity of pathologists in these institu-
tions, only limited autopsies were performed to confirm
the anatomical causes of death, except where there is
reasonable doubt.

RESULTS

        During the review period, there was a total of 6710
births, 6308 of which were live births and 402 were stillbirths. During the same period, there were 66 maternal
deaths (11.7 per 1000 live births); nineteen (28.8 percent) were booked patients and forty-seven (71.2 percent)
were unbooked patients. In the context of this study, the
booked patients were those who registered at the antenatal
clinic and had made at least three clinic visits prior to
delivery. The unbooked patients had no antenatal care in
any maternity center but were seen for the first time
because of complications at or near term, or during labor.

        Table 1 shows the incidence of maternal deaths by
age. Most deaths occurred in mothers within the ages of
20 to 34. Table 2 compares the incidence of deaths by
parity. More deaths occurred among multigravidae than
among primagravidae, whether booked or unbooked.

Causes of Maternal Deaths

        Hemorrhage is the leading cause of maternal death and
is responsible for 18 deaths (27.2 percent). Antepartum
hemorrhage claimed 6 lives while postpartum hemorrhage
claimed 12. Mortality from this cause was influenced by
parity and by the amount of blood for transfusion. This
finding agrees with the series in the Western States (8)
and in the Eastern States (12) where hemorrhage was also
found to be the leading cause of death.

        Sepsis is the next leading cause and occurred in 14
cases, 10 unbooked and 4 booked: ten cases following vaginal deliveries and 4 cases following caesarean section.

        Eclampsia is third and occurred mostly among primi-
gravidae admitted as emergencies in labor. Factors which
determined survival or death were parity, location of

Table 1.   Incidence of Maternal Deaths by Age.

Age (Years)	Booked	Percent	Unbooked	Percent
Under 15	0	0	0	0
15-19	2	10.52	3	6.38
20-24	4	21.05	12	25.53
25-29	6	31.57	13	27.66
30-34	6	31.57	10	21.28
35-39	1	5.26	5	10.68
40+	0	0	4	8.51
Total	19	100	47	100

Table 2.   Parity in Unbooked and Booked Patients

Parity	Booked	Percent	Unbooked	Percent
Primigravidae	5	26.32	13	27.65
Multigravidae	14	73.68	26	55.33
Unknown	0	0	8	17.02
Total	19	100	47	100

onset of convulsion (home or hospital), total number of convulsive episodes and type of treatment offered. The 11 deaths from eclampsia occurred among primigravidae. Hospital onset of convulsions were much easier to control than those which commenced at home. Most of those who were admitted with frank eclampsia made poor responses to standard medication and nursing care.

Obstructed labor is the fourth cause and occurred in 10 cases, 7 unbooked and 3 booked cases. Five of the unbooked patients died undelivered having obstructed labor with uterine rupture. The two other cases of obstructed labor died during emergency caesarean section. Three booked cases died; two following caesarean section for unsuccessful vacuum extraction and the third case died following spontaneous vaginal delivery of a frank stillbirth from an occult ruptured uterus.

Tetanus is the fifth cause occurring in 5 cases, 3 unbooked and 2 booked cases. All the 3 unbooked cases were multigravidae. The immunization status of the women were not known. In most of these cases, membranes had

ruptured at home in the village several days before ar-
rival at the hospital. Unsterile cloth, which had been
used to plug the vagina or lower perineum was the most
likely source of infection. Mortality from this has
claimed almost 95 percent of all the cases admitted.

Infectious hepatitis was the most important single
cause of maternal death. There were 3 deaths (4.76 percent) from this cause. Most patients were admitted
already in a state of hepatic coma. The fatal nature of
infectious hepatitis may be related to the nutritional
background of the patients.

Cardiac and pulmonary diseases caused 3 deaths (4.1
percent) indicating these as rare causes of maternal
deaths in this institution. In contrast, maternal death
from these causes are high in England and Wales. The
Ministry of Health reports on maternal death in England
and Wales covering the years 1958 to 1960, analyzed over
2,300,000 registered births and 928 deaths of women
ascribed to pregnancy and childbirth. Cardiac disease
caused 66 out of 928 deaths (7.1 percent) while pulmonary
embolism caused 132 out of the 928 deaths (14.1 percent).

Anemia caused 2 deaths (3 percent). It is the most
common major antenatal complication in this country. The
maternal mortality from anemia in this study is low
compared to the observations of Ojo and Savage (9) that
anemia accounted for 34 maternal deaths (18.6 percent) at
University College Hospital in Ibadan. Primary mortality
from this cause is rare but the anemic woman readily
succumbs to hemorrhage and infection.

DISCUSSION

It has been shown very clearly that maternal deaths
among unbooked patients far outnumber those among the
booked patients. Many factors are responsible for the
lack of antenatal care by many of our patients. First,
some patients live so far away from the hospital that they
cannot cope with the logistics of frequent clinic visits.
Second, some are too poor to afford even the meager hospital cost for antenatal care. Third, an unreasonable fear
of caesarean section exists in this society, and there are
patients who feel that participation in antenatal care
could culminate in a caesarean section. Finally, some
patients hold certain beliefs about childbirth, which they
fear might be ridiculed as superstition by hospital staff.

Table 3.   Causes of Maternal Deaths in Booked and Unbooked
           Patients.

Causes	Booked	Unbooked	Total
Hemorrhhage	2	16	18
Sepsis	4	10	14
Eclampsia	2	9	11
Obstructed Labor	3	7	10
Tetanus	2	3	5
Infectious Hepatitis	1	2	3
Cardiac Disease	2	0	2
Anemia	2	0	2
Pulmonary Embolism	1	0	1
Total	19	47	66

Maternal mortality was compiled at Ife University
Teaching Hospital Complex from January 1979 to June 1980.
Maternal mortality rate was found to be 11.7 per 1000 live
births. The rate among unbooked patients was found to be
significantly higher than those among booked. It was also
found to be higher among multigravidae. Hemorrhage was
the leading cause of death followed by sepsis and eclampsia. Causes for these alarmingly high rate of mortality
include lack of antenatal care due to some logistical
problems, poverty, fear of caesarean section and
superstition.

The establishment of adequately equipped rural health
centers and incorporation of rural midwives in the present
health care delivery system may help to alleviate some of
the problems. Educational campaign by the society of
Obstetricians and Gynaecologists of Nigeria cannot be over
emphasized.

CONCLUSION

It is interesting to note that most of the unbooked
cases in this series were first managed by quacks before
referral in extremis to the hospital. Given the approximately 300 obstetricians practising in Nigeria today, it
is clear that they alone cannot provide the necessary
care, hence quacks attempt to fill the need. Emphasis
should be laid on the role of the rural midwives in the
present health care delivery system.   It should be recognized that they are often forced to practise at a level
beyond what they had been trained for. Teaching hospitals

should take the initiative for periodic refresher courses for their training.

Providing rural health centers with well trained personnel and ambulatory service to hospitals, coupled with improvement in road network will encourage patients to seek quick medical attention in maternity centers during need.

With the introduction of free health care in this community, it is hoped that poverty would cease to be a barrier to antenatal care. Health providers should educate the public to the fact that caesarean section is not a sign of reproductive failure. Health education, including sex education should be introduced into the elementary and secondary school curricula.

The practising obstetrician should convince them-selves of the need for reduction of maternal mortality by well-timed caesarean section. Lastly, the Society of Obstetricians and Gynecologist of Nigeria should launch an educational campaign through radio, television and public symposia.

REFERENCES

1.   Akinkugke A (1972): Postpartum hemorrhage in Ife State Hospital. Nigerian Med J, 2:206.
2.   Ampofo DA (1965): West African Med J, 18:75.
3.   Balanchandonn V (1975): Maternal mortality in Kaduna. Nigerian Med J, 5:366-370.
4.   Companion to Medical Studies, 2:34, 3:14.
5.   Lawson JB and Stewart DB (1967): In: Obstetrics and Gynaecology in the Tropics, First Edition, Arnold, London, 121-185.
6.   Lucas AO: In: A short textbook of preventive medicine for the tropics, 11.
7.   Ministry of Health Report on Public Health and Medical Subjects: Report on confidential enquiries into maternal deaths in England and Wales, 1958-1960, 1967-1969. Report No. 108, 119, Hoy SO, London.
8.   Oduntan S and Odullami VB (1975): Maternal mortality in Western Nigeria. Trop Geog Trop Med, 27:313-316.
9.   Ojo OA and Savage VY (1974): A ten year series of maternal mortality rate in the University College Hospital, Ibadan, Nigeria. Am J Obst Gyn, 118:517-522.

10. Okoisor AT (1978): Maternal mortality in Lagos. A
     5-year survey, 1970-74. Nigerian Med J,
     8:349-354.
11. Olutayo O (1979): Causes of maternal deaths in
     Lagos. Medilar, 4:44-47.
12. Waboso MF (1975): The causes of maternal mortality in
    the Eastern States of Nigeria. Nigerian Med J,
    3:99-104.

FAMILY PLANNING STRATEGIES FOR THE '80s

N. Sadik

Assistant Executive Director
United Nations Fund for Population Activities
New York, U. S. A.

INTRODUCTION

The past two decades have witnessed widespread acceptance of the concept of family planning as well as innovative integrations for the delivery of information and services (1-3). Substantial declines in fertility have occurred in countries where effective family planning programs have been implemented. Achievements in this sector, however, have been far from uniform either across countries or within countries. At present there is a substantial unmet need for family planning and the number of couples of reproductive age is expected to increase by 70 percent between 1980 and 2000. During the coming decades, programs will have to address the quantitative challenge of an increased target population and the qualitative challenge of responding appropriately to the needs of this group.

This presentation surveys the family planning horizon, reviewing how the sector has evolved and identifying directions for the future. The orientation, experience and accomplishments of the United Nations Fund for Population Activities (UNFPA), in its support for the various aspects of family planning in the different regions of the world, are highlighted.

FAMILY PLANNING HORIZON

The acceptability of the concept of family planning has increased markedly during the last twenty years. Of 158 countries responding the United Nations Fourth

455

Inquiry Among Governments on Population and Development,
118 had adopted laws or policies favorable to family
planning or supporting family planning either through the
public or private sector. Of 132 developing countries, 66
have family planning programs; 35 have adopted programs
for demographic purposes, 31 for health or humanitarian
reasons. Approximately 92 percent of the population of
the developing world live in countries which support
family planning.

        A number of changes have taken place in the adminis-
trative and delivery system dimensions of family planning.
Single purpose, vertical programs have given way to more
thorough integrations in the health network. Concerted
efforts have been made to include family planning components in various development initiatives. Service delivery
systems, once wedded to the concept of a stationary clinic
staffed by highly trained medical personnel, now place
increasing emphasis on outreach services rendered by
paramedical and auxiliary workers in village locales.

        From a demographic point of view, there is ample
evidence that family planning programs have had a notable
impact. Countries which have implemented effective programs have achieved substantial fertility declines even in
the absence of advances in economic development;
Indonesia, China and Sri Lanka are cases in point.

        Over the past decade, the health and human rights
aspects of family planning have also been recognized.
Indeed one of the most significant benefits of the practice of family planning is its positive influence on the
health of women and their children, and thus on the well-
being of the entire family. In the broadest sense, family
planning contributes to family health - that is to the
mental and social well-being of mothers, fathers, and
their children - by enabling couples to achieve their
reproductive goals and therefore some measure of control
over the pattern and direction of their lives. In the
narrow sense, family planning helps to eliminate the
health hazards for both mother and infant that are associated with closely spaced pregnancies and with births to
women either too early or too late in their reproductive
cycle. The time interval between successive pregnancies
and childbirth, the age of women at childbearing, and the
number of children in the family are crucial factors known
to have a negative influence on maternal and child mortality and morbidity. Indeed most programs recognize this
contribution of family planning to health status by
linking family planning services to the maternal and child

health care delivery system and by making family planning
services available in the primary health care context.

        In view of the health and demographic benefits as
well as the human rights dimension, it is essential that
family planning be within the reach of all couples desiring such services. Yet, as we all know, this is hardly
the case. As we survey achievements to date in family
planning, the record at best is a mixed one. The finding
of the World Fertility Survey indicated that there is
still a vast unmet need for family planning. The data
from many countries show that there is a considerable gap
between those who know of at least one contraceptive
method and those who know where to obtain family planning
services, as well as a gap between the proportion of women
who know where services are available and yet, possibly
because they deem the services "unsuitable" elect not to
use them. Thus in charting the course for family planning
in the '80s, we must design and pursue strategies that
respond to the key issues of availability of services and
acceptability of services.

The Orientation of the Fund

        UNFPA's activities in the family planning sector
have been predicated on its broad mandate to promote
understanding of the population question and to extend
assistance for population endeavors in developing countries. Keenly aware of the sensitivity and complexity of
the population issue, the Fund has stressed the need for
neutrality, flexibility and innovation in its dealings
with recipient countries. UNFPA has never endorsed any
particular approach to population problems but rather, it
has provided assistance to those aspects that a requesting
country deemed important and which were within the bounds
of its mandate. During the course of its 12 year
existence, the Fund has followed two major principles in
extending assistance for population activities: that
every nation has the sovereign right to determine its own
population policy; and, that each individual couple has
the right to determine the size of its family. These
principles have been affirmed in various resolutions of
the General Assembly and were amplified in the World Popu-
tion Plan of Action (Bucharest, 1974) which held that
freedom to determine responsibly the number and spacing of
children and access to the information, education, and the
means to do so was a basic human right. In accord with its
mandate, UNFPA may support family planning programs
undertaken for demographic, health or humanitarian goals.

Experience of the Fund

        Under the rubric family planning, the UNFPA has
supported the conventional and the innovative. Under the
former, one could list: the strengthening of rural health
infrastructures to improve Maternal Child Health and
Family Planning Services; the provision of contraceptive
supplies; and, the training of medical and auxiliary
personnel. More innovative undertakings include:
comprehensive communication support for family planning
programs (Thailand); training traditional birth attendants to deliver services (Jordan, Honduras, Pakistan,
Maldives, Afghanistan); integration of family planning
into community structures (Gambia, Tanzania); and
research on cultural values and population policy
(Philippines, India, Kenya and the Dominican Republic).
The Fund has been in the forefront in calling attention to
access to family planning information and services as a
basic human right.

        UNFPA has extended assistance in family planning at
the global, national and local level. It has supported
biomedical research to improve contraceptive methods; it
has strengthened national programs; and, it has promoted
the integration of family planning into the community/
village setting. The Fund has been prudent in sensing and
respecting the variation among nations regarding the
"tempo of acceptance" of the family planning concept.
Because of its neutral stance and respect for the
sovereignty of nations on population issues, the Fund,
through activities such as basic data collection, has been
able to educate countries as to the dimensions of their
population situation and to acquaint them with the range
of policy options available. This low-keyed approach has
been responsible for introducing family planning into many
countries where it was initially viewed as an alien if not
hostile concept.

Future Challenges and Strategies

        Although the rate of population growth has slowed
down, approximately 2 billion people will be added to the
world's poppulation between now and 2000. About 90
percent of this increase will occur in the developing
countries. By the year 2000, the number of couples in
the reproductive age will be about 70 percent larger than
today's target population. If the health, demographic,
and humanitarian goals of family planning are to be realized during the coming decades, programs will have to
respond to the quantitative challenge of an increased

target population and to the qualitative challenge of
meeting appropriately the needs of this group. Family
planning strategies will have to address the following
considerations:

(a) designing programs which reflect the country- specific
    situation, level of development, extent of infrastruc-
    ture, and political and religious sensitivities;
    programs will have to be sufficiently flexible to
    permit some degress of decentralized decision-making;
(b) emphasizing the user perspective and assuring that
    program approaches are compatible with the socio-
    cultural values of the target population;
(c) increasing the density of service delivery points and
    informatin channels;
(d) improving program managment techniques; and
(e) devising ways of linking family planning with other
    development initiatives.

    In delineating family planning strategies for the
'80s and beyond, it is useful to look back on past
experience in order to identify the distinguishing characteristics of successful programs, so that these aspects
may, to the extent possible, be incorporated in family
planning initiatives in the future. Some readily identi-
fiable factors include: a high degree of political
commitments, efficient management, program interventions
closely tailored and responsive to the needs and values of
the target population, and ongoing monitoring and evaluation of program inputs. Past experience has certainly
confirmed the validity of the "community approach". The
more a program can be incorporated into community life,
utilizing existing community organizations and networks of
communication, the greater are its chances for success.
Although the merits of this apprach are widely acknowledged, its complexity is also recognized. There is no set
pattern for implementing the community approach. Indeed
it must be adapted to particular circumstances and
modified according to the needs of the locality.

    In designing and implementing programs, greater
emphasis must be placed on the user perspective. More
attention should be given to the psychosocial factors
which determine the acceptability and hence, the acceptance and use of contraception. Efforts must be made to
make services more available in outlying areas and care
must be taken to assure the quality of these services.
Improvements in contraceptive technology are essential.
On a global basis, research must be pursued to devise new
contraceptive methods that will be safe, effective and

acceptable. Such research should also investigate ways to
increase the effective use of existing techniques, including traditional methods. The United Nations Fund for
Population Activities is currently undertaking a comprehensive review of needs and opportunities in the field of
contraceptive research and development in order to discern
how it can best facilitate initiatives in this field.

CONCLUSION

        The challenge facing the family planning sector is a
formidable one - namely, to make information and suitable
services more readily available to a target population
whose size will increase substantially during the next two
decades. We at UNFPA are well aware of the magnitude of
this challenge and will assist to the extent possible
under the terms of our mandate and as permitted by our
resources.

        The world of the International Association for
Maternal and Neonatal Health, and in particular the
discussions of the scientific sessions of this Congress,
will make substantial contributions to the realization of
the humanitarian, health, and demographic goals of family
planning. We all share the vision of the day when family
planning and maternal and child health programs will be
easily available to all in need of these services and the
benefits of such programs will be reflected in improved
levels of living within the family and the community.

REFERENCES

1. UNFPA (19981): Inventory of population projects in
        developing countries around the world, 1979-80.
        New York.
2. UNFPA (1981): 1980 Report by the Executive Director
        of the United Nations Fund for Population
        Activities. New York.
3. Sadik N (1980): Family planning. Improving the
        health of women and their children. In: The
        Draper Fund Report. October.

MATERNAL AND NEONATAL HEALTH STRATEGIES IN INTERNATIONAL

HEALTH PROGRAMS WITHIN THE CONTEXT OF PRIMARY HEALTH CARE

Y. S. Kim

WHO Program Coordinator for the Philippines
World Health Organization
Western Pacific Regional Office
Manila, Philippnes

INTRODUCTION

The past decade has witnessed mounting world-wide concern about the rapidly changing family and population dynamics and their effects on health everywhere. There are still millions of people without access to any kind of health care and who are seeking out a meager existence in adverse and unstable socio-economic and political conditions, including rapid population growth.

The International Conference on Primary Health Care held in Alma-Ata (USSR) provided a forum for all those concerned with this crucial problem.

At Alma-Ata (1) and in recent World Health Assemblies (2, 3), the nations of the world have set the target of attaining an acceptable level of health for all by the year 2000, so that all peoples of the world can live socially and economically productive lives. They also endorsed the principles and approaches of primary health care as the key for achieving this goal. Underlying primary health care is the conviction that health and development are closely interrelated.

The importance of maternal and child health (MCH) within this approach can hardly be over-emphasized. The basic principles underlying the overall strategies and policies for primary health care are fundamental to the concepts of maternal and child health care: the intra-

461

sectoral approach, the need for total coverage, the participation of individual families and communities, the maximum use of existing resources such as traditional birth attendants, women's groups and school teachers, and so on.

As the major and essential part of action for maternal and child health takes place within the family, the emphasis of MCH care within primary health care must be to support community and family self-reliance, especially regarding the family's responsibilities in child-rearing, child-bearing and self-care.

FAMILY HEALTH PROGRAM RELATED TO MATERNAL AND NEONATAL HEALTH PROBLEMS

WHO works in close collaboration with the other United Nations bodies, in particular UNICEF, UNFPA, FAO, UNESCO, bilateral agencies and nongovernmental organizations concerned, such as the International Children's Center, the International Pediatric Association, and the International Planned Parenthood Federation.

WHO supports activities to promote more efficient and effective methods for the integration of maternal and child health care in all aspects of health development programs, increased community participation in maternal and child health/family planning activities, better approaches to multidisciplinary and multisectoral program development, and the inclusion of traditional practitioners in health delivery systems. The application of research findings, especially on new or adapted maternal and child health/family planning technologies is stressed.

Training

This continues to be a major part of the maternal and child health program, as part of WHO's support to national efforts in strengthening national institutions and self-reliance in health manpower development. WHO's global and regional training activities in comprehensive maternal and child health/family planning are being oriented to reflect training more appropriate to the health problems and needs of the vast majority of the population. Training will take place in regional and national institutions in developing countries.

The program of teacher-training in comprehensive maternal and child health includes activities which are

tailored to the specific needs of national programs. The
focus in all regions is on health service needs, and
priority is given to the training of those involved in
health service delivery. Emphasis is placed on activities
dealing with the synthesis of knowledge and exchange of
information on physical and psychosocial development in
childhood and adolescence, including nutritional aspects,
for use in the planning and formulation of practical
strategies for timely intervention programs. There are
six WHO collaborating centers working on this subject in
four regions.

Growth Chart

Local adaptation of the WHO "growth chart" to measure
child growth and development is also promoted. The chart
is being used as a practical tool in many areas by primary
health care workers as well as families. Studies are
carried out on the epidemiology and social implications of
low birth weight; the results will be utilized for the
development of practical intervention strategies both
during and before pregnancy in order to prevent the high
incidence of low birth weight and resulting morbidity and
mortality. WHO also is studying the feasibility at the
local level of using birth weight as an indicator for
assessing maternal health and for predicting the future
health of the child.

Breast Feeding

The WHO collaborative study on breast feeding, carried out in nine countries has provided valuable knowledge
on the patterns of breast feeding in various socio-economic groups in different regions of the world. The results
of this study are used for the promotion of appropriate
infant feeding. The second phase of the WHO collaborative
study, dealing with the quality and composition of breast
milk is in process. This program of breast feeding is
complementary to the research program in nutrition
focusing on the weaning period.

The World Health Assembly in 1981 adopted the International Code of Marketing of Breastmilk substitutes, and
WHO actively cooperates with all parties concerned in the
implementation and monitoring of the International Code at
country, regional and global levels.

Nutrition

The new focus of the nutrition activities is the

improvement of nutrition and health through action at the
community level, and as far as possible with local resources. The major thrust is to develop new knowledge and
approaches and to translate them into operational activities within the framework of primary health care. This is
done at the local level by national workers and institutions. The Organization is cooperating with countries in
four priority areas:

(a)   extending the use of nutritional surveillance
      systems;
(b)   integrating nutritional activities within primary
      health care;
(c)   applying measures to control specific nutritional
      deficiencies;
(d)   developing national multisectoral food and nutrition
      policies and programs within the framework of
      national development plans, in collaboration with
      other agencies.

Health Services Research

        Research in maternal and child health/family planning
is in line with the primary health care approach. One
example is the collaborative program on "risk approach" in
MCH care which started in 1974. By using risk indicators,
studies first establish the interrelationships between
priority health problems and communities and individuals.
This epidemiological knowledge is used to prepare new
strategies, which are then tested in "real life" before
being proposed for local or national application. Thus
the "risk approach" is a good example of health services
research in that it is action-oriented and a tool for
change in the health care system. Participation of health
administrators, health staff and the community in this
research ensures maximum utilization of the findings. In
addition, this program has a built-in component for both
training and institute strengthening.

Appropriate Technology

        The development of appropriate technology and prac-
tical guidelines relating to the management of the
complications of pregnancy and childbirth, and of specific, prevalent diseases of childhood, is also a focus of
activity. The findings of the WHO collaborative study on
the epidemiology of the hypertensive disorders of pregnancy will be followed through intervention programs,
particularly as part of maternal and child health
activities within primary health care.

Since the majority of the world's babies are born in developing countries and delivery takes place at home, a program of activities has been initiated for the development of appropriate technology for perinatal care to be applied in the home and small rural maternity units.

WHO is collaborating with 94 countries which are expanding their immunization programs in order to reduce significantly the incidence of the common infectious diseases of childhood. Special efforts are being made to train maternal and child health workers in immunization techniques in order to integrate these preventive measures in existing health services systems.

Since 1978 the Organization has been steadily expanding its activities in the field of diarrheal diseases control. In the short term, the WHO program seeks to reduce diarrhea-related morbidity, mortality and malnutrition in children through the promotion of oral rehydration therapy and improved child care practices, and to develop new tools and techniques for better control through research.

Intersectoral Programs

Technical cooperation with and among countries is promoted for the development of intersectoral programs for children and youth, the enhancement of the health and status of women and their equitable participation in development, and social support measures for the family, including organized system of day-care in factories or industrial facilities, neighborhood centers, cooperative self-help women's groups, and family-based day-care facilities for children of working parents in which older members of the family take part.

CONCLUSION

WHO pursues activities related to women and family health in collaboration with countries and relevant United Nations bodies as part of the United Nations Decade for Women (1975 to 1985).

REFERENCES

1.   World Health Organization (1978):   Primary Health
        Care, Alma Ata Report of the International
        Conference on Primary Health Care.   WHO Health
        for All Series No. 1, Geneva.
2.   World Health Organization (1980):   Towards a better
        future.   Maternal and Child Health, Geneva.
3.   World Health Organization (1980):   The incidence of
        low birth rate: a critical review of available
        information by the Division of Family Health.
        World Health Statistics Quarterly 33:3.

DEVELOPMENT OF MANPOWER FOR APPLICATION OF EXISTING

TECHNOLOGIES WHICH ARE FEASIBLE WITHIN PRIMARY HEALTH CARE

G. J. Ebrahim

Reader in Tropical Child Care
Institute of Child Health
London, United Kingdom

INTRODUCTION

Even though the term "primary health care" implies front-line or first contact care, it has a much broader meaning, the evolution of which can be traced back to the 1960s. The factors contributing to the present concept of primary health care are the following (1-4):

(a) the changing theories of development which now focus on the development of human capital as distinct from physical structures;
(b) the growing disenchantment with the hospital-based Western model of medical care utilizing expensive technologies; and
(c) the successes of several developing nations as well as of small-scale projects in achieving remarkable improvements in the health of their people utilizing alternative simple technologies.

A great deal of ill-health and mortality in the developing world is due to the synergism between infection and malnutrition. Their roots lie in the life-styles of the people. Hence involvement of the community in health-related activities has been a major innovation in many of the successful programs of health care. All these experiences hold out the hope of rapidly expanding health coverage from the present level of less than 20 percent to universal care for many developing nations.

In the context of these trends and developments, the

basic components of a primary health care program are:

(a) universal coverage especially of those made vulnerable
    because of biological, socio-economic or cultural
    reasons;
(b) community awareness of prevalent health problems and
    active involvement in their control;
(c) improved nutrition, safe water and basic sanitation;
(d) immunization against major infectious diseases;
(e) maternal and child care including family planning;
(f) treatment of common illnesses and injuries; and
(g) provision of essential chemotherapeutic agents.

POLITICAL, SOCIAL AND CULTURAL BASIS OF PRIMARY HEALTH
CARE

        Since primary health care is concerned with correct-
ing the existing disparities in health programs, there are
complex political, social and economic issues to be
addressed. There is the disparity between expenditure and
need. More than three-fourths of the health budgets of
many countries are being spent on hospitals which by their
very nature, serve the urban populations and cater for
diseases, whereas the needs are for preventive and
promotive care. There is the second disparity of resource
distribution versus population distribution. The third
disparity is between population growth which is rural and
the growth in services which is mainly urban. To correct
these disparities, governments face impossible choices.
These are the choices of reducing the gap between the
"have" and the "have-nots", that of making preferential
allocation of resources to the social periphery to ensure
full health coverage instead of hospital-based specialist-
oriented services for the elite, and that of ensuring the
necessary reforms in medical education so that the health
profession can be more supportive of auxiliaries and
village-level workers. To give an example, in Tanzania,
after a critical evaluation of health programs in 1970,
the budget allocation for hospitals was reduced by 50 to
60 percent from 1971 to 72, so that curative services came
to receive 20 to 25 percent of the total health expenditure compared to 60 percent in previous years. From 1973
to 75, allocation for hospitals was further reduced to a
low of 12 to 15 percent, and there was a simultaneous
increase in training facilities for auxiliaries. In
short, primary health care is not merely a matter of
developing a new cadre of workers, nor even of expanding
the existing services. It is more a matter of setting up
a national dialogue to create awareness and to generate

a national will which will enable the society to take a number of rather difficult decisions concerning provisions of health care.

Challenges in Training

If health services are to change their focus from rare syndromes to prevention of common illnesses, from intensive care units to rural homes and urban slums, then a new breed of health workers is necessary all through the medical hierarchy. Only then will the formal health system become supportive of the front-line workers in the community. To what extent an elitist profession can be supportive of the auxiliary and the village health worker will depend upon training in team-work, as well as the prevailing philosophical and ethical values within the profession and society. But there are certian obvious deficiencies which require immediate attention.

In the average district of a developing country, it is estimated that there will be between 75 and 100 auxiliaries and twice that number of village health workers and birth attendants. They need administrative and logistic support besides regular training and refresher courses. A district level co-ordinator or Maternal and Child Health (MCH) specialist who can provide these needs is at present lacking in most countries. Besides being a competent professional and a manager, such a person needs to have skills in communication, especially with the illiterate. One basic requirement of all programs in community health is the creation of a social framework from which such programs can draw their strength and eventaully become self-reliant. Hence one important skill of the MCH co-ordinator will be the ability to establish a continuing dialogue with the community. The long-term objective of such a dialogue will be the evolution of responsibility with eventual self-reliance for the community.

Student Selection

In all countries, student selection is based on academic performance. Entrance requirements for medical and nursing schools rarely take into account the individual's aptitude for serving the community. Secondly, there are unbreachable academic barriers between different cadres of the profession. Only a few countries have succeeded in lowering these barriers. For example in Tanzania, a rural medical aid whose basic education is only up to primary school level followed by two years of training in health sciences can qualify as a medical

assistant after short in-service training without having
to go for secondary school education. A promising medical
assistant can by-pass the entrance requirements and enter
the medical school to qualify as a physician. Several
characteristics of the primary health worker have been
identified as being essential for their success and must
be taken into account in the strategy of health man-power
development. The most important among these characteristics is the fact that the primary care worker is residing
within the community and participates in the social and
cultural life. He or she is responsible to the community
and not to a distant government official.

TRAINING

     Even though the above issues related to the objec-
tives of primary care are important, success or failure
hinges upon two vital elements, namely, the training of
the workers and the professional support they receive on a
continuing basis. Training has received a great boost in
recent years because of the development of standardized
technologies and regimens for dealing with some of the
main health problems. For example, the technology of oral
rehydration, of assessing nutrition, of prenatal care in
the prevention of low birth weight and neonatal tetanus,
and so on. At the same time there has been a marked progress in the technology of the cold chain as well as
standardization of this technology together with new developments in the manufacture of vaccines. This improvement
in our knowledge and standardization makes delegation of
health care possible to a minimally trained member of the
health team. Similar application of simplified and standardized technology in sanitation, in protection of water
supply, in agriculture and veterinary sciences is urgently
needed to bring about truly integerated development and
increased productivity.

CONCLUSION

     Training programs depend upon availability of texts.
If all the innovations are to find application at the village level, then suitable texts, well illustrated, written
in simple language and available at a price which the
trainers can afford, are an urgent need. Here is a challenge to all centers of learning. Knowledge locked up
inside libraries and expensive textbooks must be freed to
serve the masses. Science must become the handmaiden of
development and not a luxury reserved for the rich.

REFERENCES

1. Myrdal G (1971): The challenge of world poverty, a
    world anti-poverty programme in outline. Penguin
    Books, Middlesex.
2. WHO/UNICEF (1978): Final report of international
    conference on primary health care, Alma-Ata.
3. Ebrahim GJ (1981): Village health workers. In: Ma-
    ternal and Child Health Around the World, H.
    Wallace and GJ Ebrahim, Editors, MacMillan Press
    Ltd, London and Basingstoke.
4. Schuftan C (1979): The challenge of feeding the
    people: Child under Allende and Tanzania under
    Nyerere. Soc Sci and Med, 13C:97-107.

TRADITIONAL WAY OF MATERNAL AND CHILD HEALTH CARE

IN RAJASTHAN, INDIA

H. N. Mathur, P. N. Sharma, T. P. Tain

R. N. T. Medical College and
S.M.S. Medical College
Rajasthan, India

INTRODUCTION

For all ages all over India, the traditional birth attendant (TBA) commonly known as 'dai' has been playing a significant role in providing maternal and child health (MCH) services. It is estimated that there are over 6 million dais in India who attend to about 80 percent of all births (1, 2). In rural as well as in urban and semi-urban areas, people depend on them for MCH services. Although more and more health staff has been added and posted in rural areas, the dai has remained indispensable and conducts most of the deliveries even in places where lady physicians and other female health staff had been posted. Besides the traditional dai, elderly women of the house are also capable of conducting delivery. In remote villages of South India and among nomads, it is quite common to see female members and neighbors conduct the deliveries (3, 4). The traditional birth practices are dependent on the attitude and practices of the dai and hence it would be worthwhile to describe them.

PROFILE OF A DAI

Traditional birth attendants in India are invariably elderly married females with little educational background. The younger generation, though few in number and better prepared, come from barbar (nai) communities. They refuse to conduct deliveries among scheduled caste and tribes as the latter are considered untouchables. Delive-

473

ries among these communities are conducted by some elderly
women.

        To most TBAs, midwifery is a part time job. Agri-
culture and other domestic chores are the principal means
of livelihood. However, priority is given to a call for
delivery. Generally, midwifery practice is taken up by
TBAs after marriage. Before working independently, she
attends a few cases as a trainee with her mother-in-law or
her own mother or 'jethani' (wife of husband's elder
brother). The trainee TBA is exposed to various phases of
midwifery. Each dai has her own clientele scattered in
her own village or nearby locality. Usually these client-
families called 'jujmans' are passed on to the trainee
TBAs from previously trained TBAs. Encroachment on
'jujmans' by other TBAs is viewed with displeasure.

        Since dais come from within the community, they have
the confidence of the masses. Many dais have conducted
more deliveries than the lady physician or gynecologist of
that area. These factors has developed a sort of ego in
the dais which must not be hurt if their cooperation to
any program is required (5). Most of the TBAs, especially
those who have yet to receive training, have no understanding of asepis. They are blamed for high maternal,
perinatal and early neonatal mortality rates by the
medical profession. Yet, the services rendered by the dai
should be acknowledged with gratitude since they cater to
a great need of the community in the most adverse conditions of physical and social environment. The best of our
obstetricians would find it difficult if asked to conduct
delivery on a floor of a dark, ill-ventilated and foul-
smelling room. Since professionals have failed to win the
confidence of the masses, the community has still relies
upon the TBAs for the service.

NATAL SERVICES RENDERED BY DAI

Antenatal Care

        Not much importance is given to care during the
antenatal period. However, due to the close relation with
the 'jujuman', the dai comes to know of pregnancy of her
clients quite early so that when there is need for care,
she is the first to be called. Through improved education
and with medical services being made more available, the
number of women seeking antenatal care is slowly increasing. Certain 'dos' and 'don'ts' to be followed in
pregnancy are known to most of the women such as avoiding

heavy work during the first and last trimesters and
restricting coitus during these months. There are no
limitations to routine domestic work. Certain foods are
restricted during pregnancy, namely, curd, butter milk,
lady fingers, urad-ki-dal (horse bean), a type of pulp
which is very sticky. These are forbidden because it is
felt that these would cause difficulty in labor by fixing
the child in the womb. Hot tea and coffee are believed to
cause premature labor or abortion.

TBAs and the elderly women of the house are aware of
the fact that during pregnancy and lactation, nutritional
requirements are increased. However, in most families it
is customary for women to eat after all the men of the
house had been fed. This practice adversely affects the
nutrition of the women in general and pregnant women in
particular. The prevalence of anemia is quite high among
pregnant women and this contributes substantially to
maternal and child loss.

With regards to motherhood preparation, some
clothes, depending upon the economic status of the family
and the weather, are prepared in advance. Other details
of child care and her own care are learned by experience
and through advice of elderly women of the home and the
dai. For care of the child and herself, the woman
receives substantial support from relatives and friends
who are always willing to help. The TBAs estimate the
expected date of delivery by the Hindu calendar method.
She has learned by experience to judge the position of the
child, the engagement of the head and the approximate time
of delivery which is generally correct within reasonable
limits.

The government of India is laying tremendous stress
on providing antenatal care both at centers and in homes
through its maternal and child health programs, yet a very
small percentage of women, especially from rural areas
avail themselves of it.

Intranatal Care

The TBAs are generally called to conduct the
delivery or when the woman is in pain or has some other
associated complaint. TBAs have deep-rooted faith in a
God or deity and would therefore pray for safe delivery.
The TBAs do not have any delivery kit; she would thus go
bare-handed in conducting the delivery. She frequently
does a vaginal examination on the pregnant woman without
paying any attention to washing hands. The delivery is

generally conducted on the floor with the woman in labor
either lying down or in a squatting position. Traditionally the woman in labor is given rags to lie upon,
generally a gunny bag with cowdung ash spread over it to
act as absorbent for the amniotic fluid and blood. This
is done not only in poor socio-economic classes but also
in middle and higher classes. The absorbent quality of
the gunny bag and the cowdung ash makes it difficult to
assess the blood loss.

The TBAs know that enema facilitates labor but are
not versed with its technique. When complications arise,
she relies more on a male nurse than on a female staff.
Most male nurses are called to give injections of oxytocic
drugs to hasten labor or of Methergin to control bleeding.
Besides abnormally delayed labor and postpartum or antepartum hemorhage, medical assistance is also called for
eclamptic fits. Often the cases have waited too long
which contributes to the high maternal and child loss.
Mathur et al (6) observed that 33.32 percent of women
succumbed to death within six hours after admission at the
hospital.

TBAs have a limitted concept of asepsis and therefore rarely practice any type of aseptic procedure. The
cord is cut with any sharp cutting instrument made available by the household and ties the cord with a 'laccha' (a
sacred thread), both of which are not boiled. The importance of washing hands before conducting a delivery in not
realized. Washing hands and taking a bath after performing a delivery is more important. The cut end of the cord
would be dressed with any piece of linen after applying
some heated butter oil. The application of cowdung to the
cord is sometimes done. These practices are responsible
for cases of tetanus neonatorum which is frequent. Generally, the woman uses dirty discarded clothes for the
purpose of pads in the postnatal period; she takes the
ritual bath after delivery called 'Nahavan' and is given a
poor quality of bed and dirty bed covers.

In case of delayed labor the following practices are
done to hasten it:

(a) Application of pressure on the abdomen, starting with slow mild pressure by the hands and later on with
substantial force applied to push the infant. This practice is responsible for a good number of cases of ruptured
uterus which accounts for 23.39 percent of maternal deaths
analyzed by Mathur et al (6) in a teaching hospital over
a period of seven years.

(b) Application of oil or other lubricants into the vagina.

(c) Giving of some drink like hot milk or strong tea to the patient. Some also give heated sugary solution to the woman at the time of labor.

(d) Application of a hot fermentation called 'kelu' (a type of brick made of mud), on the lower abdomen in case of delayed delivery of the placenta.

The TBA, after conducting the delivery, is considered unclean and is treated like an untouchable until she takes a bath; she does not touch anyone nor any article, particularly the drinking water pitcher or kitchen utensils until after the bath.

Postnatal Care

The dai attends to the postnatal patient in a set pattern. She is aware of puerperal sepsis and advises douche with lukewarm water. In some communities, alcohol is also added to douche water. Women in the postpartum period are advised to expose their vulva to smoke generated by adding butter oil and some herbal preparations to fire. This is suppose to provide antiseptic effect. However, old rags are also used for pads and as a result the incidence of puerperal sepsis is high in home deliveries.

In the postnatal period, the dai washes the clothes of the woman, napkins and clothes of the child. She also massages the woman and the newborn every day. On an auspicious day after delivery (generally between 5 to 10 days) she gives the mother and child their first bath, this ritual being called 'Nahavan'. A feast is arranged for close relatives and friends on this day. It is only after this bath that the woman and newborn are considered touchables and are allowed to mix freely with the family. The duty of the dai to give massages and wash clothes continues for about forty days. Sometimes the postnatal work is done by one of her apprentices. In the postnatal period much emphasis is laid on nutrition when a rich diet is given the mother. Besides routine soft diet, some local food and medicines are also given. Invariably they consist of butter oil, jaggery, dried ginger, tumeric, gum acacia and 'ajvian'. It is believed that these local medicines facilitate the healing of damaged tissues and in lactation. This heavy diet wherein emphasis is given to butter oil is responsible for fat accumulation after delivery. Most of the women gain weight after delivery. Cotton belts are tied around the abdomen to keep it from bulging.

TBAs are paid for their service in cash and in kind. The charges generally depend on the economic status of the 'jujman'. Clothes and old beddings used by the mother in postpartum period are generally given to the TBAs.

CHILD CARE

The first food fed to the child after a few hours of birth is a liquid called 'Gulla' which is composed of wild herbs in sugary solution. It initiates intestinal peristalsis in the newborn. The colostrum is generally discarded and not much emphasis is laid on cleanliness. Dais are aware of smallpox vaccination, but do not administer it themselves. For minor ailments of the child, the dai or a relative in the house uses some other remedies. Hot butter oil and sometimes cowdung is applied to the cut end of the cord. Breast feeding is advised and practiced for long period. Feeding practices, personal hygiene and environmental sanitation are wanting. These, coupled with delayed and defective weaning, is responsible for the high incidence of protein calorie malnutrition.

TBAs practice abortion and some local abortifacients are known to them. It is believed that they advocate some contraceptives of their own but would not disclose their identity nor admit that they practice abortion. The community views abortion with some fear because it is believed that the dai can do much harm to the pregnant woman and child through some magic or witchcraft.

SOCIAL CUSTOMS AND RITUALS

Certain social customs and rituals are practiced in pregnancy and after delivery. The first delivery in most communities is generally conducted at the mother's house. In case of the first delivery, a prayer is offered at about 30 to 32 weeks of gestation and is known as the 8th month ceremony. This is to infuse confidence and relieve the woman of fear and apprehension associated with first delivery. Relatives and friends show their affection and happiness and invite the woman for feasts during the later months of her pregnancy.

In the postnatal period, a prayer is also offered on an auspicious day called 'Navahan', i.e. first bath after delivery . After delivery, the priest would prepare a horoscope of the child and would find out on what alphabet the child should be named.

India is a country with a large number of religions and communities. Midwifery differs from community to community, but by and large is similar with some modification. Any practice which is in use for so long a period must also have some good points. The Indian system of maternal and child health care has inherent qualities of sympathy and affection besides having the quality of rendering a service of security and tranquility. Thus, there is adequate provision of taking care of the mental health of the mother. Above all, this system is within the economic reach of the common man. The pitfalls of the system are the insufficient aseptic precautions and inability to detect risk conditions on time, which results in delayed referral. The positive and negative features of the Indian system of MCH can be summarized as follows:

Beneficial

    (a)   Quick response.
    (b)   Share and respect of patient's modesty in childbearing matters.
    (c)   Care and attention to woman's physical and mental state of health from the time of confirmation of pregnancy until 40 days after childbirth. This includes building up of physical strength and self-confidence.
    (d)   Advice on avoidance of sexual intercourse in the third trimester of pregnancy.
    (e)   Encourage prolonged breast feeding.
    (f)   Provide services in an atmosphere of cordiality, mutual trust and interdependence.

Harmless

    (a)   Wearing of amulets and charms to ward off evil spirits.
    (b)   Advice of avoidance of contacts with strangers during period of delivery and seclusion.
    (c)   Advise that women dispose of placenta in a culturally prescribed manner to avoid harm to the newborn through black magic.
    (d)   Advice to women with regards to performance of inexpensive ritual ceremonies, such as the purification bath in the 8th month.
    (e)   Treatment of mother's minor illnesses with harmless indigenous medicines.
    (f)   Treatment of child's minor illnesses with home remedies.

Harmful

    (a)   Advice to limit diet in the third trimester of pregnancy.
    (b)   Advice to avoid consuming certain locally available nutritious foods.
    (c)   Vigorous massage of woman's abdomen during the second and third stages of labor.
    (d)   Lack of asepsis in procedures adopted for delivery.
    (e)   Advice on excessive intake of 'desig ghee' (butter oil) and to lubricate the birth canal.
    (f)   Referral of seriously sick children to indigenous medicine practitioners.

CONCLUSION

    The present TBA training program launched by the government of India, if implemented in the right manner with certain modifications, can rectify many aspects of the poor quality of midwifery practice and remove its harmful practices. The dai is well accepted by the community and has access to many homes. She has developed sufficient proficiency in conducting normal labor and works with confidence. She not only conducts delivery but assists during the postnatal period. If trained and motivated to use aseptic procedures, identify high-risk mothers and refer them on time to proper health personnel, they could easily fill in the gap and prove a good non-medical supplement in providing midwifery care.

    In the progress towards urbanization and industrialization, there is danger of extinction of all traditional ways of livelihood. In India there have been family occupations. The dai profession which has been running in families has a risk of extinction. If this happens, we must strengthen our health services qualitatively, quantitatively and morally so that the communities accept them to meet the challenge of improved maternal and child health.

REFERENCES

1. Department of Family Welfare in India and the United Nations Fund for Population Activities (1979): Training of dais (TBAs) project agreement. UNFPA (Ind/78/702), New York, 6 pages.

2. Karthiyani PK (1980): Ministry of Health and Family
        Welfare, India. <u>Population Reports</u>, Series J,
        22, Johns Hopkins University Press, Baltimore.
3. Brey KH (1971): The missing midwife. Why a training
        program failed. <u>South Asia Review</u>, 5:41-52.
4. Taylor CE (1980): Personal communications.
        <u>Population Reports</u>, Series J, 22, Johns Hopkins
        University, Baltimore.
5. Mathur HN et al (1979): Analytical study of maternal
        mortality. <u>IV Annual Conference of Rajasthan
        Gynaecological Societies</u>.
6. Desk Officer, Department of Family Planning (1977):
        Letter No. 0.130, 11/1/76, New Delhi.

TRAINING AND SUPERVISION OF TRADITIONAL BIRTH ATTENDANTS

AT THE PRIMARY HEALTH CARE CENTER LEVEL

R. A. Estrada

Associate Director, Institute of Community and
Family Health
Children's Medical Center
Manila, Philippines

INTRODUCTION

The shortage of medical manpower to deliver basic
health care to the rural areas has remained a perennial
problem in many developing and even in developed countries
throughout the world. In the rural areas where 70 to 80
percent of the population reside, the people do not have
access to any system or form of basic health care. Traditional birth attendants (TBAs) have played an important
role in the present health status of women and children in
rural areas.

The World Health Organization has defined traditional
birth attendants (1) as "a person (usually an elderly
woman) who assists the mothers in child birth and who initially acquired her skills delivering babies by herself or
by working with other traditional birth attendants". They
are illiterate women who learned their skills by appren-
ticeship rather than by formal education. Rural people
have to depend on TBAs for they are the most accessible
person for the delivery of babies and folklore medicine.
Between 60 and 80 percent of births in the rural areas
are still delivered by TBAs. In some countries, they are
being replaced by young and literate trained midwife but
the TBAs continue to practice in large numbers and their
services continue to be on demand. These practising TBAs
of varying ages, limited educational levels, deeply rooted
cultural characteristics and health values, have working
experiences in health care thru the primary contact with

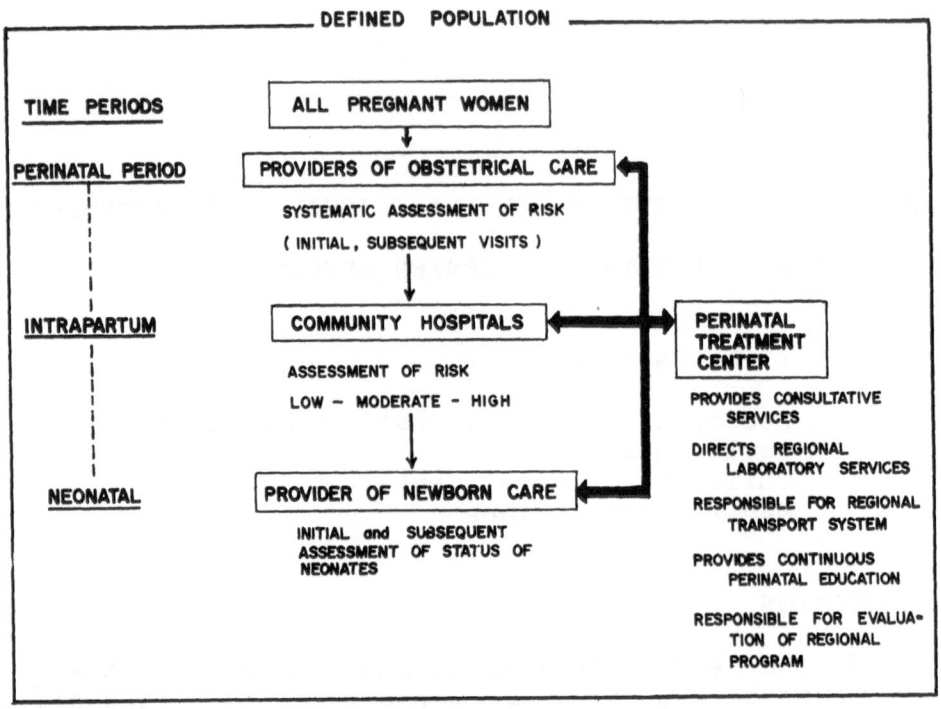

Figure 1. A model of maternal and neonatal health
           care system.

their own children as well as those of other mothers and
children in the rural areas. In some countries, mothers-
in-law or other female or even male relatives attend to
deliveries of babies and provide some form of health care
to mothers and newborns. With this outlook, we can pay
tribute also to all mothers throughout the world who are
the primary contact for health care of their children,
together with traditions, customs and beliefs of each
respective country, practised even before conception, and
through birth, infancy, childhood and adolescense.

     With regards to maternal and neonatal health care,
the new concept (2) of the "risk approach" which provides
care for the community as well as for the individual
through rational distribution of existing resources can
improve coverage and efficiency of maternal and child
health care and family planning (Fig. 1). Community
Health Workers like traditional birth attendants/mother
health workers (TBS/MHW), etc., can be provided with
adequate knowledge and appropriate skills for the early

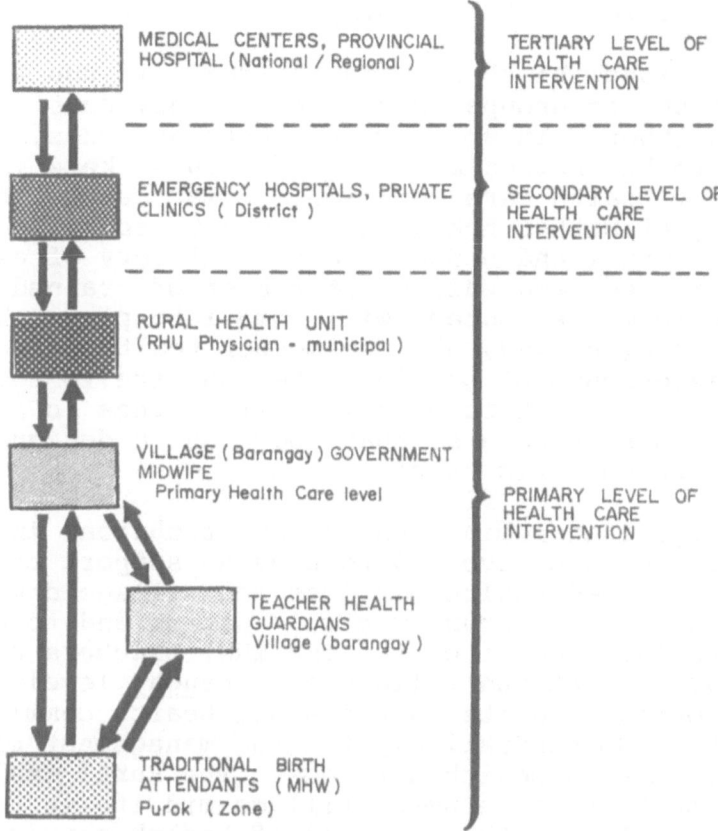

Figure 2.   Referral System

detection of high risk pregnant mothers and newborns and
obtain early referral according to the levels of risk.
Therefore some care can be provided immediately for all,
can contribute to the reduction of maternal and neonatal
mortality and morbidity and eventually to the improvement
of health status of mothers and children for a better
quality of life. A system of referrals is shown in Figure
2. For many developing countries, the utilization of
community health workers (3) who can be trained in a short
time to perform specific tasks has been envisioned for
attaining total population coverage. TBAs are found in
rural areas and are part of the local community, culture
and traditions. Moreover, they have high social standing
in the community and can exert considerable influence on
local health practices. If adequately trained and supervised, they can be the effective reforming agents in the
locality.

ROLE OF TBAs IN PRIMARY HEALTH CARE DELIVERY

Traditional birth attendants (TBAs) in the villages
are not found in groups in one area; they exist far apart
from each other. In areas where there are TBAs, they are
selected to be trained as mother health workers (MHWs) for
the primary health care approach. A TBA can be the leader
of a group of mother health workers with specific task to
perform maternal and newborn care. Delivery of essential
health services need sufficient number of trained people.
Thus, the teamwork concept will come into play. Except
for delivering babies, all the mother health workers have
had the experience of providing health care to their
children. Some mothers have more experience in some
aspects of health care so that they can be designated to
perform such specific tasks.

An organized administrative and technical infrastructure had to be evolved to provide support to the
community managed health services and village drugstore,
to promote active community participation and to ensure
continuous involvement of the TBA/MHW, teachers and students (Fig. 3). At the village or barangay level, the
village council and its captains and health committees are
responsible administratively for the management of the
community managed health services. The Rural Health Unit
(RHU) through the government village midwife is responsible technically for the delivery of health services and
training and supervision of the TBAs and MHWs. In the
restructured national delivery care system of the Philippines, one village (barangay) midwife is suppose to cover
50 to 200 households and a population of 5000. With this
population coverage, the midwife has to cover many villages, depending upon the geographical distribution of the
population. In the absence of a midwife in the village,
the TBAs or MHWs can supplement the work of the village
midwife. The trained TBAs or MHWs, being residents of the
area or zone (purok) can be called upon for assistance by
the people at any time. A model of the purok-based health
care system is depicted in Figure 4. A purok or unit of a
barangay consists of 10 to 30 households.

The recruitment and selection of community health
workers would have to be made by the community through its
village captain and health committee with assistance and
advice from the personnel who are to provide the supervision, continuing education and support.

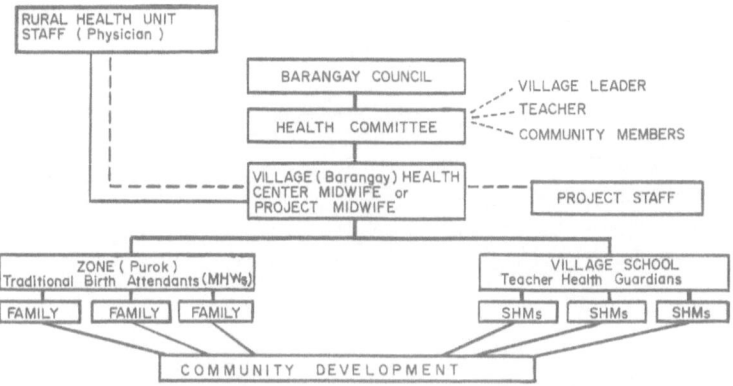

Figure 3.   Simplified Primary Health Care Delivery system
in a village (barangay).   Note: SHM = Student
Health Minders.

TRAINING AND SUPERVISION OF TBAs AND MHWs

The principle behind the TBA/MHW program is to guide
the community in mobilizing and utilizing its own resources in order to care for itself.   The aim is to make this
program an integral part of community activities and to
minimize dependence on outside support.   When possible,
the replication of new technical skills and knowledge
should take place within the community from one TBA/MHW
teaching another.   Knowledge and skill should be shared
and transmitted to one another in the zone (purok) and
village (barangay).   TBAs and MHWs should be encouraged on
a voluntary basis to provide as many services as possible
that the village requires.

In the planning and implementation of training
programs for TBAs and MHWs, the principle of functional
literacy and adult education would come into play.   In the
training of TBAs, it is important to know their characteristics.   They are adults of varying ages and limited
levels of education, with a heritage of deeply rooted
tradition, customs and beliefs.   Training should be aimed
at mastering specific tasks that TBAs are expected to
perform.

Training Program

The general purpose is to develop training programs
to teach the technical knowledge and skills that will put

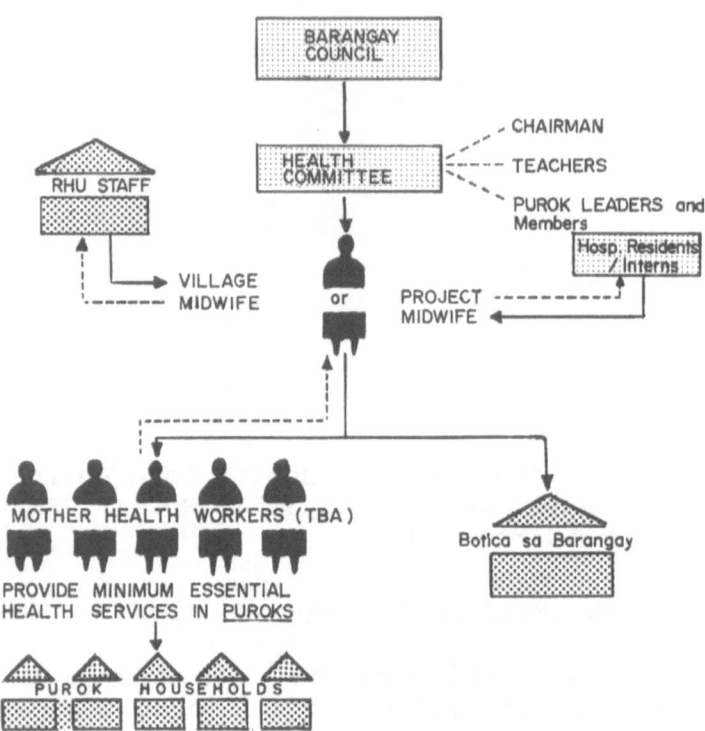

Figure 4.   Scheme of the Purok-based health care system.

into effect the expected roles and responsibilities of the
TBAs and MHWs in the delivery of essential health service
components of primary health care.

     The specific objectives are:

(a)   Training community selected TBAs and mother leaders
      as primary health care workers;
(b)   Providing the appropriate basic knowledge of essen-
      tial health service components of primary health
      care;
(c)   Developing the appropriate skills of the trainees to
      enable them to put into effect their roles and
      responsibilties;
(d)   Inculcating an awareness for needed positive change
      in attitiude towards attainment of health so as to
      make them effective reforming agents in the village.

     Selection of TBAs and MHWs.   TBAs and MHWs should
be selected by the community from among their own people.

Care should be taken to see that selection is really made by the community and not merely by its leaders. Desirable characteristics for TBAs and MHWs will vary with the range of work envisaged and with cultural considerations. Dedication and friendly personality are vital. They should be willing to render service to their fellowmen on a voluntary basis and share their knowledge and skills with others to effect self-care and self-reliance. The village (barangay), through the Health Committee and the project midwife, will select the TBAs and mother-leaders based on the required qualifications.

Trainers and supervisors. The TBAs or MHWs are accountable to the community but should be trained and supervised by a technical member of the local health service system. The government village midwife based at the primary health care center (Barangay Community Health Center) is the link between the health service system and community. She is to provide training and supervision. However, in some areas, the credibility of the government midwife is being questioned because of lack of experience and knowledge of the social and cultural conditions of the locality to be served. The trainer should be a mature midwife, should speak the dialect of the locality, be knowledgable of the socio-cultural characteristics of the people and community, should have experience in community health work and should have the potentialities for supervision. In some countries, elderly proficient TBAs have been assigned as supervisors but the problem was the creation of a hierarchy among the TBAs which involved administrative problems. The trainer's knowledge and experience should include the curriculum content as well as the principles of teaching and learning the methods of supervision. One important constraint in the training of TBAs and MHWs is the lack of experiences of midwives as trainers for this type of training program.

Supervision should be viewed as an educational process where the supervisor helps the trainees become more competent for the benefit of the people and the community. Supervision may be in the form of the supervisor visiting the TBAs and MHWs or the latter reporting periodically to the supervisor at the primary health care center. It may be for the replacement of supply or kits, which can become an opportunity for consultation and guidance and of finding out their problems and needs. The latter is preferred because it would be an opportunity for the TBAs and MHWs to meet for group discussions of problems encountered and exchange of experiences in carrying out their tasks. Continuing education as a form of super-

vision should be directed to three aspects, namely:
undertaking new or revised tasks, performing daily tasks
more efficiently, and reorienting the trainees towards
changing concepts, priorities and techniques. The key
work to educational program development is relevance to
the needs of the community. The content of continuing
education should be based on identified mistakes or short-
comings occurring in everyday practice and caused by a
lack of knowledge or skill or by wrong attitudes. Re-
training is to upgrade knowledge and skills based on
appropriate technology and scientific developments and on
the needs of the community as well as training the TBAs
and MHWs in the effective performance of their tasks.

Training Content and Curriculum. The content
should be relevant to the job functions and needs of the
community and should be limited to the minimum information
needed to perform these tasks and the rationale for doing
so. The range of services for which TBAs and MHWs need to
be trained varies with the program decided on. These will
depend on the problems and needs of the community (4). It
will cover a limited selection of varied activities in the
field of health education, such as maternal and child
health including family planning, nutrition, control of
communicable diseases including immunization, supply of
safe water and improved water storage, basic sanitation
such as proper sewage disposal and drainage, simple
curative care and first aid, and use of simple drugs and
common herbal medicine. They should be made aware of the
needed positive changes of their attitude towards the
attainment of health so as to make them effective change
agents in their communities. Training content should also
include communication, teamwork and leadership.

Instructions should be carried out in accordance with
modern teaching and learning methods and should take place
in the locality to be served. Emphasis should be on group
learning through continuous interaction between the TBAs
and MHWs, exchange of experiences, on the job traning, and
dialogue. Teaching methods would include short talks,
discussions, role playing, workshops, demonstration with
return demonstration by trainees, socio-dramas, case
presentation, and simulation games. The teaching aides
should consider the non-literacy or limited levels of
education of the trainees. Most common teaching aids used
are chalks, boards, charts, posters, flannel board, models
and actual materials. Reference books for reading should
be provided to serve as a functional literacy education
method. A constraint encountered is the lack of time
needed for quick learning since many of the trainees are

mothers with many household chores to do. Moreover, some
of them have difficulties in attending the training
sessions during planting and harvesting seasons and during
rainy season and typhoons.

        Training Methodology. Training methodology at the
primary health care center level is non-directive, dialo-
gical and experiential. The raw materials for training
would be the actual experience as traditional practitioners in child birth and folklore medicine, and as mothers
who had provided some aspects of primary health care in
the growth and development of their children based on
their own culture and traditions, practised even before
conception through birth, infancy, childhood and adolescense. Training should be simple, operational and oriented
towards the specific tasks or skills that the TBAs and
MHWs are expected to perform (5). It should be based on
clear definition of problems, the tasks to be performed
and the methods or appropriate techniques and equipment to
be used. The dialogic method of training is preferred for
practical solving approach rather than didactic instruction. Participatory training is necessary to prepare them
as change agents in the community. As change agents in
the village they would be able to respond to the needs and
to the socio-cultural conditions of the local community
life. The training process should involve the acquisition
of skills to promote relatively intangible objectives like
awareness building, a sense of community participation and
group dynamics.

        To gather baseline information, a pre-test will be
conducted to determine the knowledge of the different
subject matters to be learned and their attitudes as well
as their practices to certain extent.

        The TBAs and MHWs will conduct a survey of their
respective area (purok) of responsibility. They will
prioritize the subject matter to be discussed based on the
conceived needs of the community and of the TBAs/MHWs.
The government midwife will discuss the objective for a
particular topic before she moves to the next subject.

Group Decision about Structure of Meetings and Clinic
Rotation

        The TBA/MHW themselves will decide where and when to
hold the weekly meetings of 2 or 3 hours duration per week
for 15 months (a total of 180 hours). The training period
is staggered, depending upon the TBA/MWH's convenience and
availability of time. Meetings are held in a designated

house in the zone (purok) area or at the primary health
care center. Pertinent subject matters discussed will be
recorded in a notebook and will be checked from time to
time by the midwife.

The TBA/MWH from one zone or purok will rotate to
attend the clinic sessions once a week to know about cases
being served in the clinic and to learn some nursing
procedures such as taking weight, height and temperature,
reading blood pressure and learning minor treatment of
simple cases, first aid and use of appropriate drugs and
herbs. Medical residents and interns can provide medical
consultation and guidance in training TBAs once a week at
the primary health care center.

After 15 months of once a week dialogic training, the
TBAs will continue on the job training under the supervision of the village midwife. TBA/MHWs need training and
re-training continuously to ensure uninterrupted involvement in the delivery of essential health service
components of primary health care.

Monitoring and Evaluation

Monitoring of the training course will be the
responsibility of the trainer and other health staff.
Built-in evaluations will be conducted through periodic
reportings, observations, meetings and checking of
notebooks for the tasks or services they have rendered.

The following measures are undertaken to evaluate
training effectiveness and trainees' achievement:

(a)   Objective type test before and after training may
      show how much learning was absorbed in terms of
      ability to use and apply relevant subject matter.
(b)   Interviews, observations or questionaires relevant to
      attitude change, will show whether the training has
      modified the attitudes of TBAs with regard to subject
      matters relating to health and their tasks to be
      performed.
(c)   Client-staff relationship can be measured by
      questionaire or interview with trainees or by on-site
      observation and testimonials, criticism or
      endorsement by the clients and community.

The overall effectiveness can be measured by impact
or achievement of work objectives. Significant contribution can be attributed to training in terms of increased
capacity to meet job demands or to attain goals establish-

ed by the work role and responsibilities of TBA/MHWs.

CONCLUSION

      Training, supervision, referral, coordination with
other related health activities and evaluation should be
continuous in order to develop a long-term relationship of
the TBA/MHWs with the health care system and to effect
teamwork approach in the delivery of essential health
service components of primary health care. Volunteerism
should be promoted along with other personal qualities to
willingly share and transfer knowledge and skills to their
peers or fellowmen (mothers) in the community, thus
developing self-care and self-reliance in order to attain
a better quality of life. Every individual should assume
the responsibility of attaining health for themselves and
their family and community. This attitude will pave the
way in achieving the social goal of health for all in the
year 2000.

REFERENCES

1. WHO (1979): Inter-regional consultation on
        traditional birth attendants. HMD/NUR/80.1, Mexico
        City.
2. WHO (1979): Training in maternal and child health
        care. WHO Chornicle 33:329-333.
3. WHO (1976): New trends and approaches in the delivery
        of maternal and child care in health services.
        WHO Technical Report Series 600, Sixth Report,
        Geneva.
4. WHO (1978): Primary health care. A joint report by
        the Director General of WHO and the Executive
        Director of UNICEF. Alma Ata Conference.
5. Pasquariella BG and Wishik SM: Evaluating training
        effectiveness and trainee achievement methodology
        for measurement of changes in levels of cognitive
        competence. Manual for Evaluation, Series 8.
6. Pasquariella BG and Wichik SM: In: Methodology for
        measurement of changes in levels of cognitive
        competence. Manual for evaluation, Series 8.

UTILIZATION OF MOTHERS FOR SOME ASPECTS OF PRIMARY

HEALTH CARE IN PHILIPPINE BARANGAYS (VILLAGES)

F. Dionisio-Garcia, F. Del Mundo, and
V. Bondoc-dela Cruz

Institute of Community and Family Health
Children's Medical Center
Quezon City, Philippines

INTRODUCTION

In many developing countries as in the Philippines,
the shortage of medical manpower for delivery of health
care persists, notwithstanding all efforts to overcome
this problem (1-14). As WHO Director General H. Mahler
has emphasized: "If we do not succeed in making radical
changes, the vast majority of the world's population
will still have no access to decent health care at the end
of the century". It is evident that there is need for new
approaches for health services to be obtained in unreached
communities.

In the Philippines, as in many other countries,
there has been a tendency to depend on skilled professionals for health care but it is now clear that this is
neither feasible nor realistic. Hence, the country has
also undertaken the training of auxiliary health workers
at varied levels and with different methodology.

Youths in the community from 15 to 20 years old have
been recruited and trained to do primary health work.
After training, they have been willing to work in the
community as volunteers or with minimal compensation but
this could not go on indefinitely without any prospects
for permanent employment and progress. It is not surprising that they have began to seek "greener pastures" and
before long, hardly anyone is left in the community.

It is evident that the need in unreached and under-
priviledged communities is manpower that will be constant,
inexpensive and easily available. It becomes clear that
mothers in the household would fulfill these criteria supplemented to some extent by teachers and students in the
locality. The midwife in the restructured health delivery
system appears to be the most logical and practical person
to provide training, supervision and back-up support.

MOTHER HEALTH WORKER PROJECT

Located less than a hundred kilometers northwest of
Manila are two adjacent barangays (villages), Barrio San
Roque and Barrio Santo Niño, which are typical of remote
rural villages in the country. This is where our Institute of Community and Family Health has set up a project.
Their demography, epidemiology, economics and distinctive
profile has resulted in problems associated with lack of
essential services for health: malnutrition, ignorance,
poor environmental sanitation, large-sized families and
poverty. There are about 4,769 inhabitants in these two
villages spread in 587 household. Of the total population, children (0 to 12 years old) comprise about 25
percent, the 0 to 6 years old making up almost half of the
group. The majority of household heads have incomes below
the poverty lines. The barangay midwife, belonging to the
Rural Health Unit (RHU) of the Ministry of Health, goes to
the area once a week for ambulatory service. The immediate source of care is a traditional birth attendant in each
barangay.

Goals and Objectives

The ultimate goal of the project is to improve the
general level of health of children in the two barrios by
developing a low-cost and self-reliant health care system
which has the following objectives:

(a)   Tap and mobilize the indigenous manpower resources in
      the two communities who will serve as backbone of the
      health care system; selected mothers will act as
      first contact care providers at a ratio of one mother
      health worker (MHW) for every 10 to 15 households.
(b)   Create a two-way referral system from the home and/or
      school to the barangay health center (manned by the
      rural midwife) to the rural health unit (manned by
      the rural health physician).
(c)   Assist the community members in the identification
      and prioritization of community health problems and
      in finding ways to solve these problems.

Strategy

The basic strategy is to train selected community-interested mothers as mother health workers (MHWs) who will promote simple but essential health services in the two communities under the supervision of the project midwife and occasionally by the RHU midwife. There are 3 phases of the project:

Phase I. Regional and Community Preparation, scheduled for the first three months. Among its objectives are to have: (a) Communication channels established with local government and non-government agencies involved in health and health-related activities like the Ministry of Health, Ministry of Education, Ministry of Local Government and Community Development, Bureau of Agricultural Extension, Ministry of Social Services and Development, National Economic and Development Authority and the Rural Health Unit; to familiarize them with the project concept and to secure their support and cooperation. (b) A series of continuing dialogues in the two communities to start and create the proper environment for the health care system's acceptance and to gradually develop the community's capability in implementing and managing it subsequently. (c) The activation of the barangay health committee to become the implementing arm of the system. (d) The selection of mother trainees choosen by the community members.

Phase II. In-service Training of Mothers as Mother Health Workers (MHW), scheduled from 2 to 12 months. The non-formal training of selected mothers is done by the project midwife who acts as trainer-supervisor with support from the project staff. The dialogue method of training emphasizes practical problem-solving approach rather than didactic instruction. The trainess of one "purok" (smaller units of the barangay) meet with the midwife once a week for 2 to 3 hours at a designated house. The project midwife discusses with the trainees the objectives for a particular topic. Training subjects are prioritized according to the perceived needs by the trainees as a consequence of surveys they conducted. A standard curriculum is taught. In an example of the training scheme, a mother discussed salient features of the survey, its importance and how to accomplish the home-based family forms. A purok is divided into smaller units (10 to 15 households) under one mother trainee who survey-ed her own catchment area. She then tallies their results

and draws area maps pinpointing, through different colors,
the water supply, toilets, vegetable gardens, occupation
of household head and family planning practices. The
results of the survey are then echoed by the trainees and
discussed with their purok members. The same format is
applied to the other subject matters. After a thorough
discussion of immunization, the MHW echoes the topic to
the purok members and then arranges with the midwife or
medical staff the date of immunization. By the time the
medical personnel arrives, children with their parents
would have been gathered at one place and immunization
records filled out by the MHWs. After vaccination, the
MHW records the date, type of immunization and appropriate
measure given to the child. When the medical staff
leaves, the MHW takes charge of possible reactions
following immunization.

By the end of the 12th month, the training curriculum would have covered:

(a) Survey for home-based records;
(b) Maternal and child health including family planning
     education;
(c) DPT immunization of eligible children (0 to 6 years
     old);
(d) Finding appropriate treatment of common illness in
     the community using locally available medicinal
     plants;
(e) Identification and utilizzation of locally available
     medicinal plants.
(f) Deworming and basic environmental sanitation; and
(g) Nutrition activities like weight monitoring and food
     supplmentation which is done in coordination with the
     Catholic Relief Services, a private organization.

Phase III. "Botika sa Barangay" (Drugstore of the
village). In Barrio Santo Niño, the mother trainees,
with the help of the barangay health committee, decided to
collect two pesos per family as initial fund for the
"botika". Essential medicines were bought at cost price
and then dispensed with a small surcharge. Income from
the "botika" is used for a mushroom demonstration plot in
the community.

In Barrio San Roque, the community was loaned "seed
money" of one thousand five-hundred pesos by a private
society to start a "botika". The project had its ups and
downs but after 2 years, the loan was finally paid and
the project became viable. The pharmacy is managed on

rotation by mothers, headed by a purok leader and the
project midwife. It sells both herbal and synthetic
medicine.

RESULTS

        Out of the 39 mother trainess, there are now 37 MHWs
continuing with a staggered "iN-purok" service training.
In the areas where two trainees dropped out, the other
MHWs volunteered as replacements. Each trainee has
completed the survey of her catchment area with a map and
folder for each family serving as home-based records of
each member. The following are on-going activities of the
MHWs.

        Immunizations. In between planting and harvest
seasons, mothers are able to schedule DPT immunizations in
their respective puroks.

        Maternal and Child Care. During and after de-
liveries, the MHW assists attending midwife and give
pointers on newborn care. She emphasizes the importance
of breast feeding and proper nutrition of infants.

        Family Planning Education. With an agricultural
approach to family planning, MHWs meet with purok members
and discuss with them the importance of planning their
families. Some male members have already expressed
interest in vasectomy and other methods while a number of
mothers have chosen tubal ligation.

        Treatment of Common Illnesses in the Community.
During training, MHWs were given specific protocols for
each illness for which they made progress notes until the
child recovers. The efficacy of herbal therapy is thus
tested.

        Deworming and Nutrition Activities. Based on
parasitic infestation studies done in the past and on the
wormload profile made in the area, the MHWs conducted
deworming schedules in each purok. The MHWs weighed the
children and filled out a simple weight chart. Under the
supervision of the midwife and medical staff, they dispensed antihelminthics; lately they are trying the use of
"bunga" (betel nut), from local trees. Deworming is done
every 5 to 6 months and a fee of 25 centavos is charged
per child per treatment.

CONCLUSION

A simplified "purok" community-based health care system was initiated which mobilizes mothers for minimal but essential health services in two rural villages in the Philippines. Mothers were selected and trained on some aspects of primary health care at the purok level. They have effectively served as campaigners for immunization, nutrition and family planning activities and were readily accepted by the community to give simple and immediate management of common children's ailments. More importantly, they can be relied upon to participate actively in the continuous and permanent health care delivery in remote rural localities and make use of available indigenous materials. A reversible referral network was established complimented by a village pharmacy, which can dispense herbal and synthetic medications. It is obvious that with community involvement and active interest, the "purok" system can succeed in meeting their own health problems and needs. With an available health team (a midwife or a Rural Health Unit midwife and physician) providing back-up support at periodic intervals, of the health status of children in remote communities may be improved.

REFERENCES

1. Anderson R (1978): Health status indices and access to medical care. Am J Pub Health, 58:44-48.
2. Barrett LT (1978): The need for a focus in rural health services. Pub Health Rep, 90:349.
3. Bryant J (1967): Health and the developing world. Cornell University Press, Ithaca, New York.
4. Cauffman JG et al (1970): Community health aides. How effective are they? Am J Pub Health, 60:(10).
5. International Children's Center (1977): Children in the Tropics, ICI, Paris, p. 100.
6. Desai P et al (1968): The social background to malnutrition. Maternal and Child Care IV. 40:166-172.
7. Fielding JE (1977): Health promotion. Sound notions in search of a constituency. Am J Pub Health, 67:1082-1085.
8. Flahault D (1973): The training of rural health personnel. A crucial factor in development. World Health Organization Chronicle, 27:236-241.
9. Isely RB et al (1977): The village health committee - starting point for rural development. World Health Organization Chronicle, 31:307-375.

10. Jones S (1978): Limitations of community control of
        health facilities and services. <u>Am J Pub Health</u>,
        68:541-543.
11. Parker A et al (1967): Appropriate tools for health
        care and rural development. <u>World Health
        Chronicle</u>, 31:131-137.
12. Simborg DW et al (1978): Physicians and non-physician
        health practitioners. The characteristics of their
        practices and their relationships. <u>Am J Pub
        Health</u>, 68:44-48.
13. Terris M (1977): Strategy for prevention. <u>Am J Pub
        Health</u>, 67:1026-1027.
14. Wise HB et at (1968): The family health workers. <u>Am
        J Pub Health</u>, 58:1828-1838.

FUTURE GLOBAL CHALLENGE OF

PRIMARY MATERNAL AND NEONATAL HEALTH

H. de Watteville

Secretary General, IAMANEH
Geneva, Switzerland

INTRODUCTION

The four days of the First International Congress on
Maternal and Neonatal Health were marked by the delivery
of interesting lectures that were followed by lively
discussions. As the Congress was concluding, it was felt
necessary to determine what actions should be undertaken
for reducing maternal and neonatal mortality and morbidity. My closing remarks are answers to the two question
that were repeatedly raised during the Congress:

(a) What are the projects which are most promising
and which should be given high priority in the programs
sponsored by IAMANEH and its national sections, as well as
those of other government and non-government organizations
working in the field of maternal and neonatal health?

(b) What are the strategies for the implementation
of these projects to improve maternal and neonatal health?

PRIORITY PROJECTS

Projects should be elaborated and implemented first
of all in the following four areas: spacing of
pregnancies as a means for improving maternal and neonatal
health; treatment and prevention of obstetrical and
pediatric infections; training and equiping of auxiliary
health manpower working in a comprehensive maternal and
child health program; and investigation of the health
condition and reproductive behavior of the target population groups and evaluation of the impact selected projects

have had on maternal and neonatal mortality and morbidity.

Spacing of Childbirth

Statistical data show clearly that child spacing is
an important means of improving the health of mothers and
children. Multiparity is in itself a risk factor since
maternal mortality is lower for the second and third child
than for the first but rises sharply after the fourth
delivery. Neonatal mortality is closely linked with
maternal deaths and infant deaths are associated with
multiparity or short birth interval. The influence of
spacing on neonatal and infant mortality has been demonstrated in a WHO study in rural India. The death rates of
neonates and infants, born less than two years after the
preceding pregnancy, were more than twice as high than
those of children born after a birth interval of more than
four years. An unwanted pregnancy occurring shortly after
childbirth, or once the desired family size has been
reached, may lead to induced abortion which endangers life
and health of the expectant mother. These facts should be
known not only by physicians but also by paramedical personnel working in the field of maternal and child health.
They must encourage the mothers to participate in family
planning. Such counseling should be extended even to
remote rural areas. However, it will only be useful if
women who wish to space their pregnancies or to limit the
size of their families, have easy access to effective and
innocuous methods of fertility control. Therefore programs need to be developed for delivery of family planning
services in rural villages.

To reach this goal, not only physicians but also
paramedical personnel must obtain an adequate training in
fertility control methods and be provided with contraceptive materials. Religious, cultural, political and
technical factors must be taken into consideration when
organizing family planning services. Different methods
have to be used from one country to another, or even from
one region to another in the same country. Research for
improved fertility control methods should continue and
field trials organized for testing these methods under
various conditions should be organized. Among newer
promising developments, I would like to cite an intrauterine device which can be safely and effectively inserted
after an abortion or delivery, and also nonsurgical
sterilization by transcervical intrauterine application of
chemicals. Newly developed antihormones against gonado-
tropins or ovarian steriods may suppress ovulation or
nidation with less side effects, than those resulting from

the presently used synthetic estrogens and progestagens.
Finally, our interest should be focused on methods which
will enable women to detect their own fertile days of the
menstrual cycle.

Treatment and Prevention of Infection

Infection is one of the major causes of maternal,
neonatal and infant deaths. Puerperal and neonatal infections have become rare in industrialized countries due to
improved hygiene, healthier environment, strict asepsis
during delivery and obstetrical operations, and the use of
antibiotics in cases of threatened or evident infection.
In developing countries, the teaching of adequate hygiene
to birth attendants and expectant mothers, the improvement
of the habitat and of nutrition, are adequate preventive
measures against infection. However, it will take
considerable time to attain these goals in rural areas and
suburban slums.

One way to improve the situation in the immediate
future is to provide rudimentary training and basic equipment to traditional birth attendants (TBAs) who, in many
countries, attend childbirth of the vast majority of
women. Teaching them correct washing of their hands,
aseptic handling of the umbilical wound and perineal
tears, and disinfection of the instruments with boiling
water or antiseptic solutions, will certainly diminish the
frequency of severe and possibly fatal infections. Fur-
nishing of sterile materials for dressings, alcohol and
antiseptic soaps to TBAs would greatly contribute to the
prevention of infection at a reduced cost, than the
widespread use of antibiotics.

There is one infection which could be successfully
prevented by a vigorous campaign in the coming years, and
that is, neonatal tetanus. It is estimated that at least
500,000 newborns die every year of this disease. Vaccination of the expectant mother with tetanus toxoid will not
only protect her, but also her newborn child. Two injections during pregnancy are necessary. For women who have
already received a toxoid injection before the current
pregnancy, one single booster injection is sufficient.
Women who have been vaccinated three, or better four times
(after birth, at school, or later on), will have a lasting
titer of antibodies which is sufficiently high for
protecting them and their newborn children. The tetanus
toxoid is relatively stable; for its conservation, cool
temperature is sufficient and no cold chain is required.

Projects should be developed for vaccinating all expectant mothers against tetanus and whenever possible, all women of reproductive age. The first step in such a program would be to provide facilities for toxoid injections at antenatal clinics in peripheral hospitals and rural maternities. Progressively the campaign should reach the villages in remote rural areas. Such a campaign must include motivation of the target population by education and will need considerable managerial effort and financial investment. If interdisciplinary cooperation and financial support are developed at a national and international level, it will become possible to reduce neonatal deaths due to tetanus to a minimum.

Breast feeding protects the newborn and the infant against intestinal infection. Moreover, the transfer of antibodies with the milk will also enhance the resistance against infections of other organs. Campaigns for continuation of breast feeding and giving up bottle feeding are important in the fight for prevention of infections in the infant. Adequate mixtures of electrolytes and sugar as powder, or in solution ready for use should be given to rural midwives and TBAs for the treatment of diarrhea in infants by oral rehydration.

Training and Equipping of Auxiliary Health Personnel

Today, the vast majority of women are still giving birth without assistance of medically trained personnel. In most instances, it is a TBA who is present during childbirth and takes care of the mother and newborn during the first days after delivery. In most countries, it will take some time to train a sufficient number of midwives which would be necessary for assisting all women during childbirth. Some governments have experienced difficulties with the well-trained midwives, whom they have sent to the villages. The women in the villages distrusted the newcomers, generally originating from cities or other rural regions. Therefore, they continued to call the TBA known to them for many years.

To improve maternal and child health care at the primary level, it seems mandatory to include the TBAs in the health program. They should receive initial training followed by regular refresher courses. As a reward, they should receive a kit with basic equipment and possibly also a distinct sign (a badge or a broach), showing that they belong to the trained and officially recognized health personnel. On the other hand, they have to accept advice and supervision by better trained and equipped

midwives, since most TBAs are unable to handle successfully difficult obstetrical cases. These midwives should
preferably be recruited from the area of their future
activity. They may work in a rural maternity, or a health
center, where they can conduct prenatal and postnatal
visits, administer toxoid injections, lodge pregnant women
who need rest or special care, and attend to them during
delivery. The midwives should also pay visits to the TBAs
in the surrounding villages, refurnish them with dressing
materials, disinfectants and a few basic drugs. The rural
midwife may also render family planning services, for instance, by distributing pills and condoms and possibly also
by inserting intrauterine devices. A special task of the
rural midwife will be the detection of cases which need
transfer to a peripheral hospital, where a physician with
surgical training can perform obstetrical operations such
as cesarean section and forceps extraction.

The development of primary health care will certainly have a great impact on maternal and neonatal health.
However, one should recognize that the primary health care
scheme needs as a supplement, an efficient referral
system. There is no need to teach the rural midwives and
TBAs the diagnosis of disorders during pregnancy, or complications during labor (severe anemia, edema, accidental
hemorrhage, abnormal presentation, retracted pelvis), if
the patient cannot be transferred on time to a hospital,
where she can receive the necessary treatment. Therefore,
adequate equipment of peripheral hospitals and the creation of such medical centers where they do not yet exist,
should not be neglected even if projects for the improvement of primary health care deserve a high priority in a
comprehensive health scheme.

Special studies should be devoted to the use of
obstetrical technology at the primary and secondary health
care level. These may concern simple procedures, like the
development of scales, which can be used even by an illiterate, urinalysis (paper strips), measurement of blood
pressure and blood hemoglobin level. In peripheral hospitals, equipment for safe anesthesia should be ready for
use, easy to handle and to maintain. The development of
refrigeration and illumination derived from solar energy
would be of great value in many countries, where the high
cost of fuel are limiting the health budget available for
salaries of health manpower and for medical equipment.
Facilities for blood transfusions, or at least for intravenous infusion of blood substitutes should be available
in all hospitals, where a physician is working. Simple
laboratory tests should be possible and a microscope is

essential even in small hospitals.

To the contrary, the use of more complicated and
expensive technology, like monitoring of uterine contractions and fetal heart beat, fetal blood gas analysis and
echography, or amniocentesis, should remain restricted to
one, or a very few larger hospitals (mainly university
clinics), until the primary and secondary health care
level has become satisfactory throughout the country.

Investigations on Health Condition and Reproductive Behavior

In order to evaluate correctly the impact of new
health care projects on the mother and her child, one
should know their condition before the implementation of
the program. The first prerequisite for the collection of
reliable statistics is the use of uniform definition by
all those who contribute to the data collection. Such definitions relating to obstetrics and reproductive behavior
have been recommended by the International Fertility
Research Program (IFRP) in cooperation with the International Federation of Gynecology and Obstetrics (FIGO), and
after consultation with the World Health Organization
(WHO). The definitions are essentially based on those
used in the 9th edition of the International Classifica-
cation of Diseases (WHO). All relevant questions are
listed on a single sheet Maternity Monitoring Record,
which is suitable for computer analysis. This record has
been prepared by IFRP after consultation of competent experts and its use has been recommended by FIGO (Appendix).
A center for computer analysis of the records with rapid
feedback to the contributors has been set up at IFRP headquarters in North Carolina, U. S. A. Initial results have
been obtained by analyzing a large number of maternity
records stemming from various countries. Since the record
contains a series of questions relating to social status
and level of education, to the general health condition
and to reproductive behavior, it is possible to gain
insight on the influence these factors exert on maternal
and child health. Even though maternity records have only
been used by larger hospitals in a limited number of
countries, the analysis of the collected data has already
shown that the most important factor for lowering perinatal mortality of children born in a teaching hospital is
the number of prenatal vists (none, 1 to 3, or more than
3), irrespective of all other factors as for instance,
age, parity, level of education and social economic
status. Prenatal visits have reduced the danger for the
child, resulting from various risk factors. The creation

of prenatal clinics, which are easily accessible to a
maximum of expectant mothers, should be given a high
priority. Only if the female population is motivated to
attend these clinics by medical education, prenatal visits
will exert a beneficial influence on maternal and child
health. The risk for the outcome of pregnancy inherent in
age under 18 or over 35 years, grandmultiparity, short
birth intervals and severe anemia have also been
demonstrated with the help of the maternity records.

In the light of the encouraging results already
obtained, the use of the maternity record in all major
hospitals of a country (as it has been done for instance
in Indonesia), and the formation of centers for computer
analysis (with the possibility of rapid feedback to the
contributors), should be encouraged at a national or
regional level. The development of less expensive microcomputers may make it easier to attain this ambitious
goal. It will be most stimulating for the physicians and
personnel working in a hospital to know rapidly the
results of their efforts and to compare them with those
obtained in other similar institutions. Obstetricians and
pediatricians may adopt in their departments, methods
which have given promising results in other hospitals. So
far, the analyzed data originate from hospital deliveries
and therefore concern only a limited portion of the female
population. There is still a lack of valid information on
the prevalence of obstetrical complications, such as hypertensive disease, anemia, low birth weight and premature
labor in rural areas. The same is true for maternal and
child health at the primary and secondary health care
level as reflected in the rates of maternal and perinatal
mortality. Therefore it is mandatory to develop a simple
uniform record which can be used in peripheral hospitals
and rural maternities. At present, several studies are
under way, testing the use of a maternal record sheet, on
which illiterate TBAs can mark with a cross, the pictures,
which correspond with the facts observed, such as multiple
or single pregnancy, presentation of the fetus, size of
the baby (small, normal, big), condition of mother and
newborn (healthy, sick or dead). If TBAs could be
motivated to fill out regularly and conscientiously such
records and without hiding cases with unfortunate outcome,
even such rudimentary reporting system would probably
yield valuable information relating to obstetrical practice in remote rural areas. For demographers and health
authorities , such knowledge would certainly be most
useful, whenever elaborating programs for their future
actions. For all the above reasons, an adequate reporting
system should be included in each project aiming at the

improvement of maternal and neonatal health.

STRAGEGIES FOR IMPLEMENTATION OF MOTHER AND CHILD PROGRAMS

There exists a rich and valuable literature dealing
with the planning and implementation of maternal and child
health programs. This published Proceedings will
undoubtedly serve as a useful compendium. However, it is
difficult to tackle the gigantic task of meeting
simultanously the manifold needs for the building up of a
comprehensive and effective health scheme. Therefore,
priority should be given to selected projects likely to .
meet the most urgent needs in a given region.

In many countries, it is the lack of adequately
trained and well motivated health manpower which is
retarding the progress in maternal and child health care.
Training in public health and preventive medicine,
including maternal and child health, should therefore be
included in the curriculum not only of the medical
student, but also of the auxiliary health personnel.
Unfortunately, many university teachers of obstetrics and
pediatrics have so far shown limited interest in medical
practice at the primary health care level. They should be
made aware of their responsilities for training of future
physicians and midwives and of the importance of their
close cooperation with health authorities and epidemiologists. Fully trained midwives should not only work in
major hospitals but also be used for teaching rural midwives and TBAs and for supervising their activities in the
field. In large areas of the world, the highest priority
should be given to the inclusion of TBAs in the health
scheme by providing them with rudimentary training and
basic equipment. Often school teachers can play a useful
role by participating in the health education of the local
community. The personnel involved in maternal and child
health program could be compared to an army, where TBAs
and midwives are the soldiers in the frontline, trained
midwives and physicians are officers who help and direct
them, university teachers and health authority officials
are generals, who elaborate and implement the strategy of
the campaign, and the Minister of Health is the
commander-in-chief of this pacific army.

Health for all and specially for mothers and children
can only be secured through an interdisciplinary approach
involving not only various medical disciplines but also
several governmental ministries. The improvement of
housing and sanitation as well as the creation of

better facilities for transport and communications are all essential for adquate good health care. Education in general and specially in health matters plays also an important role in the national health programs. A major limiting factor for the implementation of maternal and child health program is funding. Only governments can finance such a program at the national level by allocating a sufficient portion of their budget to health matters. But many countries are so poor that only bilateral or multilateral cooperation among governmental and non-governmental organizations will enable them to initiate a part of their health programs.

The population of industrialized contries is in general not aware of the great distress of mothers and children in most developing countries. Humanitarian organizations should therefore undertake campaigns to inform the public on the urgent health needs in the Third World and for collecting funds which can be used for the improvement of maternal and child health care. Even if the amount of money raised is limited in comparison with the grants from governments and non-governmental organizations, such contributions may be decisive for the rapid implementation of pilot studies. Projects which have been proven successful may later be realized on a larger scale with governmental support.

Private organizations can request commercial firms, humanitarian associations (Rotary or Lions Clubs) and wealthy individuals to donate funds or materials for child health care, in the event that government cannot undertake such actions. Even in less developed countries, there are wealthy idividuals who are willing to support projects that are well designed and of proven value. In some instances, small rural communities have voluntarily participated in the implementation of a project because the villagers expect to benefit. The Japanese Association for Maternal Welfare has been able to collect large sums of money by requesting a small voluntary contribution from women during their stay in hospitals after a delivery.

The International Association for Maternal and Neonatal Health (IAMANEH) intends to affiliate with, or formulate national organizations with similar goals in as many coutries as possible. It may be expected that in the future, many more mothers and children will survive and remain healthy, provided that a global effort is made for designing and funding maternal and child health care projects.

Appendix

INTERNATIONAL FERTILITY RESEARCH PROGRAM
MATERNITY RECORD

PATIENT IDENTIFICATION: 1. Hospital or clinic no _____   2. Admission date _____
day   month   year

3. Patient's name _____   Husband's name _____
     family   first   maiden

4. Address _____

STUDY IDENTIFICATION
5. Center name _____ and number:

6. Study number: 9 0 3

7. Patient order number:

8. Delivery date:
     day   month   year

9. Registration status: 0) not booked 1) booked, patient's choice 2) referred by physician 3) referred by midwife 4) emergency 8) other _____

PATIENT CHARACTERISTICS
10. Residence: 1) urban 2) rural 3) urban slum 4) rural slum

11. Patient's status: 1) private 2) not private 8) other

12. Patient's age (completed years)

13. Patient's education: (school year completed) 0) 0 1) 1-2 2) 3-4 3) 5-6 4) 7-8 5) 9-10 6) 11-12 7) 13-14 8) 15+

14. Marital status: 1) never married 2) currently married 3) divorced 4) separated 5) widowed 6) consensual union 8) other

15. Age at first marriage/union: (completed years)

OBSTETRIC HISTORY (not including this pregnancy)
16. Total live births:

17. Children now living: number of males (8 or more = 8) number of females

18. Duration of breast-feeding of last live birth: (in months) 0) did not breast-feed 1) <3 2) <6 3) <9 4) <12 5) <15 6) <18 7) <21 8) ≥21

19. Number of stillbirths: (8 or more = 8)

20. Number of infant deaths: (less than 12 completed months; 8 or more = 8)

21. Number of spontaneous abortions: (8 or more = 8)

22. Number of induced abortions: (8 or more = 8)

23. Outcome of last pregnancy: 0) not previously pregnant 1) live birth, full term, still living 2) live birth, full term, deceased 3) live birth, premature, still living 4) live birth, premature, deceased 5) stillbirth 6) induced abortion 7) spontaneous abortion 8) other

24. Number of months since last pregnancy ended: (98 or more = 98)

25. Contraceptive method mainly used before conception: 0) none 1) IUD 2) orals/injectables 3) female sterilization 4) male sterilization 5) condom 6) withdrawal/rhythm 7) foam/diaphragm/jelly 8) other

MEDICAL DATA
26. Number of antenatal visits: (8 or more = 8)

27. Primary antenatal condition: (see code list)

28. Hospitalization required during this pregnancy: 0) no 1) yes, for condition indicated in Item 27 2) yes, for condition other than the one indicated in Item 27, specify condition

29. Tobacco smoking during pregnancy: 0) none **During part of pregnancy** (cigarettes/day): 1) 1-10 2) 11-20 3) 21 or more **Throughout pregnancy** (cigarettes/day): 4) 1-10 5) 11-20 6) 21 or more 8) cigars, pipes, etc

30. Number of previous cesarean sections:

31. Estimated duration of pregnancy: (menstrual age in completed weeks)

32. Hemoglobin at admission for delivery (to nearest gm): 1) ≤5 gm 2) 6 gm 3) 7 gm 4) 8 gm 5) 9 gm 6) 10 gm 7) 11 gm 8) ≥12 gm 9) not done

33. Rupture of membranes: **Spontaneous:** 1) <24 hrs before delivery 2) ≥24 hrs before delivery **Artificial:** 3) <24 hours before delivery 4) ≥24 hrs before delivery 5) during cesarean section

34. Type of labor: 0) no labor 1) spontaneous 2) spontaneous, augmented with artificial rupture of membranes (ARM), 3) spontaneous, augmented with drugs 4) spontaneous, augmented with ARM and drugs 5) induced, with ARM 6) induced, with drugs 7) induced, with ARM and drugs 8) other

For multiple births, code information for the most difficult delivery in Items 35, 38, 44, 46, 47 and 48 and complete a separate Multiple Birth Record for each infant.

35. Type of presentation during labor: 0) vertex, occiput anterior 1) vertex, occiput transverse or posterior 2) frank breech 3) footling breech 4) complete breech 5) brow/face 6) transverse lie 7) compound 8) other

36. Anesthetic administered: 0) none or psychoprophylaxis only 1) analgesic, systemic or inhalation 2) local 3) paracervical/pudendal 4) spinal/epidural 5) general 6) 1 and 2 or 1 and 3 7) other combination 8) other

37. Episiotomy: 0) none 1) midline 2) midline, with extension 3) midline, with hematoma 4) mediolateral 5) mediolateral, with extension 6) mediolateral, with hematoma 8) other

38. Type of delivery: 0) spontaneous 1) outlet forceps 2) vacuum extractor 3) mid- or high forceps 4) manual rotation 5) breech extraction 6) cesarean section 7) destructive procedure 8) other

39. Primary injury during labor and/or delivery: 0) none 1) vulva 2) vagina 3) perineum 4) cervix 5) uterus 6) rectum 7) bladder 8) other

40. Primary complication of labor and/or delivery: 0) none 1) prolonged/obstructed labor 2) placenta previa 3) placenta abruptio 4) hypotonic uterine contractions 5) hypertonic uterine contractions 6) hemorrhage 7) retained products 8) other

41. Secondary complication of labor and/or delivery: 0) none 1) prolonged labor 2) cord prolapse 3) hypotonic uterine contractions 5) hypertonic uterine contractions 6) hemorrhage 7) retained products 8) other

42. Duration of labor: (in completed hours) 0) none 1) <2 2) 2-6 3) 7-12 4) 13-18 5) 19-24 6) 25-48 7) over 48

43. Attendant at delivery: 0) none 1) nurse 2) qualified midwife 3) student nurse/midwife 4) paramedic 5) medical student 6) general physician 7) OB/GYN physician 8) other

44. Birth weight: (gm; 9988 or more = 9988)

45. Sex of infant(s) born at this delivery: number of males (write number of each) number of females

46. Apgar score: 9) not done at 1 minute (8 or more = 8) at 5 minutes

For Items 47-48, use the following codes: 0) normal or stillbirth with no apparent pathology 1) fetal distress during labor 2) minor malformation 3) major malformation 4) respiratory distress syndrome 5) isoimmunization 6) neonatal sepsis 7) trauma 8) other (for codes 2, 3, 7 and 8, specify)

47. Primary fetal/neonatal condition, specify _____

48. Secondary fetal/neonatal condition, specify _____

49. Death of fetus/newborn: 0) none 1) antepartum, one 2) antepartum, two or more 3) intrapartum, one 4) intrapartum two or more 5) postpartum, one 6) postpartum, two or more 7) combination 8) other

50. Primary puerperal condition: 0) normal 1) fever requiring treatment 2) bleeding requiring treatment 3) urinary tract infection 4) mastitis 5) phlebitis 6) dehiscence 7) death (complete Death Report) 8) other

51. Maternal blood transfusion during hospitalization: 0) none 1) yes, before delivery 2) yes, during delivery 3) yes, after delivery 4) 1 and 2 5) 1 and 3 6) 2 and 3 7) 1, 2 and 3

52. Number of nights hospitalized this admission before delivery: (8 or more = 8)

SPECIAL STUDIES
53. _____

54. _____

55. _____

Complete these items at time of discharge:
56. Number of nights hospitalized this admission after delivery: (8 or more = 8)

57. Female sterilization: 0) none 1) before this delivery 2) at cesarean section 3) immediately after delivery 4) same day 5) 1-2 days later 6) 3-4 days later 7) 5-9 days later 8) 10 or more days later

58. Number of additional children wanted: (8 or more = 8)

59. Contraceptive method planned or provided: 0) none 1) IUD 2) orals/injectables 3) female sterilization 4) male sterilization 5) condom 6) withdrawal/rhythm 7) foam/diaphragm/jelly 8) other

    1

Recorder's name _____

PLEASE AIRMAIL TO: International Fertility Research Program, Research Triangle Park, North Carolina 27709 USA

MAT 001 12/78

ANTENATAL CONDITIONS
(Refer to manual, Item 27)

Numbers in parentheses refer to codes in WHO International Classification of Diseases 9th edition

00 None
99 Unknown

Hemorrhage per vagina
01 Threatened abortion (640.0)
02 Placenta previa (641.0, 641.1)
03 Placenta abruptio [premature separation] (641.2)
04 Rupture of the marginal sinus (641.8)
05 Antepartum hemorrhage associated with coagulation defects (641.3)
06 Other and unspecified antepartum hemorrhage per vagina (641.8, 641.9)

Hypertensive disorders
07 Preexisting hypertension (642.0)
08 Preexisting hypertension with superimposed preeclampsia or eclampsia (642.7)
09 Hypertension of this pregnancy (642.3)
10 Preeclampsia (642.4, 642.5)
11 Eclampsia (642.6)
12 Other hypertensive disorders and isolated symptoms of preeclampsia (642.9, 646.1, 646.2), specify____

Amniotic cavity and genitourinary tract disorders and infections
13 Infection of amniotic cavity (658.4)
14 Lower urinary tract infections (646.6)
15 Acute pyelitis/pyelonephritis (590.1)
16 Chronic pyelitis/pyelonephritis (590.0)
17 Nephritis, nephrotic syndrome and nephrosis (580-583, 590)
18 Pelvic inflammatory disease (614.8, 614.9)
19 Urinary-genital tract fistula (619.0)
20 Other infections or disorders (646.6, 647.2), specify____

Cardiovascular and respiratory disorders
21 Varicose veins of legs, vulva and vagina (671.0, 671.1)
22 Phlebitis or thrombophlebitis (671.2)
23 Phlebothrombosis (671.3)
24 Congenital cardiovascular disorders (745-747)
25 Rheumatic heart disease (390-398)
26 Acute respiratory conditions (460-466, 480-487)
27 Chronic obstructive lung disease and allied conditions, nontubercular (490-496)
28 Other cardiovascular and respiratory disorders (648.6, 460-519.9). specify____

Blood disorders
29 Iron deficiency anemia (280)
30 Other deficiency anemias (282-283)
31 Sickle-cell anemia (282.6)
32 Thalassemia (282.4)
33 Other anemias and blood disorders (285), specify____

Diseases and disorders of pelvic organs
34 Tumors of the body of the uterus (654.1)
35 Incompetent cervix (654.5)
36 Ovarian cysts and benign ovarian tumors (620.0, 620.1, 620.2, 620.8)
37 Other abnormality of shape or position of uterus and neighboring structures (654.4)
38 Other and unspecified abnormality of cervix, vagina and vulva (654.6-654.9)

Fetal problems
39 Rhesus isoimmunization (656.1)
40 ABO and other isoimmunization (656.2)
41 Fetal distress (656.3)
42 Intrauterine death (656.4)
43 Intrauterine growth retardation (656.5)
44 Previous malposition, successfully converted to cephalic (652.1)
45 Other known or suspected fetal condition affecting management of pregnancy (655, 656.6, 656.8, 656.9)

Fetopelvic disproportion
46 Abnormal or contracted pelvis (653.0-653.4)
47 Large or abnormal fetus (653.5-653.7)

Other complications of pregnancy
48 Hyperemesis gravidarum (643)
49 Threatened premature labor (644.0)
50 Polyhydramnios (657)
51 Oligohydramnios (658.0)
52 Other complications of pregnancy (640-646, 650-679), specify____

Infectious and parasitic disease
53 Rubella (647.5)
54 Other viral diseases except respiratory (647.6), specify____
55 Tuberculosis (647.3)
56 Malaria (647.4)
57 Syphilis (647.0)
58 Gonorrhea (647.1)
59 Bilharzia [schistosomiasis] (120)
60 Gastrointestinal parasites (120-129), specify____
61 Other bacterial infections or parasitic diseases (001-136.8), specify____

Gastrointestinal disorders
62 Appendicitis (540-542)
63 Noninfective ileitis and colitis (555-558)
64 Cholecystitis and cholelithiasis (574.0-574.5, 575.0, 575.1)
65 Rectovaginal fistula (619.1)
66 Other gastrointestinal disorders (531-579.9), specify____

Malignant neoplasms
67 Breast (174)
68 Cervix (180)
69 Lymphatic and hematopoetic (200-208)
70 Other (140-208.9), specify____

Benign neoplasms
71 Other neoplasms (210-229) [except as in code 34], specify____

Neurologic disorders
72 Cerebral palsy (343)
73 Encephalitis (062-065)
74 Epilepsy (345)
75 Paraplegia (344.1)
76 Other neurologic disorders (320-359), specify____

Endocrine disorders
77 Hyperthyroidism (240-242)
78 Hypothyroidism (243-244)
79 Diabetes mellitus, preexisting (250)
80 Diabetes mellitus, gestational (648.0)
81 Parathyroid disorders (252)
82 Adrenal disorders (255)
83 Other endocrine disorders (240-258.9)

Mental disorders
84 Psychosis (290-299), specify____
85 Neurosis (301-316), specify____
86 Mental retardation (317-319)
87 Alcohol dependence (303)
88 Drug dependence (304)
89 Pica (307.5), specify____

Malnutrition
90 Avitaminosis (264-269.2)
91 Other malnutrition (260-269)

Musculoskeletal system disorders and injuries
92 Bone and joint disorders of back, pelvis and lower limbs (part of 711-719; 720-724; part of 725-738)
93 Internal injury to chest and pelvis (860-869)
94 Trauma involving abdominal injury (868)
95 Other musculoskeletal disorders and injuries (part of 710-739 and 800-999), specify____

Poisoning
96 Poisoning and toxic effects (960-989), specify____

Other disorders
98 Other, specify____

CONTRIBUTORS AND PARTICIPANTS

Adeoye, C. O., M.D., Department of Obstetrics and
    Gynaecology, Faculty of Health Sciences,
    University of Ife, Ile-Ife, Nigeria.

Apelo, Ruben A., M.D., Professor of Obstetrics and
    Gynecology, College of Medicine, University of
    the Philippines; Office-in-Charge, National
    Family Planning Office, Ministry of Health;
    Comprehensive Family Plannng Center, Lope de
    Vega St., Sta. Cruz, Manila, Philippines.

Arellano, Remedios G, M.D., President, Maternal
    and Child Health Association of the
    Philippines, Metro Manila, Philippines.

Aviado, Domingo M., M.D., Co-Editor of Proceedings;
    Adjunct Professor of Pharmacology, University
    of Medicine and Dentistry of New Jersey, Newark;
    President, Atmospheric Health Sciences, Inc.,
    PO Box 307, Short Hills, New Jersey
    07078, U. S. A.

Awan, Asghari Khanum, M.D., Ph.D., Professor of
    Maternal and Child Health; Chairman, Maternity
    and Child Welfare Association of Pakistan,
    MCH House, 30-F, Gulberg-11, Lahore, Pakistan.

Azurin, Jesus, M.D., Minister of Health, Metro
    Manila, Philippines.

Baens, Jose S., M.D., Chairman, Department of
    Obstetrics and Gynecology, University of the
    Philippines, Metro Manila, Philippines.

Banzon, Amparo, M.D., National PHC Coordinator,
    Ministry of Health, Metro Manila, Philippines.

Bautista, M. S., M.D., Department of Obstetrics and
    Gynecology, University of the East, College of
    Medicine, Quezon City, Philippines.

Begum, S. Firoza, M.D., Professor and Head of
    Obstetrics and Gynaecology, Galimullah Medical
    College; President, Bangladesh Association for
    Maternal and Neonatal Health, 3/10, Block-A,
    Lalmatia, Dacca 7, Bangladesh.

Bernard, Roger P., M.D., MSPM, Director of Field
    Epidemiology, International Federation for
    Family Health, 22 Avenue Riant-Parc,
    1209 Geneva, Switzerland.

Bondoc-Dela Cruz, Vilma, M.D., Institute of Community
    and Family Health, Children's Medical Center,
    11 Banawe St., Quezon City, Philippines.

Chelli, Mohammed, M.D., Professor and Head,
    Department of Obstetrics and Gynecology,
    University of Tunisia, Tunis, Tunisia.

Concepcion, Mercedes B., Ph.D., Dean, Population
    Institute, University of the Philippies, Metro
    Manila, Philippines.

Cho, Young W., M.D., Professor of Pharmacology and
    Medicine, Director of Clinical Pharmacology Unit,
    University of South Alabama School of Medicine,
    Medical Science Building, Mobile, Alabama 36688,
    U.S.A.

Cuyugan, Carmelita B., M.D., University of Santo
    Tomas Hospital, Manila, Philippines.

Del Mundo, Fe, M.D., Co-Editor of Proceedings;
    President, First International Congress on
    Maternal and Neonatal Health; Professor
    Emeritus of Pediatrics, Far Eastern University,
    College of Medicine; Founder and Director of
    Children's Medical Center; 11 Banawe St.,
    Quezon City, Philippines.

Del Rosario, Santiago, M.D., President, Philippine
    Obstetrical and Gynecological Society,
    Metro Manila, Philippines.

De Watteville, Hubert, M.D., Secretary General,
    IAMANEH, 11 rue d'Italie, CH-1204, Geneva,
    Switzerland.

Diamante, A. N., M.D., Department of Obstetrics and
    Gynecology, University of the East, College of
    Medicine, Quezon City, Philippines.

Dionisio-Garcia, Fe, M.D., M.P.H., Institute of
    Community and Family Health, Children's Medical
    Center, 11 Banawe St., Quezon City, Philippines.

Doctor, V.S., M.D., Department of Obstetrics and
    Gynecology, University of the East, College of
    Medicine , Quezon City, Philippines.

Dominice, Andre, Ambassador and Vice-President,
    IAMANEH, Geneva, Switzerland.

Ebrahim, G.J., M.D., FRCP, DCH, Reader in Tropical
    Child Health, Institute of Child Health,
    University of London, 30 Guilford St.,
    London WC1N 1EH, United Kingdom.

Esquerra, Aquilino B., M.D., Department of Obstetrics
    and Gynecology, University of the East, College
    of Medicine, Quezon City, Philippines

Estrada, Remedios A., M.D., M.P.H., Associate Director,
    Institute of Community and Family Health,
    Children's Medical Center; 13 Pitimini, San
    Francisco del Monte, Quezon City, Philippines.

Fayad, Mohammed, M.D., President, Egyptian Society of
    Maternal and Neonatal Health, 1103 Korniche Nile
    St., Garden City, Cairo, Egypt.

Fernandez, Josefina V., M.D., Medical Director, JVF
    Hospital, Dagupan City, Philippines.

Foege, William H, M.D., Assistant Surgeon General;
    Director, Centers for Disease Control,
    Department of Health and Human Services,
    Atlanta, Georgia 30333,   U. S. A.

Fukuiya, T., M.D., Department of Obstetrics and
    Gynecology, School of Medicine, Keio University,
    35 Shinanomachi, Shinjuku-ku, Tokyo 160, Japan.

Furuya, Hiroshi, M.D., Professor of Obstetrics and
    Gynecology, Juntedo University, c/o Family
    Planning Federation of Japan, Inc., Hoken Kaikan
    Bekkan, 1-1 Ichigaya Sadohara-cho, Shinjuku-ku,
    Tokyo 162, Japan.

Gabr, Mandough, M.D., FRCP, Minister of Health,
    Professor of Pediatrics, University of Cairo;
    Cairo, Egypt.

Genuino, Aurora Salegumba, M.D., FAAP, FPPS, FAACP,
    Department of Pediatrics, University of the
    Philippines, College of Medicine - Philippine
    General Hospital, Manila, Philippines.

Gomez, Trinidad A., M.D., Vice-President, Maternal
    and Child Health Association of the Philippines;
    President-elect, Medical Women's International
    Association, Metro Manila, Philippines.

Gutierrez, Ernesto, M.D., Chief, Anesthesiology
    Section, University of the East Ramon Magsaysay
    Medical Center, Metro Manila, Philippines

Iizuka, R., M.D., Department of Obstetrics and
    Gynecology, School of Medicine, Keio University,
    35 Shinanomachi, Shinjuku-ku, Tokyo 160, Japan.

Inciong, Minerva B., M.D.,Executive Director,
    Nutrition Foundation of the Philippines,
    Metro Manila, Philippines.

Ines-Cuyegkeng, Elena, M.D., Co-Editor of Proceedings;
    Executive Director, Association of Philippine
    Medical Colleges, University of the Philippines
    College of Medicine, 547 Pedro Gil St.,
    PO Box 593, Manila, Philippines.

Jahan, Farida A., M.D., Research Coordinator,
    Bangladesh Fertility Research Programme,
    Dacca, Bangladesh.

Jahan, Shawkat, M.D., Assistant Registrar, Department
    of Obstetrics and Gynaecology, Dacca Medical
    College Hospital, Dacca, Bangladesh.

Jhaveri, C.L., M.D., FACS, FICS, Professor of
    Obstetrics and Gynaecology; President,
    International Federation for Family Health;
    Consulting Obstetrician and Gynaecologist,
    Hospital for Women, Jayadeep, 224 Lady Hardinge
    Road, Matunga, Bombay 400 016, India.

Kamal, Ibrahim, M.D., Professor of Obstetrics and
    Gynecology, Faculty of Medicine, University of
    Cairo, Cairo, Egypt.

Kanakura, Y., M.D., Department of Obstetrics and
    Gynecology, School of Medicine, Keio University,
    35 Shinanomachi, Shinjuku-ku, Tokyo 160, Japan.

Kawakami, S., M.D., Department of Obstetrics and
    Gynecology, School of Medicine, Keio University,
    35 Shinanomachi, Shinjuku-ku, Tokyo 160, Japan.

Kawana, Takashi, M.D., Associate Professor, Department
    of Obstetrics and Gynecology, Faculty of Medicine,
    University of Tokyo, 7-3-1 Hongo, Bunkyo-ku,
    Tokyo, Japan.

Kessel, Elton, M.D., M.P.H., Founder and Senior
    Consultant, International Fertility Research
    Program, Research Triangle Park, North Carolina
    27709, U. S. A.

Khan, Atiqur Rahman, M.D., Chief, Population Planning
    Section, Planning Commission, Dacca, Bangladesh.

Kim, Taek II, M.D., Ph.D., Director, Korean Institute
    for Family Planning, 115 Nokbun-Dongg,
    Sudaemun-ku, Seoul, Korea.

Kim, Yong Sung, M.D., WHO Programme Coordinator for the
    Philippines, PO Box 2932, Manila, Philippines.

Laufe, Leonard E., M.D., Medical Director, Internationl
    Fertility Research Program, Research Triangle,
    North Carolina 27709, U. S. A.

Leedam, Elizabeth, Executive Secretary, International
    Confederation of Midwives, 57 Lower Belgrave
    Street, London SW1W OLR, United Kingdom.

Lopez, Guillermo, M.D., Director, Corporacion Centro
    Regional de Poblacion, Carrera 6A, No. 76-34,
    Apartado Aereo 24846, Bogota, Columbia.

Lorenzo, Conrado Ll., Jr., M.D., President and
    Executive Director, Population Center Foundation,
    Metro Manila, Philippines.

Macalino, P. D., M.D., Department of Obstetrics and
    Gynecology, University of the East, College of
    Medicine, Quezon City, Philippines.

Mathur, H.N., M.D., Assistant Professor of Community
    Medicine, R.N.T. Medical College, 22 Subhash Bose

Nagar, Facing B.N. College, Udaipur-313001,
Rajasthan, India.

Morisada, M., M.D., Department of Obstetrics and
Gynecology, School of Medicine, Keio University,
35 Shinanomachi, Shinjuku-ku, Tokyo 160, Japan.

Nirapathpongporn, Apichart, M.D., Chief Medical
Officer, Medical Department, Population and
Community Development Association, 8 Sukhumvit
12, Bangkok 11, Thailand.

Okai, Rhoji, M.D., Department of Obstetrics and
Gynecology, School of Medicine, Keio University,
35 Shinanomachi, Shinjuku-ku, Tokyo 160, Japan.

Omran, Abdel R, M.D., Dr.P.H., Professor of
Epidemiology, Carolina Population Center,
University of North Carolina at Chapel Hill,
407 Pittsboro St. 253H, Chapel Hill,
North Carolina 27514, U. S. A.

Ofosu-Amaah, S., M.D., Professor of Pediatrics;
Chairman, Department of Community Health,
University of Ghana Medical School, Accra,
Ghana.

Oteyza, E. N., M.D., Department of Pediatrics,
University of the Philippines College of
Medicine - Philippine General Hospital,
Manila, Philippines.

Pagorogon, R. R., M.D., Department of Obstetrics and
Gynecology, University of the East, College of
Medicine, Quezon City, Philippines.

Pine-Tanesco, L., M.D., Department of Obstetrics and
Gynecology, University of the East, College of
Medicine, Quezon City, Philippines.

Puqiu, Xie, M.D., Chief, Department of Maternal and
Child Care, Shanghai First Hospital of Maternal
and Child Care, 536 Chang Lu Road, Shanghai,
People's Republic of China.

Ramos, M. M., Jr., M.D., Department of Obstetrics and
Gynecology, University of the East, College of
Medicine, Quezon City, Philippines.

Ransome-Kuti, O., M.D., FRCP, Professor of Paediatric

and Primary Care; Director of Institute of Child
Health and Primary Care, College of Medicine,
P. M. B. 1001 Surulere, Lagos, Nigeria.

Ratnam, S. S., M.D., Professor of Obstetrics and
Gynaecology, National University of Singapore,
Kandang Kerbau Hospital for Women, Singapore
0821, Republic of Singapore.

Ravenholt, Rei T., M.D., M.P.H., Director, World
Health Surveys, Centers for Disease Control,
Washington Office, Room 8-65 Parklawn Building,
5600 Fishers Lane, Rockville, Maryland 20857,
U. S. A.

Rigor, Eustacia M., M.D., Secretary, Maternal and
Child Health Association of the Philippines,
Lungsod ng Kabataan, Metro Manila, Philippines.

Rochat, Roger W., M.D., Director, Family Planning
Evaluation Division, Center for Health Promotion
and Education, Centers for Disease Control,
Atlanta, Georgia 30333, U. S. A.

Robles, Emma, M.D., Assistant Director, National
Family Planning Office, Ministry of Health,
Metro Manila, Philippines.

Rosales, Vicente, M.D., Director, Institute for the
Study of Human Reproduction, University of Sto.
Tomas, Metro Manila, Philippines.

Rushwan, Hamid M.E., M.D., President, Sudan Fertility
Control Association, Department of Obstetrics
and Gynaecology, Faculty of Medicine,
PO Box 102, Khartoum, Sudam.

Sadik, Nafis, M.D., Assistant Executive Director,
United Nations Fund for Population Activities,
220 East 42nd St., New York, New York 10017,
U. S. A.

Sanada, Koichi, M.D., Executive Director, Japanese
Association for Maternal Welfare, 1-2,
Ichigayasadohara-cho, Shinjuku-ku, Tokyo, Japan.

Santos-Ocampo, Carlomagno, M.D., President,
Philippine Society of Anethesiologists,
Metro Manila, Philippines.

Santos-Ocampo, Perla, M.D., Chairman, Department of
Pediatrics, University of the Philippines;

President, Philippine Medical Association,
Metro Manila, Philippines.

Sastrawinata, Sulaiman, M.D., Professor of Obstetrics
and Gynecology; Chairman, Coordinating Board of
Indonesian Fertility Research, Hasan Sadikin
Hospital, Jl. Pasteur No. 38,
PO Box 238, Bandung, Indonesia.

Senanayake, Pramilla, MBBS, DTPH, Ph.D., FRSH, Medical
Director, International Planned Parenthood
Federation, 18-20 Lower Regent St.,
London SW1Y 4PW, United Kingdom.

Sharma, P. N., M.D., D.P.H.), Professor and Head,
Community Medicine, R. H. T.Medical College,
Udaipur-313001, Rajasthan, India

Shiraki, Kazuo, M.D., Professor of Pediatrics,
Faculty of Medicine, University of Tottori,
Tottori, Japan.

Sin, Jaime Cardinal, His Eminence, the Archbishop of
Manila, Manila, Philippines.

Sureau, Claude, M.D., Chaire de Clinique Obstétricale
et de Physiopathologie de la Reproduction,
Université René Descartes (Paris V), Faculté
de Médicin Cochin, Clinique Universitarie
Baudelocque, 123 Boulevard de Port-Royal,
75674 Paris Cedex 14, France.

Surjaningrat, Suwardjoho, M.D., Minister of Health and
Chairman of the National Family Planning
Coordinating Board, Jalan Let. Jen. M. T.
Haryono, PO Box 186 JKT, Jakarta, Indonesia.

Suskind, Robert M., M.D., Chairman and Professor of
Pediatrics, University of South Alabama School of
Medicine, Mobile, Alabama 36688, U. S. A.

Takahashi, T., M.D., Department of Obstetrics and
Gynecology, School of Medicine, Keio University,
35 Shinanomachi, Shinjuku-ku, Tokyo 160, Japan.

Tain, T. P. (M.D., M.P.H.), Professor of Community
Medicine, S. M. S.Medical College, Jaipur,
Rajasthan, India.

TombyRaja, R.L., M.D., Associate Professor of Obstetrics

and Gynaecology, National University of Singapore,
Kandang Kerbau Hospital for Women, Singapore 0821,
Republic of Singapore.

Trussel, R. R., OBE, ChM, FRCOG, Professor of Obstetrics
and Gynaecology, St. George's Hospital, University
of London Medical School, Cranmer Terrace, London
SW17 ORE, United Kingdom.

Tyrer,Louise B., M.D., FACOG, Vice President, Medical
Affairs, Planned Parenthood Federation of America,
810 Seventh Avenue, New York, New York 10019,
U. S. A.

Valdes, C. B., M.D., Department of Obstetrics and
Gynecology, University of the East, College of
Medicine, Quezon City, Philippines.

Viravaidya, Mechai, Secretary-General, Population and
Community Development Association, 8 Sukhumvit 12,
Bangkok 11, Thailand.

Wagatsuma, Takashi, M.D., Head and Chief Consultant,
Department of Obstetrics and Gynaecology, National
Medical Center Hospital, 1 Toyamacho, Shinjuku-ku,
Tokyo 162, Japan.

Walker, James, M.D., Professor of Obstetrics and
Gynaecology, University of Dundee Medical School,
Dundee, Scotland.

Wickramasuriya, K.P., M.D., Medical Officer, Family
Health Bureau, Ministry of Colombo Hospitals and
Family Health, 213 De Saram Place, Colombo 10,
Sri Lanka.

Wong, Vivian Chi-Woom Taam, M.D., MB, BS, Senior
Lecturer, Department of Obstetrics and
Gynaecology, University of Hong Kong,
Consultant, Queen Mary Hospital, Hong Kong,
British Crown Colony.